Contents

Infertility Counselling

Edited by
Sue Emmy Jennings

b

**Blackwell
Science**

> ## Dedication
>
> This book is dedicated to all people who have problems with realizing their desires, in particular for fertility.

© 1995 by
Blackwell Science Ltd
Editorial Offices:
Osney Mead, Oxford OX2 0EL
25 John Street, London WC1N 2BL
23 Ainslie Place, Edinburgh EH3 6AJ
238 Main Street, Cambridge,
　Massachusetts 02142, USA
54 University Street, Carlton,
　Victoria 3053, Australia

Other Editorial Offices:
Arnette Blackwell SA
1, rue de Lille, 75007 Paris
France

Blackwell Wissenschafts-Verlag GmbH
Kurfürstendamm 57
10707 Berlin, Germany

Blackwell MZV
Feldgasse 13, A-1238 Wien
Austria

First published 1995

Set by DP Photosetting, Aylesbury, Bucks
Printed and bound in Great Britain by
Hartnolls Ltd, Bodmin, Cornwall.

DISTRIBUTORS

Marston Book Services Ltd
PO Box 87
Oxford OX2 0DT
(*Orders*: Tel: 01865 791155
　　　　 Fax: 01865 791927
　　　　 Telex: 837515)

North America
　Blackwell Science, Inc.
　238 Main Street
　Cambridge, MA 02142
　(*Orders*: Tel:　800 759-6102
　　　　　　　617 876-7000)

Australia
　Blackwell Science Pty Ltd
　54 University Street
　Carlton, Victoria 3053
　(*Orders*: Tel: (03) 347-5552)

A catalogue record for this title is available from
the British Library

ISBN 0–632–02445–3

Library of Congress
Cataloging in Publication Data is available.

Foreword

As assisted reproduction techniques become ever more complex, and increasingly successful, the desire of couples to try to have a baby has grown, when once they would have had to accept that there were to be no children, or adopt, or foster. Indeed, it has grown rapidly, and the difficulties of coming to terms with infertility, with the implications of treatment that may help to alleviate it, and with the implications of treatment that includes gametes which have been donated by others, are only now becoming clear to us. We have an emotional minefield in what is still a difficult, scientifically fascinating, sometimes experimental field. And we have conflicting desires between halves in a couple, or individuals and their wider families, over human reproduction, its meaning and its necessity in order to be considered a real person – whether male or female.

It is into this area of emotional eggshells that counsellors in the field have to walk. Counselling has to be offered by every centre offering treatment licensed under the Human Fertility and Embryology Act. In many cases – though not all – the counsellor is an integral part of the team which provides the treatment. Yet she (or he) has a complicated relationship with the clients. For there is an assumption, and often an acknowledgement, of confidentiality. But in the course of that confidential exchange, a counsellor may hear something that would lead her to think that this couple might not be the most suitable of parents for a child. And, under the HFE Act, the 'welfare of the child' has to be taken into account.

These are not the only difficulties facing infertility counsellors. Infertility counselling is a new speciality. Its exact requirements are not yet absolutely clear. Its early practitioners are people with strong, but not always congruent, views. The practice of in vitro fertilisation itself goes through changes. There are scientific advances with which to be familiar, a counselling qualification to be attained, a specific series of areas of concern to be examined. Then there is the tender, difficult task of getting to know individuals and couples, gaining their trust, and going through with them some of the pain, and hope, and loss.

This volume begins to do just that. With contributions from a variety of specialists, excellently edited by Sue Jennings, it deals with many of the major questions, and answers some of the most commonly voiced concerns. It will be of enormous use: to counsellors themselves, to doctors and nurses and others involved in the field, and indeed to the patients and their families themselves, whose interests are best served by the provision of high quality, very professional, well informed counselling.

Julia Neuberger

List of Contributors

Prue Bakpa is a registered nurse and midwife, and is Nurse Coordinator at the Rowan Clinic, The Royal London Hospital, Whitechapel.

Eric Blyth BA, MA, CQSW is Principal Lecturer in Social Work at the University of Huddersfield.

Robert Bor BA, MA, DPhil, CPsychol, AFBPsS, UKCP is a registered family psychotherapist, a family therapist and clinical and counselling psychologist; he is Senior Lecturer in Counselling Psychology at the City University, London.

Jean Campbell RATh is a Fertility Counsellor and Art Therapist at the Rowan Clinic.

Marilyn Crawshaw BSc(Soc), CQSW, MA is a practising social worker and a Tutor in Social Work at the University of York.

O. Djahanbachkh MD, MPhil, FRCOG is Reader in Obstetrics and Gynaecology in the Academic Department of Obstetrics and Gynaecology of the Royal London Hospital.

Len Doyal BA, MSc is Senior Lecturer in Medical Ethics at the London and St Bartholomew's Medical Colleges.

Hilary Everett Dip Soc Sc is a social worker in the Gynaecology Unit of St Bartholomew's Hospital.

J. G. Grudzinskas BSc, MB BS, MD, FRACOG, FRCOG is Professor of Obstetrics and Gynaecology, London Hospital Medical College, Whitechapel.

Jennifer Hunt MA, CQSW is Senior Infertility Counsellor at the Hammersmith and Royal Masonic Hospitals, London.

Sue Emmy Jennings PhD, Dip Soc Anthrop RDTh(UK) RDT(USA) is Senior Research Fellow and Consultant Fertility Counsellor, The London Hospital Medical College, Honorary Fellow of the Roehampton Institute and Visiting Professor at New York University.

A. B. Kadva MB, BS, LRCP, MRCS, MRCOG is a clinical Research Fellow in the Academic Department of Obstetrics and Gynaecology at the Royal London Hospital.

Sammy Lee BSc, PhD, FRSH, FIMLS was formerly a Counsellor at the Rowan Clinic and is currently working at the Hale Clinic in London.

Elizabeth Lenton BSc, PhD is Senior Lecturer in Reproduction Endocrinology at the University of Sheffield and director of the Sheffield Fertility Centre.

A. M. Lower BMedSc, BM BS, MRCOG is Lecturer in Obstetrics and Gynaecology and Subspeciality Trainee in Reproductive Medicine at the London Hospital Medical College, Whitechapel.

Alexina McWhinnie MA, PhD, Cert Soc Stud, AIMSW, AAPSW is Senior Research Fellow in the Department of Social Work, University of Dundee.

Roger Neuberg FRCOG is consultant Obstetrician and Gynaecologist and Director of Infertility Services at Leicester Royal Infirmary.

J. Q. Norman-Taylor MBChB, MRCOG is Lecturer in the Department of Obstetrics and Gynaecology at the Chinese University of Hong Kong.

Paul Pengelly is a Senior Marital Psychotherapist at the Tavistock Marital Studies Institute, London.

E. Saridogan MD is Clinical Research Fellow in the Academic Department of Obstetrics and Gynaecology, The London Hospital Medical College.

Isobel Scher BAMA is a clinical psychologist and family therapist and Lecturer at the Family Therapy Clinic, University of Cape Town, SA.

Robert Silman L ès L, BSc, MB BS, PhD is Senior Lecturer in Reproductive Physiology at the London Hospital Medical College, Whitechapel.

Acknowledgements

Firstly, I must thank all the contributors for working within the guidelines and deadlines, and also, all the people with whom I have talked informally, including the clients and patients themselves.

I must thank all the people in my own department, the Academic Unit of Obstetrics and Gynaecology, who have allowed this book to take precedence over my other activities. I also appreciate, despite budgetary constraint, that the London Hospital Medical College endorses both the practice of art therapy and dramatherapy and its teaching to medical students.

Finally, I must thank Melanie, Martha and Pauline for all their secretarial backup in the complex world of computers.

Sue Emmy Jennings
1994

O wind of Tizoula, O wind of Amsoud!
Blow over the plains and over the sea,
Carry, oh, carry my thoughts
To him who is so far, so far,
And who has left me without a little child.
O wind! Remind him I have no child.

O wind of Tizoula, O wind of Amsoud!
Blow away that desire for riches
That sends our young men away
And makes them forget the girls they've married, their mothers,
And the old ones left in the village.
O wind! Remind him that I have no child.

Berber woman's song

Introduction

The counselling of people with fertility problems is a newly emergent specialism within the counselling field as a whole. Traditionally, such counselling has been done by doctors and nurses and has been seen as the giving of advice, the discussion of treatment options or the comforting of distress. Doctors and nurses have felt themselves to be the right people to provide appropriate counselling because they have medical knowledge and therefore hold the necessary information with which to advise patients. Indeed, the several dictionary meanings given to the word 'counsel' make it understandable that the medical professions could regard themselves as counsellors in this context:

(i)   advice, especially formally given;
(ii) consultation, especially to seek or give advice, or
(iii) to give advice to a person on social or personal problems, especially professionally;
(iv) to assist or guide a person in resolving personal difficulties.

The Concise Oxford Dictionary, 1990

However, developments during the last two decades have expanded our understanding of counselling and consequently extended the range of professionals and volunteers engaged in its practice. A profession of counselling has emerged in its own right, together with various counselling specialisms, such as marital and bereavement counselling, and there are now special requirements for counsellors who work in educational, pastoral, medical and industrial fields.

There is continuing debate as to the differences between counselling and psychotherapy, particularly when counselling is described as 'psychodynamic' or 'psychoanalytically orientated'. More recently, the counselling professions have separated out the idea of 'counselling skills' and counselling itself, a distinction which is not necessarily accepted by professionals other than counsellors themselves. Additionally, there are an increasing number of theoretical frameworks for counselling which include 'person-centred', 'rational-emotive', 'transactional analysis', 'feminist', 'gestalt' and 'personal construct'.

Many of these variants started as new approaches and alternatives to psychoanalysis and psychodynamic psychotherapy.

Within this elaborate and sometimes confusing counselling maze grows a recent specialism, that of the infertility counsellor, which is the focus of this book. As can be seen from the varied approaches and styles of the authors, there is no one view of the practice of the infertility counsellor, nor indeed is there agreement as to who should undertake such practice, and with what training.

Definitions of counselling

In their *Code of Ethics and Practice*, The British Association of Counselling defines counselling as follows:

> The overall aim of counselling is to provide an opportunity for the client to work towards living in a more satisfying and resourceful way. The term 'counselling' includes work with individuals, pairs or groups of people, often, but not always, referred to as 'clients'. The objectives of particular counselling will vary according to the client's needs. Counselling may be concerned with developmental issues addressing and resolving specific problems, making decisions, coping with crisis, developing personal insight knowledge, working through feelings of inner conflict or improving relationships with others. The counsellor's role is to facilitate the client's work in ways which respect the client's values, personal resources and capacity for self-determination.
>
> (BAC Code of Ethics and Practice for Counsellors, Section 3.1)

A briefer definition is stated by G. Brearley and P. Birchley in their book *Introducing Counselling Skills and Techniques*:

> 'The use of skills that enable a client to recognise and identify his [sic] own problems, and the ability to help the client find his own solution or resolution' (p. 15).

However P. d'Ardenne and A. Mahtani in *Transcultural Counselling in Action* (p. 12) offer their own brief definition which allies counselling to psychotherapy:

> In our working model, counselling has many of the components of short-term psychotherapy, that it is a relationship aimed at facilitating the process by which clients change their feelings, understanding and behaviour.

There are many more variations in the definition of counselling within the different theoretical perspectives and indeed within the professional bodies for counsellors and psychotherapists.

The counselling relationship

There appears to be agreement that, whatever the focus or theoretical underpinning, counselling (like psychotherapy) is a relationship through which change and understanding can be facilitated. Furthermore, it is generally accepted that the counsellor/client relationship should not be confused with other role relationships, (such as the doctor), and that its basis is respect, trust and confidentiality.

However, even this needs a caveat, since it is a contemporary Western perspective. Other cultures do not necessarily designate a separate person as 'the counsellor', and counselling may be built into other culturally important healing roles such as shaman, midwife, ritual specialist or even a senior member of the family. Counsellors therefore need to be especially careful when counselling people from different ethnic, class or geographical backgrounds from their own, so that different cultural beliefs and practices are respected and not denigrated and the right of people to consult their 'own' counsellors respected. Whatever their value system, clients must have the counsellor's respect, and an understanding that the counsellor's values will not be imposed on them.

Clients must also be able to trust the professional integrity of the counsellors. This is stated in the codes of ethics and practice of all counselling, psychotherapy and arts therapies organizations and their practising members have to abide by them.

One major issue in relation to trust is that of confidentiality. Clients must be clear when they come for counselling who will be party to their disclosures. Some practitioners claim that there should be 'total confidentiality' and that this should not be broken unless clients themselves give specific permission. Most counsellors would agree that confidentiality must be maintained except when there is a danger to the client or others, or when discussing their client work in professional supervisions (which is considered further below). The issue of confidentiality takes on a particular nuance in infertility counselling, where there may be problems relating to potential harm to an unborn child.

Supervision

It is accepted that all practising counsellors and psychotherapists need supervision from a professional supervisor. This is quite separate from any managerial supervision or trainee supervision that may also be required. Supervision is a safeguard both for the client and the counsellor because it enables the counsellor to deal with any 'blocks' or feelings of being overwhelmed (for instance) which may be triggered by the client's disclosures. As far as possible, supervision prevents the counsellor's personal bias getting in the way of the client's issues. A skilled supervisor will enhance the counsellor's practice and enable the counsellor to make use of personal understanding, in the same way that he or she is helping the client.

Infertility counselling

All the issues referred to briefly above need to be taken into consideration when people with fertility problems undergo counselling. The Human Fertilisation and Embryology Authority (HFEA) state in their Code of Practice that three sorts of counselling must be available at licensed treatment centres. These are: support counselling, implications counselling and therapeutic counselling. The Code states, on p. 29:

> Centres *must* make implications counselling available to everyone. They should also provide support or therapeutic counselling in appropriate cases or refer people to sources of more specialised training outside the centres.

Implications counselling enables clients to consider the implications of proposed treatment for themselves, their family and any children born as a result of treatment. While this must be available, it is important to note that the Code states that 'no-one is obliged to accept counselling' (p. 28, HFEA Guide).

It is also important to remember that infertility counselling, as described by the HFEA Guide, is counselling which relates specifically to the infertility itself. Support counselling, however 'aims to give support at particular times of stress, e.g. when there is failure to achieve a pregnancy' (p. 28, HFEA Guide). Therapeutic counselling 'aims to help people cope with the consequences of infertility and treatment, and to help them resolve the problems which these may cause. It includes helping people to adjust their expectations and to accept their situation.' (p. 29, HFEA Guide.)

Indeed, I was challenged several times because I wanted to include a chapter which focused on the counselling of people who wanted to terminate a pregnancy, and on those who wished to limit their pregnancies. How does termination link with the counselling of people with fertility problems? In some ways, the author of Chapter 9 answers this question herself when she says that termination and infertility are the two extremes of the continuum of life and that she feels at ease working with all people on this continuum, wherever they may be.

I would like to add that termination counselling can occur directly within the infertility setting. Clients often blame themselves for having had a termination of pregnancy and see their infertility as a punishment. Termination counselling may well occur a long time after the actual event, especially if there was no counselling available at the time, and there are many issues of guilt and conflict to be addressed, especially when the client concerned may not have told their current partner. In addition, there also the more unusual cases. I was once asked to counsel a gynaecologist who had just enabled a woman to conceive through assisted conception; the same woman then returned to him to request a termination. The gynaecologist initially thought she had fears about a possible abnormal birth. The woman, however, made it clear that she only wanted to test her fertility, and since she now knew she was capable of pregnancy, she wanted a termination as she did not actually want a child. The gynaecologist concerned therefore needed non-judgmental time in order to reflect on the many facets both of the situation and his feelings.

There may well be people attending infertility centres with other existing problems and who therefore need referral to outside organizations – for example for marital counselling, family therapy, alcohol dependency counselling and so on. The HFEA's concern, however, is for those people embarking on infertility investigation and treatment and for the provision of distinctive counselling for these people. When people first come for counselling/psychotherapy they need support, and part of their explorations will be about the implications of their life decisions, within the context of a therapeutic relationship. So it is possible to have the elements of support, implications and therapeutic counselling within a single session.

Implications counselling becomes a rather more prescriptive intervention in that it relates to decision-making about the infertility treatment itself, and the HFEA specifies the sorts of issues that counsellors should invite clients to consider, for example:

(a) the social responsibilities which centres and providers of genetic material bear to ensure the best possible outcome for all concerned, including the child;
(b) the implications of the procedure for themselves, their family and social circle, and for any resulting children;
(c) their feelings about the use and possible disposal of any embryos derived from their gametes;   (p. 30).

The guidelines for implications counselling cover over two pages of the HFEA document, with less than a page for support and therapeutic counselling together. This illustrates just how important this aspect of the treatment is thought to be, but it also shows how it can lead to the confusion of understanding of what counselling is. *The counsellor here is taking on a prescribed role with a stated agenda, in a relationship where most counsellors argue that the client should state the agenda so that they are enabled to discuss what is troubling them.*

We need to keep this in mind when looking at the specialism of infertility counselling and how it is focused within the investigation and possible treatment of infertility problems.

How independent is infertility counselling?

Within the HFEA debate, there has been much discussion concerning the degree of independence of infertility counsellors, and what is actually meant by 'independent'. The updated Code of Practice says that 'the skill mix of clinical, nursing, counselling and scientific staff should reflect the requirements of the work undertaken at the centre' (p. 3). It further states that counselling should be distinguished from the giving of information or the normal relationship between clinician and client, who may be offered treatment, or is offering to donate gametes, which includes giving professional advice or assessing people 'in order to decide whether to accept them as a client or donor, or to accept their gametes and embryos for storage ...'   (p. 28).

It would seem that an ideal situation is one where the counsellor is part of the professional team, with a special remit to cover the three areas of counselling outlined above. Nevertheless, in many centres this is not the case: for example part-time counsellors may come in specifically to see clients by appointment and have no presence in the team, or clients may be handed some names and addresses and encouraged to go for counselling. In fact, a counsellor's presence in the team can ensure that the treatment discussions are far-reaching, and can soften the impact of technology in this highly personal area.

Confidentiality in infertility counselling

The HFEA states that any information obtained from potential donors or clients must be kept confidential unless disclosure is authorized by law.

If a member of the team has a cause for concern as a result of information given to him or her in confidence, he or she should obtain the consent of the person concerned before discussing it with the rest of the team. If a member of the team receives information which is of such gravity that confidentiality *cannot* be maintained, he or she should use his or her own discretion, based on good professional practice, in deciding in what circumstances it should be discussed with the rest of the team.   (p. 16).

Not all counsellors are asked to undertake assessment of potential donors and clients, therefore the direct assessment may not apply to them. However enshrined in infertility counselling legislation is a moral imperative for counsellors to disclose any serious concerns about potential parents and the welfare of children. It is very important that the infertility counsellor has appropriate supervision in order to deal with such sensitive and sometimes contentious issues of confidentiality.

Professional Training

The various professional bodies that regulate counselling, psychotherapy and arts therapies have requirements of training for professional membership. If one considers, for example, the training and practice requirements for the British Association of Counselling, the British Psychological Society, the British Association for Dramatherapists and the British Association of Art Therapists, there are similarities in hours and duration. An average would seem to be about 1 000 hours of taught course, practical application and supervision, though not all the organizations expect these to be at a postgraduate level.

Addresses of some professional organizations are found in Appendix 3 and Appendix 4 which list training requirements and approved training courses in these fields, as well as to which codes of ethics and practice members must adhere.

The Training of Infertility Counsellors

There is currently extensive debate concerning the appropriate training for people who undertake infertility counselling. The problem has been addressed by a multidisciplinary working group set up by the HFEA, whose recommendations were published in 1994.

At the moment there is only one training course which offers a Diploma in Fertility Counselling; this is offered by the London Hospital Medical College and has been running since 1990. The course formed the basis for the recommendations of the British Association for Infertility Counsellors (BICA) for specialist counsellor training, and these were further elaborated by the HFEA working group.

The Code states:

Unless it is engaged only in research, a centre should ensure *either* that at least one of its staff has a Certificate of Qualification in Social Work or an equivalent qualification recognised by the Central Council for Education and Training in Social Work, or is accredited by the British Association of Counsellors, or is a Chartered Psychologist, *or* that a person with such a qualification is available as an advisor to counselling staff and as a counsellor to clients as required.   (p. 5).

This statement is a little curious because it does not state that the professional people listed above must be trained counsellors, apart from those accredited by the British Association of Counselling. Many people with social work training or Institute of Chartered Psychologists membership do not have qualifications in counselling, and the list excludes, for example, people who are professionally trained in the several psychotherapies or dramatherapy or art therapy. The training requirements are very similar in all the main professional organizations which have practitioner membership and codes of ethics and practice.

A survey which was carried by HFEA as part of their documentation of training needs demonstrated that those people who were designated infertility counsellors in different licensed centres came from a wide variety of backgrounds. It is generally agreed that all infertility counsellors must at least have basic training in counselling skills, with specialist training in infertility counselling, especially in relation to understanding the welfare of the potential child. Whether in the future there will also be a requirement for them to have a counselling or psychotherapy qualification remains to be seen, but is not currently envisaged in the recommendations in the HFEA Code of Practice.

Counselling and the public debate

The environment in which counselling has to function has undergone many changes in recent years. Assisted conception and the technology of reproductive medicine have made rapid advances during the latter half of the twentieth century, to the extent that technology has outstripped the legal and ethical framework within which such medical treatments can be regulated. These developments have resulted in much public controversy and media outcry over 'Frankenstein babies' or 'supermarket mothers', and these emotive issues have often been distorted. There is currently much conflict over the treatment of older women and whether there is a 'natural' cut-off point after which fertility treatment should not be allowed to continue or begin.

The HFEA guidelines

Within its broad guidelines, the HFEA has sought to provide a framework for consideration and clinics have subsequently formed their own policy and protocols, subject to the monitoring of their own ethics committees. However, this situation has now changed with the advent of the current purchaser-provider economy, and Health Authorities are now giving their own guidelines for funding treatments. Some authorities will not fund infertility treatment under any circumstances; others will not fund treatment of older or single women; and still others will only fund people who are not only in settled heterosexual relationships but where there are no previous children to either partner. This has provoked some people to move into a different area, or to transfer into the private health sector where a greater range of treatments can be bought, often at high cost.

The debate continues, but it would seem that for some time to come funding bodies will set their own criteria as to what treatments they will finance; the regulation of infertility will therefore be less in the control of the ethics committees of infertility clinics.

The scope and limitations of this book

This book is the work of a multidisciplinary group of professionals who are linked in various ways to the counselling of people with problems of fertility. It is the first book of its kind to look at the practice of this specialist form of counselling and at the wider issues surrounding it. The contributors' backgrounds and work are many and various and their approaches to the subject vary enormously; this is inevitable in such a new specialism, and the practice of counselling is a constantly re-defining field.

The individual chapters of the book reflect the contrasts of the multiprofessional team who may well be working in a treatment centre for infertility. The individual counsellors, psycho-, arts and family therapists, social workers, doctors, as well as representatives from law and ethics, nursing, and embryology all have their own perspective on the issues involved.

Not everyone for example accepts the separation of counselling from counselling skills, and others include advocacy as a part of counselling. There are also differing views on the ethical and legal implications of medical technology in relation to infertility treatments. While guidelines are provided through a code of practice, specific matters should be left to the discretion of individual counsellors. Perhaps the most interesting development in this field is that it has brought together these disparate groups of people who otherwise would not be in communication with each other.

All the contributors are directly involved in the infertility field, whether as HFEA inspectors or infertility clinicians and counsellors or lecturers to medical and social work students on infertility. Additionally the authors of Chapters 5, 6, 8, 10, and 17, (Pengelly, Bor, Jennings, Blyth, Hunt, and McWhinnie) and Julia Neuberger, who wrote the foreword, are all members of the HFEA working group on Training of Infertility Counsellors.

Conclusion

This introduction has outlined the general field of counselling and looked at problems of terminology, as well as discussing the specialist practice of infertility counselling. Issues of supervision, confidentiality, independence and the multiprofessional team, and infertility counselling training have been explored as a backdrop to the book as a whole. The editor takes full responsibility for the views expressed in this section, as do individual authors for their chapters.

Please note that when the specific gender of both clients and therapists is indicated, it reflects the actual practice; otherwise gender-free language is used throughout.

Sue Emmy Jennings
Stratford-upon-Avon, September 1994

Part I
Infertility Counselling in Practice

In this section there are several perspectives on infertility counselling, each illustrated with actual case-history material. In chapter 2 (Bakpa) the nurse's role and its limits are explored, as well as the concept of the nurse-counsellor. In Chapters 3 (Crawshaw), 4 (Lee), 5 (Pengelly) and 6 (Bor and Scher), the authors write about practice in relation to gender and relationships, so that the themes of 'women', 'men', 'the couple' and 'the family' have various theoretical perspectives as well as a practical focus. In Chapters 7 (Campbell) and 8 (Jennings) the authors take us into the field of art therapies – both visual art therapy and dramatherapy – and their important contribution to infertility work. Finally in this section in Chapter 9 (Everett), the related areas of both termination and limitation of fertility are addressed, enabling a counsellor to place the concept of 'infertility counselling' or 'fertility counselling' in some perspective.

Chapter 1
Infertility Counselling and Medical Diagnosis

Sue Emmy Jennings and Sammy Lee

Introduction

There is no doubt that many people at some stage of their lives seek advice, guidance, counselling or therapy in relation to their fertility. People make decisions to have children or to prevent conception or to terminate a pregnancy. Having decided to have children they may find that they do not conceive (an estimated 1 in 10 people, and some clinicians say 1 in 6) and so they seek medical assistance. People's feelings, conflicts and decisions about procreation lead many to seek some kind of counselling help.

Infertility counselling is a specialist form of counselling associated specifically with the provision of medical treatment for infertility. It has become increasingly important as the medical technology surrounding many treatments has developed. Infertility counselling is seen as protecting both the client, whereby people can make informed decisions about proceeding with treatments, and also the unborn child, so that decisions are not made which can adversely affect the welfare of the child. To make an informed decision, people need to have adequate information, and professional advice, as well as having implications counselling, both before giving consent to treatment and after consent has been given, (HFEA Code of Practice 1993, pp. 28–33; also see the general introduction of this book). It is generally considered that the provision of services should not all be carried out by the same member of staff; but there is also an argument for continuity in client care – for example where nurses are the people recognized by clients and to whom they turn for information and support.

The HFEA also requires that there is provision for clients to have support counselling as well as therapeutic counselling when appropriate. Support counselling is seen as the support given to people who may be unsuitable for treatment, or for whom the treatment has not resulted in a 'take-home baby', for example, and it is often recommended that such people might join support groups (see Appendix 3). The HFEA also states that:

Centres should ensure that, as part of their training, all staff are prepared to offer emotional support at all stages of their investigation, counselling and treatment to clients who are suffering distress.
(p. 32)

There seems a natural progression from support counselling to therapeutic counselling and the HFEA Code goes on to state that

Procedures should be in place to identify people who suffer particular distress and to offer them, as far as is practicable, therapeutic counselling with the aim of helping them come to terms with their situation . . .   (p. 32)

There are therefore two main strands to the provision of infertility counselling: one that enables people to make an informed decision which takes into account the welfare of those concerned; and the other that gives support and therapeutic counselling when people experience distress in relation to the success or otherwise of their fertility treatments.

The medical context

Once counsellors grasp the medical aspects of infertility treatment fully, their clients will be better served during their work together, whether they are dealing with support, therapeutic intervention or the implications of donor insemination treatment.

Male infertility

Male infertility is a challenge for the 1990s. During the 1980s, more and more specialists came to realize that male infertility accounts for up to 50% of all diagnoses of infertility. About 30% of all cases seem to involve male factors only, whilst 20% of cases include male infertility amongst other factors.

Over the years, reproduction technology has developed at breathtaking speed. However, understanding of male infertility has essentially remained in the dark ages. What is male infertility? The traditional method of assessing male fertility has been the semen analysis. In most hospitals in the UK this meant a simple count of sperm numbers. In some hospitals a cursory subjective figure for the motility percentage was also given. More recently, some of the better laboratories give an analysis of the percentage of abnormality rate as well as subjectively analysing the quality of sperm movement.

How may we diagnose male infertility?

Diagnosing and treating mechanical problems

Before moving on to diagnosis, it is necessary first to consider absolute male infertility, or *azoospermia* – meaning literally no sperm, a condition arising as a consequence of the absence of testicular function. This may be revealed by biopsy or a blood test. High levels of follicle stimulating hormone (FSH) may indicate primary testicular failure. Occasionally azoospermia is due to absence of the vas (the cord connecting the testis to the urethra). This may sometimes be corrected surgically; and nowadays a procedure involving surgery may be able to recover sperm directly from the testis – using a method involving direct biopsy, or else by means of microsurgical epididymal sperm aspiration (MESA). The other surgically correctable reason for azoospermia is vasal or epididymal blockage, a condition which may sometimes be successfully overcome. All these conditions may be diagnosed by vasography, a procedure that relies on X-ray analysis and dye injection.

Where sperm are present, but in low numbers or low motility, it is sometimes possible to determine the cause of the condition. Partial blockage of the vas or epididymis may be the reason, but, more commonly, a varicocele (varicose spermatic vein) is present. Somehow this engorged vein is associated with low sperm count and motility: the mechanism for this is unknown, but there is speculation that the varicocele may raise the temperature of the scrotum locally, thereby reducing the function of the testes. Nevertheless, ligation of the vein may often result in a return to normospermia (normal sperm levels). Here also a blood test may reveal much: low FSH and luteinizing hormone (LH) levels indicate hypogonadism, a condition which may respond to drug treatment. Low testosterone, associated with low motility may also respond to hormone replacement therapy.

Problems in carrying out research into male infertility

If all the above have been tested for and excluded, and even though we may still not understand the underlying pathology, we usually have to work with what we've got: the diagnosis is traditionally limited to semen analysis. Semen analysis tells us little about sperm function, which might explain some of the problems of research in this field, and since semen analysis is inaccurate for diagnosis, so far most studies attempting to assess treatments of male infertility have been basically flawed. Since no-one has been using the same yardstick when doing research, we are rarely comparing like with like and this has meant that medical opinions on male infertility vary enormously. Some of these opinions have been based on myth rather than fact. To receive a diagnosis of male infertility can therefore be a shocking experience, not only because of the social stigma still involved, but also because those who often must seek a second and third opinion find themselves becoming increasingly confused, isolated and frustrated because of the conflicting information and opinion available.

How to define sperm function?

The best yardstick of fertility is provided by the study of sperms from proven fertile donors. Counts and motility are always good in these circumstances. However, even when dealing with apparently fertile donor semen, caution is required. In one clinic that I worked in, over a one-year period, 21 different donors were used. At the end of the year, with donor *in vitro* fertilization (IVF) producing success at approaching a 20% delivery rate per cycle, we discovered that 10 of the 21 donors had provided all the pregnancies. Indeed, seven of the eleven failures had been used more than three times each! An excellent example that count and motility assessments are not enough, since all 21 samples had excellent count and motility; and moreover these samples regularly achieved >50% fertilization rates in IVF cycles involving their use.

However, if we accept that proven fertile donor samples (ones known to have achieved pregnancy and deliveries) have demonstrated sperm function, then we may be justified in using such samples as a yardstick which may then be used to assess the samples of males from infertile couples. What parameters might then provide the best yardstick? In my experience, one of the best quantitative methods of testing sperm function is that of mucus penetrability. Briefly, this test assesses the sperms' ability to migrate through mucus. It is an objective test, being quantitative because we are able to measure the distance that the sperm are able to penetrate. When eleven proven fertile donors were identified and subjected to the test, the mean penetration distance was found to be 39.2mm (± 2.3SE, n = 11). Using the test for 44 male patients (where the female partner was investigated, and no problem detected), the mean penetration was just 19.6mm (± 1.7SE, n = 44), a significantly lower penetration distance ($p < 0.01$, Student's t-test). This test is therefore clearly useful in assessing sperm function or dysfunction. Having established the value of the test, the efficacy of the test had to be further studied. Results have previously been published (J. Erian and S. Lee, 1990) and demonstrated that men with a sperm migration distance of less than 11 mm did not achieve fertilization, even with treatment. Above 25 mm distance, results with treatment approached 75%, indeed all the spontaneous pregnancies occurred amongst this group. Men whose sperm penetrated in the interval 12–24 mm seemed to be the ones most likely to benefit from treatment.

Mucus testing to detect reduced sperm function

The work with cervical mucus penetration as a test of sperm function also revealed an interesting finding. Since the use of frozen-thawed semen samples for donor insemination (or DI) (the advent of AIDS has necessitated the quarantining of samples before use), many clinics throughout the world have reported a reduction in success rates, from about 10% to 5%. It was postulated that the downturn was due to the effects of freezing and thawing, and if this was so, we would expect frozen-thawed samples to reveal reduced sperm function. Therefore, using the migration test, the fertile donor samples mentioned above were tested after both freezing and thawing, and the mean reduction in sperm migration distance was found to be 36% ($p < 0.05$, Student's t-test). It seems clear, therefore, that the reduced success rates of DI after the adoption and use of frozen-thawed samples may be directly attributed to the effect of freezing and thawing on the functional capability of the sperm samples. It is interesting to note that despite the reduction in DI success rates, IVF success rates with frozen-thawed samples remains undiminished. This is probably due to the routine use of sperm preparation in IVF. Thus IVF-type sperm preparation seems capable of overcoming the deleterious effects of storing semen samples.

Therefore, the use of intrauterine insemination with prepared sperms should produce improved results in all DI cycles. Future use of this method of assessing sperm function will help to improve semen assessment and to ensure patients obtain better information and diagnosis and consequently clearer options regarding treatment will be possible.

Does the male equivalent of menopause exist?

Let us conclude by considering one final aspect of male infertility: at least 30% of men attending clinics in which I have worked have *secondary infertility* – and these are not men who have had vasectomies (which is another story!). These are men, with usually only one previous child (often conceived spontaneously), and generally suffering subsequently involuntary infertility of over five years duration. I have come to the conclusion that these men represent a subgroup of male infertility, in other words, a population of men demonstrating the clear incidence of age-related reduction in fertility in men – until now, a phenomenon mythically dismissed by male experts.

I was alerted to this possibility by the fact that all the men in this category were over 37 years of age. Using the migration test, 22 men were recruited for the study and all were tested. The cut-off age was 37 years; men younger than this were tested against men older. Not one man over 37 achieved a migration distance better than 30 mm, whilst

50% of the younger men did (though the semen analysis results for men in both groups were not significantly different). The migration distance difference was significant ($p < 0.05$, Chi-squared 2×2 table test). As far as I am aware this is the first clear demonstration of an age-related decline in fertility in men and the results are important for at least two specific reasons. Firstly, I believe that it shows that men's fertility does decline with age, just as women's does. The idea that man is able to defy reproductive decline, unlike woman, has been perpetrated and perpetuated by men; in my travels, I have heard many specialists state that men's fertility did not drop off with time, interestingly, all these specialists have been men! Perhaps one of the reasons for the persistence of the myth has been our inability to define sperm function. The second reason for the importance of these results is that they are clearly an interesting group of men to study. Do men with secondary infertility experience different feelings from men with primary infertility? Since they all have one child, is their perception of infertility different? I feel that a study on the group along these lines would be most fruitful. Setting up a meaningful study will almost certainly be difficult, but very worthwhile. I see a priority here in terms of future research possibilities!

Female infertility

How may we diagnose female infertility?

Like the section on male infertility, this part should not be considered as a comprehensive treatise on female infertility. Rather, it offers an introductory overview, geared in particular to giving counsellors of clients with infertility problems a grasp of the relevant subjects. Readers should expect to do further study of their own.

Sexual reproduction

When looking at fertility, the obvious place to start is to consider what happens in the 'normal' course of events. Sperm are normally deposited at the cervix in hundreds of millions. The sperm that arrive at the ampulla, the site of fertilization, must have undergone an epic journey through the cervical mucus, across the uterus and through the Fallopian tube. The few thousand sperm that arrive at the ampulla must therefore be an elite subgroup of sperms, the sperm 'troopers'. The poorer sperms, whether they be abnormally shaped or less motile, are lost mainly in the cervix and in the further journey up the female reproductive tract.

How do things go wrong?

The female cycle: the hypothalamus-pituitary-ovary-uterus axis. The hypothalamus is an area in the brain which fulfils many functions, some of which we are only just beginning to understand, though nevertheless, its role in controlling the output of sex hormones is well known. The hypothalamus releases a substance called GnRH which causes the pituitary gland to release FSH (follicle stimulating hormone) and LH, the sex hormones that together stimulate the ovary and produce ovulation (the release of an egg). Under the influence of FSH and LH, the ovary makes oestrogen, a hormone which is particularly important during the follicular phase (the part of the female cycle occurring prior to ovulation). Once the oestrogen level crosses a certain threshold, it feeds back to the hypothalamus, which produces a large surge of LH released from the pituitary. This causes ovulation to occur within 24–48 hours. The oestrogen also has a strong effect on the uterus, during the follicular phase, causing the lining of the womb to proliferate by the growth of tissue and new blood vessels. After ovulation, progesterone becomes the important hormone. Its main action is to maintain the endometrium (womb lining), ensuring a receptive environment for the fertilized egg to implant into. The time following ovulation is called the luteal phase. Luteal phase insufficiency means that progesterone levels are too low or drop disastrously at too early a stage.

Anovulation is a common cause of infertility in women. Up to 20% of all cases of infertility in women are caused by ovulatory failure. Sometimes this is caused by low levels of the sex hormones LH and FSH, which in turn results in low oestrogen and progesterone levels. At other times the LH and FSH levels may be normal, but the oestrogen level may nevertheless remain low because the ovary may not be responding properly, which will also mean a low progesterone level. It is also possible for LH, FSH and oestrogen levels to be normal and for the progesterone level to remain low – the hypothalamus which controls pituitary release of LH and FSH is unable to respond to the rising levels of oestrogen for some, as yet, unknown reason. In some women anovulation is manifested by high FSH levels indicating primary ovarian failure. Often these women may have Turner's (XO) syndrome (see glossary), and in a few unfortunate cases they have normal chromosomes, but for unknown reasons undergo the menopause prematurely. Anovulation may also be caused by hyperprolactinaemia, or excessive production of prolactin – this is how contraception is achieved in most nursing mothers as the hormone prolactin normally induces the breasts to produce milk, and is also able to suppress ovulation.

Oligomenorrhoea: ovulation can sometimes be variable or occasional.

This may be due to some of the above-mentioned reasons, but is more commonly caused by 'PCO' or polycystic ovary syndrome. This is a condition revealed by abnormal LH levels in the blood, and also by high androgen (male hormone) levels. In serious cases anovulation (or amenorrhoea) may occur.

A common test of ovulation is a day-21 progesterone test. Any value less than 30 nM is supposed to indicate an absence of ovulation. These days, in my opinion, the best way of detecting amenorrhoea is to utilize follicular tracking with ultrasound. This entails the use of ultrasound to monitor the development of follicles on the ovary. Scanning might be carried out on days 2, 5, 9, 11, 13 and 15 of the patient's menstrual cycle, depending on its normal length. In this way, we can be sure that follicles develop normally, and then rupture, allowing the oocytes (eggs) to be released. There is some data that shows progesterone to be a poor indicator of ovulation – some 25% of cases may be inaccurate, compared with tracking (S. Lee and L. Mascarenhas, unpublished data).

Tubal blockage: this accounts for about 15% of all infertility. One of the most common causes of tubal blockage is pelvic inflammatory disease. Other mechanisms may also cause blockage, but the key to this condition is that the egg almost never reaches the womb, since its passage is blocked.

Non tubal-related infertility: unexplained infertility accounts for 30% of all cases of infertility. Despite routine investigations, no obvious reason can be determined and this may indicate the presence of 'occult factors'. For example, despite a normal sperm count, there may be an absence or low numbers of functional sperms, or indeed the same may be true for the eggs. This is the most common diagnosis in cases of infertility.

Endometriosis: this has a 5% incidence. Here, uterine tissue is found in the abdomen, on the outside of the uterus or on the ovaries. Endometriosis does not always cause infertility, but it is still commonly associated with involuntary infertility. Modern research suggests that endometriosis may be caused by or related to immunological disorders. In my experience, severe endometriosis (for example, profuse presence in abdomen, especially on one or both ovaries) requires attention (drug or laser) before infertility treatment can begin.

Morphological: an abnormal pelvic anatomy may contribute greatly to infertility. Fibroids in the womb, severe retroversion or torsion of the ovaries or tubes due to pelvic adhesions, etc. may all contribute to difficulties.

The diagnostic regimen

Bearing in mind the diagnoses mentioned above the following guidelines might be used for initial investigation. Physical examination is vital, in order to ensure that the overall anatomy is as it should be. Following a detailed history, an arrangement for a day-21 blood sample should be made. In the case of anovulation, a blood sample may be taken at any time and an arrangement made for follicular tracking (in the old days, progesterone and oestrogen challenges would have also been arranged, but are not so commonly used now). The hormones whose levels should be tested are FSH, LH, progesterone, prolactin and testosterone. These tests will reveal any reasons for anovulation and provide information on the endocrinal state of the female patient.

Further tests will follow at different times depending on the age, duration of infertility and the urgency of the couple to achieve pregnancy. Tubal patency should be proven as a matter of priority. There is some controversy though as to the timing of such tests. An early test avoiding surgery is the use of X-ray, also called the hysterosalpingography test. A dye is passed into the womb and its passage is monitored by X-ray. A newer method of this test is being developed whereby instead of X-ray, ultrasound is used. Laparoscopy reveals more information, since a visual inspection of the anatomy of the pelvis can also be carried out at the same time as the tubal patency test (dye spill) is administered.

At least two blood tests should be carried out initially, with a three-month gap in between. Thereafter, following the initial diagnosis and treatment, blood and tubal patency tests should be carried out after every 12–24 months.

Chapter 2
The Nurse and Infertility Counselling

Prue Bakpa

You yourselves know how valuable a woman is in illness, being there to help a sick person.
Demosthenes

Speaking from the physician's or surgeon's point of view, the best nurse is she who can subordinate her own ideas of treatment to the medical attendant.
Lancet, 1879

Introduction

In this chapter, I am concerned with the relationship of the practising infertility nurse to the counselling process, rather than with the role of nurse herself as counsellor. The traditional and contemporary roles of the nurse, and the pivotal position she occupies at the interface between doctor and patient, are discussed briefly. Many of the skills that are used by counsellors are in fact part of the repertoire of the nurse, and this chapter seeks to clarify the difference between such counselling skills and the practice of counselling. Common difficulties in practice, such as role boundaries, are discussed; a strong case is made for the availability of a multidisciplinary team which, ideally, should include both nurses and counsellors, as well as medical specialists and scientists.

I have referred to the nurse as 'she' throughtout this chapter, in order that sentences and grammar are less cumbersome and also because, in 1994 in Great Britain, the majority of nurses remain women.

Nursing, unique among professions in 1994, is still viewed by the majority of people as 'woman's work'. Numerically, women dominate the profession, though, significantly, they no longer dominate hier-archically – male nurses now occupy many senior posts in all aspects of nursing.

For thousands of years, it has been accepted that the essence of nursing is inherently understood by women; women being the 'natural' subordinates and carers – of children, elderly relatives, parents, husbands and, of course, patients. Nursing skills, so long equated with womanly attributes, have been correspondingly undervalued, mis-

22

understood, degraded, feared and dismissed. Nurses today continue to battle against the attitudes of colleagues in the health professions; this includes women who, of necessity, have had to embrace 'male' values in order to succeed. The nurse may often be seen by colleagues as subservient, rather than equal and complementary; useful in a 'handmaiden' role, but useless as a colleague with whom to have an equal dialogue or exchange of ideas and expertise.

In a health-care environment which is now orientated towards cost, efficiency and other parameters of the business world, nursing skills cannot readily be properly costed: they are invaluable and immeasurable in market terms.

The nurse, in the struggle to professionalize nursing, has often embraced the discipline of counselling. With its fluent and vocal 'spokespeople', its academic language, its jargon, its articulate endorsement of the qualities of care and respect for people which are integral to nursing, counselling is a useful vehicle for nurses seeking to enhance their status and credibility and validate aspects of their job. It provides a whole new language which properly describes the communication skills which have so long been undervalued and yet are inherent within the role of the professional nurse.

But nurses are not primarily counsellors. I think it is fairly widely recognized now that good nurses use counselling skills, for example, giving respect to each patient, employing careful listening, open questioning, summarizing the patient's story, observing the patient minutely, understanding the patient's behaviour in context and so on. It is also recognized that good nurses and good counsellors often share very similar personal qualities, not least that highly unbusinesslike commodity – compassion. However, if nurses are to be counsellors in the full sense of the word, they must embark on post-professional training, as described elsewhere in this book.

The HFEA, as the government agency set up to interpret and enforce the Human Fertilisation & Embryology Act 1990, is the authority responsible for inspecting and licensing all fertility clinics in the UK. It arranges for a small team of experts to inspect each clinic annually and this includes inspecting the counselling provision.

Many nurses working in the field of infertility feel they have sufficient counselling skills. Their medical colleagues may well support them strongly in this claim. One of the 'problems' about counselling, is that most health professionals think that they are good at it. Many nurses believe that the counsellor role is inherent in their routine daily work; a role that can be adopted in all situations or woven into any nursing procedure. Usually, nurses are talking about the skills which humanize the technical business of nursing and make it unique and special.

Counselling, though, is also special, and it needs to happen in a special place. Most nurses do not have the opportunity to be uninterrupted with a patient for more than a few moments, however skilfully they manage their time. That immediately places limitations on how free-ranging a conversation can be, how much emotion and feeling can be explored and displayed and raises issues about privacy and confidentiality.

It is no denigration to say that the nurse uses counselling skills but is not a counsellor; this is rather about recognizing the worth of complementary disciplines. If a nurse or doctor is privileged to work with highly skilled counsellors they may begin to see where nursing ends and counselling begins.

Counselling, as the term is used to describe a profession, does not consist of advice-giving, opinion-giving, information-giving or offering practical help, nor befriending. The task of counselling means, rather, giving 'the client an opportunity to explore, discover and clarify ways of living more resourcefully and towards greater well-being'. What is more, the counsellor 'agrees explicitly to offer time, attention and respect to another person/persons temporarily in the role of the client'. (These definitions are provided by the British Association of Counselling.)

The ultimate goal of the counsellor is to help the client achieve autonomy. To empower the client and to be able to 'let go', to watch as the client makes his or her own choices and decisions and puts them into action. For the counsellor to be in need of the client's dependence, awe, gratitude or any of the other emotions which the client may bring to sessions, is inappropriate and may be counter-productive to the therapeutic process.

The counsellor must be able to unravel the client's story, to summarize and reflect back clearly, to focus on specific points, to clarify certain issues, to clearly define conflicts and opposites, to identify and challenge blind spots. The counsellor's clear perception of the 'duality' likely to be found in many clients can illuminate otherwise chaotic or confusing patterns.

Case history of Ms A

Ms A was efficient and successful in her career and was cool and brisk in her dealings with clinic staff; she accepted the need for implications counselling prior to embarking upon donor insemination treatment, in her usual business-like way.

During the ensuing counselling session, the counsellor noticed Ms A's underlying anxiety, picked up in a number of clues revealed in body language, such as a constant fiddling with her fingers. The counsellor was able to explore with Ms A her need to be in control and very busy in order to cope with inner feelings of helplessness and grief. The counsellor was able to prepare Ms A for her treatment and support her afterwards when treatment failed. Ms A declined a final medical appointment but requested a final counselling session and came 'just to cry'.

Whereas the counsellor recognized the duality in this patient, the nurse, in her traditional role, may see this patient as coping well and have no time to explore this further. In fact, in this case, the counsellor was able to alert nursing staff to Ms A's underlying feelings, without breaching the confidential nature of the discussions, and the nurses' insight and understanding thereby grew and they were able to establish a warm and open relationship with Ms A during the course of her treatment.

Of course, clinicians need to have faith in the skills of the counsellors with whom they work. Counsellors need to possess some very sterling personal qualities and to have undergone rigorous training – short correspondence courses are not enough!

Without a deep-rooted liking of, and interest in, humankind, there would be little motivation to pursue the lengthy process of becoming a skilled counsellor. From this 'love' of people comes the counsellor's ability to be a real person for the client; not merely an automaton parroting the standard counselling responses, but a warm, sincere and genuine person who is open and who is there for the client during the course of the session.

As Egan (1990) says in *The Skilled Helper*, 'genuine helpers do not take refuge in the role of counsellor'. They are not essentially needy people in terms of their interaction with clients. Egan also says 'relating deeply to others and helping are part of their lifestyle, not roles they put on or take off at will'. In layman's terms, Egan is describing a 'loving' person.

Counsellors are trained to examine their own beliefs and value systems and to recognize the process of transference of feelings in themselves and others. Most people would not be good at remaining truly impartial in such an emotive field as fertility without such training. If the counsellor does not understand what has motivated her to become a helper, what embarrasses her, what distresses her and so on, how can she be sure that her interactions with clients are not distorted by her own prejudices and conditioning, background and education, life-experiences and encounters? It is vital that counsellors examine though not necessarily change all their assumptions about class, education, male and female roles, race, religion, sexual orientation, speech and so on.

Chaplin (1988), in *Feminist Counselling in Action*, says 'learnt social attitudes such as "females should be passive and caring while males should be aggressive and competitive", are as deeply buried in the unconscious as our early personal experiences. Ideas about a male God with ultimate power over everything have a profound effect on our unconscious feelings about men and women and about fathers and male authority figures in particular' (p. 9). It is essential that the skilled helper recognizes in what way and how much of such social conditioning she has absorbed or to assess his or her view of these ideas.

All counsellors have to learn their trade and formal supervision is a professional requirement for all counsellors and trainees. The supervisor acts as a sounding board, and highlights inconsistency, cautions and affirms, and generally safeguards the good practice of the counsellor. Without supervision, the counsellor has no opportunity to share the minutiae of her encounter with the client and check that she has not slipped into unhelpful interaction.

A skilled counsellor also requires breadth of vision – by this, I mean the ability to observe clearly, to truly see the world outside one's own small and probably fairly homogenous circle; to cast one's net wide when gaining knowledge and experience and to be interested in all people everywhere. Furthermore, to be interested not in a purely academic way, but to be in tune with ordinary lives and popular culture.

Integration of the nurse and the counsellor working together

Practical ways in which the nurse can influence the clinical team in viewing counselling as complementary to, rather than a distraction from, fertility treatment are listed here, and considered below:

(1) Schedule regular team meetings, at which both the clinicians and counsellors are present.
(2) Draw the team's attention to the HFEA Code of Practice and the legal requirements to offer counselling as well as the HFEA's recognition of different types of counselling – implications, support and therapeutic.
(3) Draw up clear treatment plans which include counselling.
(4) Ensure that clearly written literature is available describing the treatment plan.
(5) Ensure that counsellors are present at case conferences and at times in the working week when treatment decisions are made.
(6) Use positive, clear language when referring to counselling.

Regular team meetings

Both the clinical team and counsellors should be present so that an understanding of each other's disciplines may develop and some consensus on treatment plans may be reached.

The counsellor's role must be endorsed by the team and its most senior members if counselling is to be truly effective. The senior nurse has a vital role to play here in keeping the channels of communication open, mediating and promoting understanding between colleagues.

The HFEA Code of Practice describes 'independent counselling'. I see this as meaning counselling which is independent of the treatment-givers, (i.e. doctors and nurses) rather than independent of the clinic team as a whole. To be outside the clinic team would leave counsellors isolated rather than independent, and counsellors must surely be part of any multidisciplinary fertility clinic team; their training and professionalism ensures their 'independence'.

The counsellor's role within the team may not just be client-focused. Counsellors have a very healthy influence on colleagues, for example in addressing the needs of other professionals in the way they show care and appreciation, challenging doctors', and nurses' concepts of 'success' and 'failure', challenging ideas of what is a 'good' or 'nice' patient (or whether such terms are relevant. Nurses and doctors so often expect patients to be good, grateful, and compliant, and in fertility clinics especially most patients seem to be on very best behaviour. Patients often disclose to counsellors that they feel the need to 'act up' to doctors in order to get the desired treatment; that somehow by being 'good', the treatment will be successful. Counsellors can help the team to see 'difficult' patients in context and can explain patients' anger or hostility as expressions of grief, anxiety.

However counsellors cannot, of course, influence anybody if they are not part of the team, or if they are geographically removed and only communicate by means of the occasional letter or memo.

Counselling protocol

The nurse can draw the team's attention to the HFEA Code of Practice and the legal requirement to offer counselling to patients as well as the HFEA's recognition of different types of counselling – implications, support, therapeutic (see Chapter 1).

Although the ideal may be to have all patients participate in counselling as part of their treatment, many centres do not have the resources to offer this, and compromises may need to be made. In such a case it would therefore be necessary to decide, in consultation with the whole team if possible, on where counselling resources were best directed. In some centres, for instance, implications counselling is mandatory for any couple contemplating receipt of donor eggs or donor sperm, or surrogacy, or wishing to become a donor of gametes or a host mother. Implications counselling might be offered, but not scheduled in the treatment plan for other treatments, such as IVF or ovulation induction.

In other centres, support counselling may be emphasized for those treatments considered particularly stressful. Very often, the technically fairly 'simple' treatments such as donor insemination or ovulation induction may, if not immediately successful, induce great stress which is protracted over many months and is compounded by successive negative pregnancy tests.

I have noticed a good deal of hostility to the Human Fertilisation & Embryology Act because it attempts to regulate the way in which doctors, in particular, work and to impose restrictions on what has been previously standard practice. I have heard one doctor declare, outraged 'How can this Act help? I have a close relationship with my patients. I know what's best for them. Why doesn't the government stop interfering. This is increasingly becoming a nanny state'. In the next breath, the very same doctor voiced similar outrage, that as a team, we had decided to treat a single woman with donor sperm. In other words, in this doctor's view the state should lay off and leave the doctor to impose his or her moral values on patients.

Treatment plans

The nurse will, it is hoped, be able to use her knowledge positively to influence the design of treatment plans, which include counselling. This enables counselling to be seen from the outset as an integral part of treatment and gives some sort of time-scale to treatment. Clinicians and patients alike will then have a clear time-frame for planning purposes, and it will become clear that the counsellor is able to function more effectively because proper time for counselling has been built into the plan from the start rather than thrown into the equation as an after-thought.

In a well-designed treatment plan (see Fig. 2.1), the counsellor does not hold up the medical consultation or treatment process, but rather enhances it because the patient is more confident, receptive and better informed and, what is more, once treatment commences, is more likely to be fully committed to it.

Week 1	Week 2	Weeks 3–5	Week 6	Week 7	Week 8
Doctor	Nurse	Counsellor	Doctor	Nurse	Counsellor
Initial medical assessment	Information-giving – legal – practical – technical aspects of treatment	Implications counselling session Optional follow-up	Finalize treatment details	Detailed information-giving – drug regime & timetable	Support counselling offered

Fig. 2.1   Example treatment plan for donated ovum recipient.

Case history of Mr and Mrs C

Mr and Mrs C are undergoing IVF, with back-up donor sperm. The implications of using donor sperm as a back-up in IVF can be thoroughly and effectively explored once the client couple have received clear information about the legal, practical and technical aspects of their treatment. The nurse, in giving information must be aware that Mr & Mrs C need to know the following:

- exactly what IVF involves
- the time-frame within which IVF might take place
- the various scenarios in which donor sperm might be best used, i.e. possible number and quality of eggs and the likelihood of getting good sperm from Mr C
- the embryologist's attitude to making choices on behalf of Mr and Mrs C – as many embryologists see this as outside their remit and expect patients to have made their own choices prior to egg collection (it is advisable, therefore for couples to be in possession of full information)
- the law regarding non-mixing of husband and donor sperm
- the law regarding the potential needs of a child to know of its origin
- the law regarding records of the couple's identity, donor identity and pregnancy outcome
- the law regarding the legal parenthood of the child in relation to use of husband and/or donor sperm
- possible/probable outcome if donor sperm is used i.e. the reality of having a part 'donor' child.
- why counselling is an important part of infertility treatment
- the centre's legal duty to address the welfare of potential children and any existing children the couple may have.

The nurse who understands the counselling process will be able to prepare Mr & Mrs C effectively for the counselling session or sessions which follow. The nurse's information-giving can draw in some of the implications of legal requirements. This will then give the nurse the opportunity to describe the way the counsellor might be able to help the couple to think through implications arising from these so that Mr & Mrs C find their own solution and understand more clearly why counselling is offered.
For example:

Nurse   If this treatment is successful and you have a baby as a result of the donor sperm, the law says that the child might have a need to find out about being born from donor sperm when it reaches the age of 16 or 18. The HFEA will keep all the information about your pregnancy very securely but, in the future, should the child request, the HFEA will be obliged to answer 'yes' or 'no' to the question 'was I born from donor sperm'? This does not mean that you *have* to tell your child that it is born of donor sperm. This is your decision and many couples decide to keep this secret. Of course, if a child knows nothing of this, it will not be able to ask the HFEA the relevant questions. But there may be difficulties in keeping with a life-long secret especially if a few other people close to you already know about your plans to have this treatment. It is important that you cast your mind forward to when your child will no longer be a baby but will be a questioning young adult, and make your decision about whether to tell your child about the donor sperm, having considered all these things very carefully. The counsellor has a great deal of experience in talking with people about this and I think you may find it helpful to talk through your thoughts with her.

If you decide that you might like to know more about how to tell your child about the donor sperm, the counsellor will be able to give you some ideas on how to handle this.

The decision you reach is entirely yours. The important thing is that we (the centre) have alerted you to all the implications of your treatment and have helped you to the decision which is right for you.

In this conversation, the nurse has linked counselling to the whole treatment process and has clearly demonstrated its relevance.

During the information session, the nurse is able to focus the patient's attention on the reality of what is offered. Sometimes, clinicians assume that fertilization of eggs at any cost, *must* be what the couple would choose; there may be covert pressure on the couple to 'go for' what is scientifically possible. The nurse may need to shift the focus back to what the couple really want. Again, he or she can recommend the counsellor's potential contribution here.

This is where mandatory implications counselling written into treatment plans is so valuable. With it the patient/client couple do not feel singled out for counselling, rather it is seen as an integral part of the treatment, and is presented in the clinic literature as such. Some couples remain hostile to the idea of counselling and I often explain that the counselling is not a test or an assessment but a way for us, the clinic, to be sure that we are offering them what they really want not what we presume they want.

If counselling is scheduled to take place before an information-giving session, it will usually be seen as a preliminary or support session. In my experience, implications counselling only works if the facts have been delivered first. The implications of treatment spring from the patient's attitude towards these facts.

Literature

Clearly-written literature should be available for colleagues and patients and helps ensure that protocols are adhered to.

You may find it helpful to ask members of your patient support group to put suggestions on how clinic literature might be improved to ensure that its language is accessible to everyone. Remember too that a translation service is often needed in order to provide the literature in appropriate minority languages.

The counsellor's participation in decision-making

Medical staff in the context of infertility treatment may see their sole aim as the conception and birth of babies and the speedy 'processing' of a couple towards that end. With regard to some complicated treatment, how often have other professionals heard a doctor (or nurse) say 'let's get on with it, let's just do it'?

By contrast, the counsellor's aim may be to slow things down; to give the clients time and space to reflect and absorb what is happening or going to happen to them; to offer support; or to explore implications effectively.

It may turn out that, when space and time are given, the client's apparent aim of having a baby at almost any cost masks other needs, which need to be met or at least addressed first.

For instance a woman who is grieving but unable to express that grief; she may be mourning lost youth or a previous abortion or miscarriage, or the death of parents – any number of things. She may need to acknowledge her loss before she can feel committed to motherhood. Or a man may play a dependent role within a marriage and is in fact deeply ambivalent about his wife having another real baby to mother and divert attention from him.

Counsellors may become superfluous within a clinical setting if their expertise is not fully acknowledged; if there are no established channels by which the counsellors' observations can be fed back into the treatment process; or if the counsellors' opinions, when voiced, are dismissed or undermined. What is the point of the grieving woman or the ambivalent man exploring feelings with a counsellor, deciding that more time is needed before treatment commences and the counsellor being unable to relay such expressed needs back to the treatment team; or, if they do, being unheeded and the treatment ploughing on regardless. The usual consequence of this sort of muddle is that the treatment fails, often because the patient is unable to comply.

Use of language

The nurse should use positive, clear language, and should avoid diminishing the counselling role by using phrases such as: 'pop in and have a quick chat with the counsellor on your way out'; or 'I suppose you could always have a chat with the counsellor if you really want to . . .'

Conversely, jargon should also be avoided – such as: 'perhaps you would like to share and explore some of your deeper feelings around this issue'. Such phrases sound fine to those used to 'counselling-speak' but do not initially mean much to the average patient or colleague.

Making referrals

Nurses have to make appropriate referrals to counsellors for both support and implications counselling. They cannot do this unless they understand what counselling is and how the process differs from what the skilled listener has to offer.

Introducing the idea of counselling to a patient can be difficult. It means the nurse facing the fact that she must hand over to another professional, and that she is suggesting to the patient that something serious enough is going on to need specialist help, other than medical. Many patients react with dismay at the suggestion of counselling, say such things as:

- 'Are you suggesting I am mad?'
- 'But I like you and trust you, nurse. I would rather talk to you.'
- 'I have done lots of homework; I already know exactly what this treatment involves.'
- 'I don't like people to see me upset.'
- 'I'll only feel worse if I talk about it.'
- 'It seems like such an indulgence.'
- 'I don't want it to look as if I can't cope.'

The nurse may need to work hard to help the patient understand that there is the possibility of a skilled person willing to listen and talk with them for an uninterrupted hour. Most patients need to be given permission to take up this offer and most need the counselling demystified.

Examples of stress signs which may alert the nurse to a need for further therapeutic or support counselling include:

- the patient mentions isolation, e.g. having no friend or relative in whom to confide
- the patient no longer feels able to communicate effectively with or confide in their partner
- the patient is persistently unable to comply with treatment e.g. late for appointments, forgets to follow the drug regime correctly, getting confused over instructions, etc.
- the patient is unable to find adequate time for treatment, perhaps totally committed to a career and unable to slow down, while still remaining highly anxious to pursue treatment
- the patient mentions feelings of despair, panic and may describe symptoms of anxiety attacks, or 'going mad'
- the patient mentions feelings of overwhelming anger, or behaves in a very angry way with clinic staff
- the patient appears unable to contemplate any break between

courses of treatments e.g. is desperate to hurry into the next treatment cycle of IVF as the previous one finishes.
- the patient appears unresponsive, or unkempt e.g. may have a problem with personal hygiene, in which case the nurse should question possibility of depression

Examples of what the nurse might say on observing any of the above symptoms include the following:

- 'This may be a good time to look at these stresses you have told me about. Why not see a counsellor just once and see how you feel'?
- 'The counsellor does not just listen, but offers practical and useful ideas for helping you through this difficult time.'
- 'You seem to be very alone with all this. It can really help to have someone to talk to who will be understanding and helpful.'
- 'This may be the time to unwind and take some time for yourself. Perhaps you just need to slow things down a bit and put yourself first.'
- 'Your counselling helps us, as a team, to feel sure we are offering you the treatment that you really want and not one that we think you want.'

There are lots of ways to say the same thing. The skilled nurse will adjust her introduction of counselling to the situation and to the patient. Some patients are 'therapy-literate', others are highly 'therapy-resistant', with all shades in between.

The skilled and experienced fertility nurse is highly perceptive and will possess a well-honed intuition about her patient's emotional state. She will probably have a clear idea of the nature of the conflicts or emotional turmoil affecting those of her patients she refers to her counsellor colleagues, and will hopefully be able to write a detailed and enlightening referral report. She may also have a good idea of the way in which the counsellor will need to work with the patient and where that work will eventually lead. But the nurse is not in a strong position to undertake that work herself.

Case history: Mrs B

Mrs B is 34 years old and a shop assistant. A cheerful, very well dressed woman, she appears to have a good marriage. She underwent one cycle of IVF (on the NHS) two years ago after which she was not pregnant. During the planning of the second cycle, she telephoned the nurse-coordinator of the fertility clinic to say that she was 'too busy with work' to go through treatment.

The nurse's first task was to take the pressure off, reassuring Mrs B that treatment could continue whenever her work allowed. But the nurse, knowing the patient a little and remembering that, formerly, her career had not seemed to be a priority in her life, sensed that Mrs B might be trying to find a plausible reason for not going ahead for treatment. The nurse kept the pace of the conversation fairly gentle and slow and asked one or two questions (N.B. this is a highly edited version of a much longer conversation:

Nurse How have you been feeling since the last treatment?

Mrs B It hit me pretty hard. I had no idea I could feel so bad.

Nurse Yes, these treatments are very tough on you.

Mrs B To tell you the truth, I thought I was going to go mad and now I'm beginning to get these awful attacks. I just can't breathe and it's really horrible. I thought I would be OK by now but the treatment was six months ago. I just don't know what to do with myself.

Nurse You are not alone in suffering like this after treatment. You are not going mad, but having a very understandable reaction to a very difficult situation. These breathless attacks must be frightening for you. Have you told anyone else how bad you are feeling?

Mrs B Well, my husband knows I suffer with nerves but he doesn't know what to do and I try to make light of it. I can't tell anyone else.

Nurse I'm so glad you have told me this. You know it can be very difficult to bear this all on your own. Many other patients have described the same feelings. In fact, it is often because you 'coped' so well with the treatment that the grief and sadness comes out in this way and, like all griefs, it can take a long time to subside. There are very skilled and sympathetic counsellors here who will understand so well what you have just told me and would be able to give you some very solid support. Talking to someone can really help you to understand why you are feeling like this and give you a sense of a light at the end of the tunnel. My advice is that you give the counselling a try.

It is a measure of the nurse's skill and experience that she is able to judge when people need more time. It would have been so easy for her to 'deal' with Mrs B very briefly, arrange her next IVF cycle for a few months time and wish her a swift 'Goodbye'.

The nurse used many counselling skills during the course of this conversation: listening, open questioning, gentle probing, reflecting back, summarizing.

Mrs B took up the offer of counselling with relief. Nine months later, she was still seeing the counsellor every two to four weeks. On first impression, she appeared as cheerful and well-presented as ever, but admitted to the nurse that 'without the counsellor, I would have been under the wheels of a tube train'. Throughout this time, she remained insistent that the next IVF cycle should be planned for a date in only a few months' time. Each time the treatment was imminent, she felt unable to go ahead. This happened three times.

It took approximately one year of therapeutic counselling before Mrs B could begin to admit that she did not want to go ahead with IVF again; that the emotional cost was too great. It took a little longer, all the time with her counsellor's support, before she could admit to her husband and all the other people who she perceived as having a vested interest in her treatment, that not only did she not want IVF but that she was not sure that she wanted a child.

As a nurse, I need to feel that vulnerable patients, such as Mrs B, are 'safe'. It takes a great burden off the nurse to know that a skilled colleague is offering the sort of expertise which supports patients through emotional crises and helps them to move on towards 'the light at the end of the tunnel'. A nurse is unable to offer this long-term support within his or her normal daily routine. Most fertility clinics are frantically busy, as are the nurses and doctors who work in them, so it is usually the counsellor who has the specific time to take the patient on this sort of 'journey'.

Of course, many counselling sessions in fertility work involve brief interventions of maybe one or two sessions. However, the HFEA Code of Practice draws a distinction between implications counselling, support counselling and therapeutic counselling. The majority of patients will probably not require the long-term therapeutic counselling taken up by Mrs B, but the HFEA clearly recognizes the need for this sort of counselling in a proportion of patients.

The case of Mrs B illustrates another 'problem' with counselling, in that, often the most skilled and protracted work and sometimes the very best work, has no specific medical payoff or treatment result.

In Mrs B's case, there was no way of recording her resolution towards childlessness as a medical success. In fact, in the clinic's audit, this case could be seen in purely negative terms, appearing as a financial deficit; public money available for an IVF treatment cycle which the clinic was unable to spend for more than a whole financial year while the patient 'dithered'.

It is vital that counsellors have some mechanism, perhaps regular staff meetings, by which they can describe this sort of work to other members of the team and convey something of the nature of the therapeutic process. It is important that the team understands the concept of therapeutic counselling and that it measures the outcome as a positive success for the clinic. As described earlier in the chapter, the nurse may play a vital role here in facilitating this sort of communication between counselling and medical staff.

Combining the roles of nurse and counsellor

If the two roles of nurse and counsellor must be combined, it is essential that the patients or clients understand which 'hat' is being worn – counsellor or nurse. You should not begin an *ad hoc* counselling session when a patient begins to open up just as you have finished giving an injection or visiting him or her on the ward. That is the time for the traditional nursing skills of supportive and empathic listening and then appropriate referral to a counselling colleague, or perhaps to yourself as counsellor, in a scheduled session.

It is very easy, when embracing a new discipline, to behave like the newly converted with a tendency to interpret guidelines rigidly as solid rules and an over-enthusiasm for the jargon of a new discipline. This should be avoided if a counsellor is not to alienate sceptical colleagues. It is important to retain your sense of humour and irreverence, as it makes the rules the counsellor does insist upon all the more meaningful.

As a nurse-counsellor, you should insist upon the following conditions in order to carry out your counselling work:

● wearing your own clothes rather than a uniform
● no interruptions – inform colleagues what you are doing (N.B. hospital culture of the same space belonging to everybody needs to be changed in this respect)
● a separate room in which to counsel which is different from the one in which you practise as a nurse
● do not perch on a couch in a treatment room surrounded by needles and syringes, with colleagues blissfully unaware of the session in progress and blundering in every now and again, and then expect your client to 'open up'.

The combination of the role of nurse and counsellor may put the professional and client into a difficult conflict because the nursing process and counselling process must be separated out.

I find it almost impossible to expect clients to share things with me as a counsellor, to talk openly about their fears and misgivings about treatment, procedures, etc. when I am also the person who is going to be treating them. Here, the difficulty is in reconciling the different aims of counsellor and nurse. Wearing both hats, as nurse and counsellor, is very difficult, if not impossible, to do well. Counselling training certainly enables one to be a better nurse and a better administrator because the nurse then understands so much better the boundaries between the disciplines.

Conclusion

It is vital that nurses acquire and then hone their counselling skills. Post-basic counselling training endorses for nurses the worth of what they have always done. Validating respect for the client, acting as client advocate, using listening skills and trying to understand what the client is really saying. These are aspects of the nurse's professional role which should not be eroded by the 'accountants' model' of health care. As all good nurses know, caring for the human spirit is as important in the healing process as caring for the human body. So many hospital clinics are not solely therapeutic places for patients but are politically potent places where clinicians/managers, with their own agendas, all too easily see counselling as an optional extra, something which clutters the streamlined, cost-effective and technological approach to health care. It is difficult to fight this attitude. Nurses, conditioned as they are to be good at listening, not just to patients but to colleagues, are very unused to being listened to.

In this chapter, I have addressed issues relating to the nurses' and counsellors' roles, and the spheres of experience of counselling skills and the counselling process. I maintain that, in most cases, it is not appropriate for nurses to counsel in the way understood by professional counsellors and psychotherapists as this leads to a blurring of boundaries and confusion between roles.

However, I maintain that the nurse has a crucial role within the clinic team (not as one of the usual stereotypes beloved by the media and traditional male doctors) but one in which the well-being of the patient is truly enhanced; thereby enabling the best decisions and treatments to be implemented.

Chapter 3
Offering Woman-Centred Counselling in Reproductive Medicine

Marilyn Crawshaw

Introduction

This chapter examines some possible impacts of gender in shaping our reactions to fertility and parenting and suggests ways of better understanding its interaction with other social forces. It outlines a feminist counselling model and also examines tasks for grief-work with individual women coping specifically with pregnancy loss, including abortion, miscarriage, stillbirth, infertility, subfertility and also adoption. It stresses the need to better understand women's experience of their relationship with their unborn child and to reverse the trend to think of mother and child as separate entities. Finally, it suggests models for helping patients in addition to counselling.

Growing up male or female helps shape our approach to life in general and to parenting in particular. Women have an image of themselves in relation to mothering; men in relation to fathering regardless of whether or not they actually perform that role at any time in their lives. The gender experience of our social and emotional world obviously influences us as users of reproductive health services and as providers. 'Gender' is here taken to mean what can be seen as socially imposed dichotomies of male and female roles and attributes.

In this chapter, I describe the feminist counselling models which I use in my work as a social worker in a maternity & gynaecology unit in a busy northern District Hospital. The chapter starts by looking at the extent to which women and men appear to have gender-specific reactions to fertility and to parenting. Current literature on the links between the development of a female psyche and women's societal position is then considered. In the final part of this section, the impact of pregnancy on women is considered.

Having set the scene, a feminist model of counselling is outlined which focuses on work with women coping with pregnancy loss, but which also has wider applications. The tasks in counselling are explored within this framework.

In the final section, conclusions are drawn about the effectiveness of feminist fertility counselling and about therapeutically helpful approaches within reproductive health services for all women and couples.

Setting the scene

Many of the women using counselling services are referred via the nursing staff (including the midwives) or the medical staff. Some are routinely seen as part of a pre-agreed service delivery, for example women coming for abortions. Some women refer themselves or are referred by family, friends or outside agencies.

Not all women and couples requesting social work help use our counselling service, of course, as it is not always appropriate. Some find our other skills and services more helpful – such as supportive listening, advocacy, liaising with other professionals and agencies, or benefits advice.

Counselling is a term which is anyway widely used to cover a multitude of differing encounters. I use it here as defined by the British Infertility Counselling Association (BICA), namely: '. . . a process through which individuals and couples are given an opportunity to explore themselves – their thoughts, feelings and beliefs, in order to come to a greater understanding of their present situation and to discover ways of living more satisfactorily and effectively'.

Part of the social worker's task is to help assess the client's needs and consider with them the most appropriate way of helping. A useful paper by Ken Daniels (1992) provides a basic framework for assessment of psychosocial needs in the reproductive medicine area.

The interactive nature of 'life experiences'

Whether or not men and women's experience of, and approach to, life is biologically or socially determined, it is undoubtedly true to say that there are gender differences in all cultures. Women are one of the groups in our society that tend to experience some (apparent) structural disadvantages. These can adversely affect women's images and expectations of themselves, and other people's images and expectations of them.

By focusing on gender in this chapter, it is not intended that gender is thereby taken to be the dominant oppressive experience for women. Indeed, it is crucial to try and recognize the interplay between the various oppressive experiences that an individual woman may encounter in order to better understand both her emotional make-up and her use of any helping service.

Thus, characteristics other than gender may, either separately or in conjunction with gender, also affect the patterns that women's lives take. These might include ethnic identity, disability, class, age and sexuality.

Parallels can be drawn between different forms of oppression but they have to be treated with caution. The bases of differing oppressions may be similar ideologically if one accepts that they are socially constructed, but the overt explanations may differ. For example, sex discrimination may be based on anatomical difference, whereas racial discrimination may be justified on grounds of ascribed personality characteristics.

The routes through which people receive and transmit messages about themselves, however, occur in three main ways regardless of the particular type of oppression a person may encounter, namely:

- personal – through individually experienced negative attitudes and behaviour
- cultural – from the ideas and beliefs prevailing in our society, reflecting the dominant social group's belief
- institutional/structural – from society's institutions which can be seen as largely constructed on the basis of the assumed superiority of one viewpoint.

The issue which affects the counselling process most is the extent to which people take on beliefs and develop an internal representation of themselves based on the messages they have received about themselves as a 'type' as well as an autonomous individual. The pattern of any service delivery (including medical as well as counselling services) is also affected by received impressions and messages. Professionals need to be aware of this. If people do not believe they have a right to certain services and if providers assume certain groups of people will not use services or will only use them in certain ways, the organization of the service may reflect that.

There are commonalities in the experiences of people who face discrimination and are oppressed but there are also specificities relating to the particular nature of each. For example, women may identify with each other in certain aspects of their relationships with men and within families, but black women may find that their particular experience of being on the receiving end of racism limits the extent of that identification. Indeed, in certain circumstances, black women may identify more closely with black men in their common experience of racism. This has led Audre Lorde and Bell Hooks to insist that 'to deal with one (gender) without even alluding to the other (race) is to distort our commonalities as well as our differences' (Phillipson, 1992).

Iris Singer (1993) has suggested a way of understanding these commonalities and differences and their relevance to counselling. In what she calls the 'intercultural therapy space', Singer says that we need to identify what the key likely influential experiences are for each client according to characteristics (e.g. gender, ethnic identity, disability); and what experiences are likely to relate to the particular problem that they are seeking help with (e.g. infertility, abortion, stillbirth). Under each of these groupings, the counsellor and client can identify key psychosocial variables that are known to characterize reactions to that state and then identify the extent to which that individual client may be displaying or using those. The counsellor and client may then look at what is common between these groupings, and therefore likely to be mutually reinforcing within the individual client's makeup, and what is specific.

Counsellors can benefit from identifying and managing the experiences and variables that they themselves bring to the counselling relationship (or are perceived by the client to bring), and which affect the power differentials within it. Singer (1993) usefully employs the work of Jafar Kareem in this (Kareem & Littlewood, 1992). Kareem coined the terms 'status contradictions' and 'status congruence' to describe what to look for. For example, status contradictions occur where the client and counsellor are of different ethnic identity or different gender. If the counsellor has the more dominant status, this will potentially increase the existing counsellor-client power differential further. Where the counsellor is of what is deemed to be the less powerful identity, the 'status contradiction' factor needs to be managed. Where counsellor and client share an identity in major areas (e.g. both black and both women), a status congruence may be said to exist. However, Kareem suggests that vigilance needs to be paid by the counsellor to the client's perception of the amount of congruence that exists. Although the counsellor may assume congruence, the client may in fact find that other attributes such as differing class, lifestyle etc., make identification difficult.

In both scenarios, the congruence or contradiction can have the effect of distorting the counselling if they remain unrecognized. Thus for example female counsellors may find themselves avoiding challenging female clients in order to preserve the sense of shared identity; white counsellors can avoid challenging black clients in their desire to avoid accusations of racism.

The remainder of the chapter focuses more specifically on gender experiences, starting with fertility and parenting.

Gender-specific reactions to fertility and parenting

Women are usually centrally preparing for motherhood from their earliest conscious days (Belotti, 1975; Sharpe, 1985), whether or not they eventually take on that role. Their major psychosocial role as caretakers is traditionally passed down through the maternal line (Rich, 1984). Certain attributes are usually emphasized in women including nurturing, cultivating emotional sensitivity, recognizing the vulnerability of others and placing others' needs before their own.

The centrality of women's reproductive status to their identity is manifest in much of their adult activity and is arguably a major factor in their lower earning potential and reduced career opportunities. Women are less likely to do full-time work outside the home and are more likely to earn less than their male partners. They take greater responsibility in contraception, have major responsibility for childcare, and do the bulk of housework. In the event of a marriage breaking up, a woman is likely to remain the main carer for any children, and will generally be poorer than their ex-partner (EOC, 1992; Oppenheim, 1993).

A woman in a lower socioeconomic group is more likely to experience miscarriage, premature labour, stillbirth, or giving birth to a child with a congenital malformation or of a low birth-weight (Oakley *et al.*, 1990). Black women and women with disabilities in the UK are disproportionately represented in lower socioeconomic groups.

Although society purports to value motherhood highly, it is actually currently seen as low-status work and carries few obvious material rewards. For certain groups of women, society appears to value their entry into motherhood even less: there is some evidence that black women are discouraged from becoming pregnant because their pregnancies will produce more black people (Williams, 1987); proportionately more black women than white women have abortions (Bryan *et al.*, 1985). Women with disabilities may find themselves meeting hostile reactions when they embark on parenthood or seek help with becoming pregnant (Brice, 1993); and lesbian women were not favoured as potential mothers in the parliamentary debate on the Human Fertilisation & Embryology Bill.

As mothers, women have additional attributes ascribed to them which reinforce their likely newly acquired economic dependence on either their male partner or the state. Their social status is determined by their relationship to others (husbands, fathers and children). They are portrayed in contradictory lights as mothers. At times, they are identified with children as being in need of protection, as naïve, innocent and incapable of the same standards of adult behaviour as men. At other times, they are seen as antagonistic to children, unable to act in children's best interests and in need of regulating or monitoring.

Jalna Hanmer and Daphne Statham (1988) have shown that there is a concept in British society of a 'fit mother' but no equivalent of a 'fit father'. Miriam David similarly found that messages about the desirability of particular 'types' of mothers and nuclear families are increasingly embedded in social policies (David, 1986). Thus, at the time of writing, interpretations of what a fit mother is owe more to society's current needs than to considerations of good child care. The fit mother concept offers a compliant model against which to measure an 'unfit' one.

People who are already in the socially legitimate role of parent are less likely to identify accurately the strength of the desire and reasons for wanting to become parents than those who are still trying. Studies of people who are experiencing infertility or sub-fertility are therefore of particular help in pointing to possible gender-specific emotional reactions to parenting.

A recent study by Arthur Greil, a therapist and himself a member of a couple unable to conceive children, led him to conclude that; 'husbands and wives interpret, respond to, and give meaning to physical symptoms and physiological conditions ... 'but ... infertility is not to be thought of as a static condition with psychosocial consequences, but as a dynamic, socially-conditioned process whereby couples come to define their inability to bear their desired number of children as problematic and attempt to interpret and correct this situation' (Greil, 1991). He suggested that a couple's experience of being involuntarily childless is shaped by the ideology and social structure of the society in which they live including:

- nature of medical technology in that society
- functions and social value of marriage and children in that society
- beliefs about the importance or not of blood relationships
- ideas about the relative contributions of men and women to the process of conception and childrearing
- general theories about the causes and cures of health problems.

In the UK, a study carried out in Sheffield by Jim Monach (1993) similarly concluded that there were strong social pressures on people to become parents, but only within clearly prescribed kinship networks. He concluded that: 'Perceptions of marriage are still almost inextricably interwoven with expectations of child-bearing'.

Monach's work is particularly interesting here in that he looked at gender-specific reactions as one major aspect of his study. Part of the study involved recruiting 30 couples from referrals to a specialist infertility clinic and interviewing them over a five-year period. At all stages, Monach found that men and women had different experiences, with pronatalist pressures bearing more heavily on women (1993, p. 108). Men were much less involved than women in attending clinics (1993, p. 80); and there were differences in their willingness, over time, to admit to feeling upset. At the outset, both men and women expressed similar feelings. However, over time the men were increasingly less likely to admit to continuing feelings of distress while women were increasingly more likely to identify such reactions.

Women spoke of distress, guilt, bitterness and of wishing to fulfil the role of mother. Men linked their infertility to a threat to their virility more than to their inability to become a father. Women were more likely to feel that they had 'let their man down' than feel that their femininity was threatened (1993, p. 118). Women talked about deep and lasting hurt and personal pain while men talked about their wife's distress, their own diagnosis, or the process of the investigation. None referred to failing to fulfil the husband role.

Men, at every stage, were less likely than their female partners to have confided in any group within their social network (including friends, family, work) confirming other findings of men's reduced likelihood of confiding personal matters to others (1993, p. 120).

Monach suggests that this relates to women's internalized role-model of how they think they should be coping, and to the greater social acceptability of women expressing their feelings and to the lesser social significance for men of the loss of the parenting role.

Given my earlier suggestion that women define themselves more centrally as mothers than men do as fathers, Monach's findings appear to support that view. Thus, most men, employed or not, see fatherhood as one of a range of adult roles that they expect to occupy. Many women see motherhood as their main or exclusive adult role.

Counsellors need to be aware of the extent to which they too are operating within all these constraints.

The development of the female psyche

Many therapists are agreed that girls and women are more likely than boys and men to have feelings of low self-esteem. Many women report feeling emotionally deprived, that something is missing and that no-one cares centrally for them (Eichenbaum & Orbach 1983). Women are more likely than men to suffer from depression, thought by many to be a manifestation of anger turned in on to the woman herself, rather than expressed outwardly. Women are more likely than men to engage in self-harm activities including eating disorders and attempted suicides (Gorman 1992) while men are more likely to engage in outwardly violent behaviour aimed at some external apparent cause of their 'disease' or affliction.

The phenomenon of women displaying an outward coping self while experiencing an inner needy self is what I have elsewhere called 'dislocated reality' (Crawshaw 1988). Hence, women can find greater difficulty than men in achieving a congruity between their outer and inner worlds and a centred sense of self – a belief in their right to consider their own needs alongside those of others instead of always putting others first. Some therapists believe that this is related to mothers' problems with allowing their daughters to achieve and maintain a healthy emotional identity separate from themselves. (I use the term mothers here to include the varying patterns of mothering that occur, while assuming the predominance of women in the 'mothering' role. Although many of the theories used concentrate on the typical white western model of an individual woman and child, I have assumed my adaptions of them to also apply to variations around the western model such as the child who has several female parenting figures.) Because of the different gender of mother and son, it is suggested that mothers are better able to allow their sons to separate off from themselves. This then enables males to believe at an emotional level that they are an 'OK person', with a right to have needs and a right to have others to respond to those needs (Eichenbaum & Orbach, 1987; Ernst, 1987; Lawrence, 1992).

In my view the danger of such an analysis is that it can appear to collude with the notion that men achieve sound emotional health while women inevitably grow up needy and neurotic. That would be true if such analysis confined itself to early mother-infant relationships alone, but it does not. Instead it emphasizes the need to overlay early experiences with ongoing life experiences. It is then possible to see that the ongoing emotional neediness of females contributes to their reduced ability to allow their daughters to separate. But the extent to which that is problematic in their lives is also affected by their ability to view themselves either more or less positively through received messages from other sources.

Similarly, males are affected by their ongoing emotional and social interactions. Boys, and later men, tend to have their physical and emotional needs met by mothers and sisters before they are aware of them. They therefore develop an expectation of entitlement, but no pattern of recognition, acknowledgement or nurturing of their own or others' emotional needs. So they too are cut off from their emotional needs, but in a different way. It is this which contributes to the sorts of difficulties that we associate with males and which make them more disposed to be violent, to commit crime, to sexually abuse others, and to be less emotionally aware.

If one thinks of the mother/child ability to achieve separation as a line of continuum, then the theory allows for relationships to reach varying points on that line. There is therefore a tendency for daughters to find it more difficult than sons to separate but this will be less of a problem for some daughters and more of a problem for some sons. In other words, it allows other factors to move into the equation.

Working with women does not mean trying to help them better emulate men. It means helping them to better connect with themselves and find ways of developing a more intact sense of self and an improved internal representation of that self with which to negotiate the outside world.

In the search for ways of achieving this with women, I have found concepts from the work of Eileen Aird (1985) and Jean Anyon (1983) especially useful. They believe that it is crucial to help women see that, even as adults, they can continue to develop emotionally and creatively while at the same time preserving and indeed validating aspects of their femaleness which have previously been discredited as unhealthy or infantile. The so-called female values of sharing, caring and concern for human relationships can be reframed as positive and desirable so that women can sustain them constructively and not at the expense of their own well-being.

Anyon believes that the female psyche has an ability to 'accommodate' externally received messages about the 'correct' way of being as a woman. Alongside this, she says that women maintain an 'inner non-subordination' to this view if it does not accord with their felt experience about themselves. If recognized and validated, e.g. in counselling, this internal non-subordination can be harnessed to creatively resist damaging external messages and allow constructive reframing to take place. She suggests that women can only achieve this inner resistance once their dependency needs are met to the extent that they become able to put themselves at the centre of their emotional stage in a way that has proved impossible before. In using this concept in my counselling, I believe that some constructive changes have resulted, and discuss them in more detail later.

The impact of pregnancy

In pregnancy, many women are consciously aware of their own experience of being parented as they prepare for becoming a parent themselves – and within that they look predominantly to their own experience of being mothered as that is the particular role that they will play. Many of their judgements about what to aim for and what to avoid in their new role are based on those past experiences.

When women become pregnant, identification with the mothering images and experiences of their infancy and childhood are enhanced. Object representations of their own mother as mother may now become self-representations of themselves as a potential mother. Their foremost psychological challenge over the course of the pregnancy is to reconcile the mother and the infant within their psyche. Maternal identifications may fuel their nurturant capabilities while infantile identifications may threaten them with profound neediness and dependency yearnings – the two need to be reconciled if a pattern of 'dislocated reality' is not to be repeated.

Entry into motherhood can block or at least dampen the urge to achieve emotional separation from one's own mother. If a woman has not dealt with this before entering motherhood, then her chances of dealing with it will be lessened as she re-enters the domain of the early-infancy mother/child relationship, even though she is the mother this time. In particular, for women facing difficulties in attaining motherhood through infertility, miscarriage and so on, the inner neediness resulting from incomplete separation may become more insistent, and may in part explain the greater distress that women showed in Monach's study.

However, our image of mothering is also influenced by what our society tells us that we should expect – and we all have a shortfall in our 'mothering', for which we are more likely to blame our mothers as the physical manifestation of that image, instead of the invisible 'mother image-makers'. Even women who have been better able to move along the mother/child separation continuum have been influenced in growing up in this country or elsewhere, or within differing cultures within the UK itself.

Irving Leon (1990) suggests that many women experience greater happiness in a first, wished-for pregnancy than in actual motherhood. They anticipate that the child will give them unprecedented bliss. This investment in an unborn child is not surprising, given the usual human shortfall between experience and image. However, it makes the negotiation of the actual relationship with the born child more problematic because it is inevitably less than perfect. Additionally, the mother has to negotiate this relationship according to her own internal representation of herself and also of course according to the gender of the baby.

In pregnancy loss (including abortion), with adoption or in giving birth to a child with a disability, women may experience what has been called 'narcissistic wounding' (Leon, 1990: p. 11), or having a sense of their own maternity being damaged. Women with an already impaired sense of self-esteem can feel, on delivery of such a child, especially confirmed in their view that nothing positive can come from them, that the child is a reflection of themselves and that they must therefore reject it, or that they are not good enough and will damage the child in some way if they try to parent it.

Many women experience a tremendous drive to get pregnant again quickly following a pregnancy loss. This is popularly thought of as the need to produce a replacement baby and therefore to be discouraged as unhealthy and potentially inhibiting of grieving. For me, this has never seemed an adequate explanation of women's reactions at this stage. Leon suggested that it may instead be an adaptive wish to repair one's sense of damaged maternity (1990: p. 77). In exploring that idea with women in counselling, I have found it to be much closer to what many feel. They describe their longing to be pregnant again – and for it to 'go right this time'; 'to try again and have a happy ending this time'. In my experience, women do not want to replace their baby – indeed they are often busy trying to 'reclaim' their baby from professionals who seem much more intent on denying it than they do! What women do want to replace is their experience of themselves as being unsuccessful in completing a pregnancy and producing a healthy baby, and they want to replace it with positive experiences.

Unintended pregnancy loss can sharpen a woman's awareness of her feelings about herself and her body but it can also reveal a conflict between her reproductive nurturing role and her non-domestic role. Men do not usually experience heightened bodily awareness during their partner's pregnancy and are less likely to experience role conflict.

The role conflict may be further heightened between the time of this loss and any subsequent pregnancy. Women are more likely than their male partners to be pressured to reveal their plans for further pregnancies because of implications for their paid work. They may find themselves marginalized, as colleagues act on an expectation that the women will withdraw in an ensuing pregnancy. Women report feeling that they now belong to neither world (Hey *et al.*, 1989 p. 151).

Similar findings are reported by women undergoing fertility investigations and treatments. Women talk about limiting their expectations of themselves in their work and in their careers but also feel marginalized and in limbo once they reveal their fertility state publicly (Monach, 1993; Pfeffer & Woolett, 1983).

Just as unplanned pregnancy loss can have an impact on women's roles and functioning, so can planned pregnancy loss. Abortion is sometimes seen as a challenge to motherhood as the socially approved female destiny. Women talk of being aware of this both in their internal representations of themselves and in the reactions of others (Davies, 1991; Dana, 1987; Pipes, 1986). This is further complicated when the abortion follows a diagnosis of a fetal abnormality. Here, the social acceptability of the action may be increased but some 'tainting' of the female image remains (Hey *et al.*, 1989).

Unplanned pregnancy can lead to a crisis in which women experience conflict between their internal and external worlds (Bishop, 1992). The conflict may be between the private and public meaning given to sexual mores; between the meaning of motherhood and single-parenthood; between being dependent and independent; between being a mother and having a career; between personal and social success and failure; between thinking about one's own life and that of a potential life. Even planned pregnancies will involve women in an awareness of such conflicts in varying degrees.

Mother or fetus at the centre?

Conflict also occurs in another area which is of central concern here – between the way that women are seen in relation to their unborn children by women themselves and by medicine and medical science.

I am regularly asked how I can offer counselling to one woman coping with abortion at ten o'clock and to another woman facing infertility at eleven. The question illustrates the extent to which our society splits off the unborn baby from the woman carrying it. For me, the woman is at the centre of each piece of work, not the fetus or longed-for child, and thus I do not experience a conflict.

Within reproductive medicine, there is an increasing tendency to marginalize women both in the literature and in the development of services (Raymond, 1987; Spallone, 1989). The terminology and style employed sometimes make it tempting to think that babies grow in a vacuum somewhere! Recent major reports about pregnancy – related developments have either not referred to women at all (Clothier Report, 1992) or only as parents to born children (Warnock Report, 1984). There have been cases in the USA where women have been forced through the courts to undergo Caesarian sections; and the fetal rights lobby has extended into post-delivery situations too.

A collection of women's experiences brought together in a book by Hey *et al.* (1989) is especially helpful in illustrating how important it is to remember that pregnancy and pregnancy-related developments are experienced by women in their bodies. In listening to women in this way and centrally taking account of women, it is obvious that we need to comprehend the relationship between the unborn child and its carrying mother or between the baby to be conceived and the potential carrying mother in order to better understand the emotional and social sig-nificance of reproduction.

In Hey's accounts, the women have each experienced different aspects of pregnancy loss and conclude that they are not necessarily mutually opposed ethically, politically or emotionally (although indivi-dual women may at times have experiences that relate to these divisions, at times, as social and socialized beings).

By denying the critical importance of the relationship between mother and unborn child or between potential mother and child to be conceived, there is a danger that our socialized expectations of this relationship become distorted. This has a reinforcing negative effect on women by further increasing the distance between their internal reality and external expectations of the mother/unborn child relationship. The role of the counsellor and of the health services in reversing this is of paramount importance for developing a more therapeutically healthy environment for women.

It is now time to turn to a more detailed look at the application of all of this to counselling.

Issues and principles of feminist counselling

All counselling models subscribe to the belief that the counsellor must have enhanced self knowledge so that he or she can identify where his or her own emotional material in the interaction begins and ends (roughly). The counsellor is thereby better able to help the client to move forward. (The counsellor has a right to work on his or her own problematic emotional material of course, but must negotiate the space and attention for that away from the counselling relationship with the client.)

Mainstream counselling makes use of the idea that people develop an internal representation of themselves which informs their sense of self-esteem. Some people have a more negative internal representation than others, and this is determined in part by their response to the key interpersonal relationships that have been available to them. People with experience of very damaging relationships are likely to develop a 'filtering' system which makes them later distort even positive messages into negative ones which better fit their internal sense of themselves. This makes it imperative for counsellors to get alongside their clients to try and understand what meaning the client makes of such experiences and received messages and to try and establish a relationship through which constructive change can be achieved by the client.

What is unique to a feminist-informed model?

Unlike most mainstream theories which concentrate solely on inter-personal relationships, feminist therapy centrally states itself to be political; it has an explicit world view and as such is likely to arouse antagonism. Luise Eichenbaum and Susie Orbach (1987) have said that: 'Feminist therapy does not simply "tack on" women's issues to therapeutic practice ... it profoundly affects the structure and the understanding of the therapeutic dialogue. It reframes the terms of the therapy relationship.'

Within this framework, there is a tremendous variety of therapeutic explanation and style of working, but each feminist-informed model subscribes to the view that counsellors need to understand and take account of the inner, the interpersonal and the external worlds.

Counsellors develop styles which deepen their understanding and which they have found to effect change or enable their clients to come to terms with major crises a little better. An awareness of gender issues, and their interplay with other life experiences such ethnicity, sexuality, able-bodiedness, class and so on is introduced centrally into the counselling experience. For me, it is feminism and feminist counselling that makes sense and has a meaning and that is why I continue to explore and develop it.

Feminist therapy affirms women's capacity to make constructive changes once their inner needs have been positively recognized and better addressed than previously. It acknowledges that women's capacity for change is also affected by wider societal forces over which they have no control, beyond the improvements that come through their own ability to better manage them. Counselling *per se* cannot change cultural and structural forces, it works on the personal level.

Following a crisis such as pregnancy loss, many women's previous coping mechanisms collapse, albeit temporarily. They need a therapeutically helpful external environment to 'look after' them during this time, but do not always need counselling. Acknowledgement of their inner need may be enough to enable them to rebuild their coping strategies constructively along similar lines. They will necessarily incorporate into such strategies the new knowledge that they may gain about themselves through this new experience. A helpful environment may be provided by family, friends, self-help groups and sensitive health and other professionals who can offer attentive listening and support.

This process of being nurtured in a positive environment may lead to increased awareness of the ways in which their gender experience has negatively impacted on the way that they deal with life, and they may make constructive changes for themselves.

Women who need counselling to help with the rebuilding are those whose previous coping mechanisms cannot be reassembled within an acceptable time-scale or where the crisis unleashes previous damage which is too great to be tackled alone and where the woman herself decides that she needs to change and wants to use counselling to achieve that. Counsellors like myself who offer a support service as well as counselling are well placed to recognize which is the more appropriate service to offer.

The starting point in establishing a counselling relationship is when the woman client perceives that the counsellor wants to help, to work alongside them in their difficulties; the woman wants to believe the motivation is altruistic and that the contact will be helpful, but at the same time, she may be afraid of it. A consideration of women's psychosocial role allows us to understand that women often feel that they shouldn't expect to be helped; or that as they're not sure that they deserve help so may sabotage it; or that they're beyond help. Female clients can tend to take responsibility for insensitive, unhelpful helping. Counsellors need to recognize this and to avoid colluding with it, instead concentrating on enabling the woman to believe in the right to have her needs met constructively.

In counselling in reproductive medicine, it is often a loss which precipitates the counselling to start – be it a pregnancy loss through miscarriage, stillbirth or abortion; the loss of anticipated parenting through infertility and sub-fertility; or the loss of social parenting as a result of deciding to place a child for adoption.

A feminist counselling model of grief-work

This section focuses on outlining a feminist-informed counselling model which I have found helpful in my work around pregnancy loss and loss in this wider sense.

There are many books written about bereavement counselling. Among the best known are those by Colin Murray Parkes (1986) and William Worden (1991) and I have adapted their work to suggest the following main stages in the grieving process.

The initial stage is characterized by feelings of shock, disbelief, and numbness. The woman may then try to blot out, deny or ignore the fact that the loss is happening to her. She may experience overwhelming feelings such as guilt, anger and hostility. The woman typically goes through times of 'searching' for the unborn baby that she has lost, or for the baby she has placed for adoption, or for the baby that she wanted to conceive. This searching gradually moves on to a search for her lost identity or for ways to regain control or meaning in her life.

The final stage is when the woman is able to face the reality and understand it as a loss. Denial is broken, so conflict can pass; she does not forget but moves towards accepting. She recognizes the changed circumstances, revises her representational models and redefines her goals in life so that she does not have to remain in a state of suspended growth.

In practice the process is rarely, if ever, linear, and women move in and out of these states within an overall progression. This delineation is best used as an aid for counsellors and clients in identifying the stages that may need to be negotiated.

Many of the feelings associated with pregnancy loss are not dissimilar to those associated with other grief reactions (Jennings, 1991). Bereaved people everywhere often experience a sense of the futility of living, that life has lost its meaning. But there are crucial additional feelings in reproductive loss. In their work about infertility, Diane and Peter Houghton (1987) talk about 'unfocused grief' when describing the loss of a longed-for child, the thwarting of love and experiencing of 'genetic death'. This feeling is present throughout pregnancy loss whereby the grief is not only for the baby lost but also for all that the baby could have meant to the parent. This includes the lost future with this baby for them as an individual, as part of a couple, as a family and as part of an extended family and social network.

Studies by both Mira Dana (1984) and Simon Bishop (1992) also found that women facing abortions at around the time of confirmation of pregnancy or when a fetal abnormality was diagnosed (i.e. before abortions are even performed) were often in a state of early grief or anticipatory grieving, Similar descriptions apply to women who have been told that they are about to miscarry, or that their baby has died *in utero* (Kohner & Henley, 1992; Leroy, 1988).

In my practice, I have identified other grief reactions. Loss of 'innocence' is widely experienced as women lose any belief they had that as such a loss could never happen to them, it cannot possibly exist. Women experience strong feelings, including sadness and rage, that they will never again contemplate or have a pregnancy which they can approach in that innocent way.

Envy is another powerful emotion and is often followed by shame. Many women feel ashamed and guilty at having envious feelings. They try to suppress them or turn their 'destructive envy' in on to themselves. Women are often afraid that they will somehow damage the person they feel envious of through such feelings. When encouraged to give words and expression to the feelings within counselling, they gain enormous relief. The counsellor can help a woman see that this is a common response, and that she needs to connect with those feelings for her own sake, that it is herself that she will harm if she doesn't, and that she does not 'deserve' to be harmed. The counsellor can help the woman make such feelings more manageable and give the woman the crucial message that she will not be rejected or destroyed as a result of sharing these 'wicked' thoughts.

Case history:

Lynne, 28, felt consumed with envy on hearing from her mother that two old school friends of hers were pregnant within weeks of Lynne undergoing a therapeutic abortion at 20 weeks pregnant, after being told that her unborn baby had a serious abnormality. Lynne told me about their pregnancies in counselling and I suggested that she might have uncomfortable feelings about them. She told me that she was afraid that she might somehow transmit a 'death wish' onto those pregnancies. This also opened up the opportunity for her to share with me her inability to tell her mother or husband how she felt. Holding her back was a mixture of thinking that they would reject her for being so awful and that it would lead to them telling her how she had deprived them of their child and grandchild. But it also allowed her to say how angry she was that neither of them had realized how she might feel; and how she had felt so guilty at having such 'selfish' thoughts that she had been trying to suppress her anger.

Feelings of envy are regularly expressed to me by women about other women from apparently diametrically opposite groups. Thus, infertile women envy fertile women; mothers envy non-mothers; mothers with one child envy those with more. Women who have suffered stillbirths and women who are infertile have written about their intense feelings of jealousy towards those with successful pregnancies (Kohner & Henley, 1992; Houghton & Houghton, 1987). It has been suggested that jealousy is a part of 'wanting'. Following pregnancy loss, the wanting can continue for a long time. For some women, the wanting may never be fulfilled with a longed-for child and, for them, they may need to move on to 'a necessary sadness' (Kohner & Henley, 1992 p. 77) before their feelings of envy and shame can become less intense.

A woman experiencing pregnancy loss may also have a heightened sense of feeling somehow to blame, of feeling a failure. This baby was a part of her, growing inside her body and connected with her, consciously or unconsciously, in a way that cannot be replicated in her male partner. She may feel that her body has let her down but she may also feel that she *is* her body, and her self-image of her body is thereby damaged.

Case history

Jane, 32, had not enjoyed her pregnancy. She had hated the change in her body shape and the resulting immobility. She had longed to get back to her pre-pregnancy size when she thought that she could be more herself. The stillbirth of her daughter left her feeling dreadful, especially when she found herself looking longingly at baby dresses and fantasizing about dressing her daughter up in them. In counselling, we explored the meaning of body shapes and clothes for Jane and she connected up many messages from her own childhood and from her relationship with her partner about the importance of physical appearance. Jane started to work out for herself what shape and appearance she felt comfortable with on the inside as well as the outside.

Many women in western society already feel uncomfortable with their bodies (Orbach, 1993, Chernin, 1984). Their grief experience brings an added sense of failure and what Erving Goffman has called a 'spoiled identity' (Goffman, 1963) which here incorporates body and self. Additionally, the source of that shame and spoiled identity becomes distressingly public through the public involvement of the medical world into the experience.

Women often link this sense of failure with previous messages of failure received over the years e.g. 'I've failed again'; 'why me?'; 'nobody understands'. This sense of failure may be illuminating for locating and redressing sources of earlier emotional damage if counsellors ask women where and from whom they have felt similar feelings in the past.

Case history

Julie, 19, placed her baby for adoption shortly after birth. She had felt a failure most of her life. Her young mother had been unable to manage her and soon abandoned her to her grandmother's care; her grandmother had died when Julie was a turbulent 13 year-old and she blamed herself for the death; she was unable to settle in a string of foster homes and had already had one abortion prior to this pregnancy. She felt that she did not deserve to keep the baby and would anyway emotionally damage him if she cared for him. Her periodic bouts of depression and unsettled life-style confirmed her in her decision to let her son go but, with support, she did care for him while in hospital and visited him prior to placement; and she still maintains occasional written contact with the adoptive parents through me. Counselling did not effect major changes for Julie, but it helped her develop a more positive view of herself as a mother and a woman than she started with. She did some initial work about her feelings of guilt about 'causing' her mother's desertion and her grandmother's death. I remain hopeful that she will return to counselling to move further forward in the future.

Not uncommonly, women find that their impaired body and self image leads them to resurrect negative feelings about previous pregnancies, previous abortions, and previous sexual encounters which now take on new self-punitive meanings. Those around them, including health professionals, frequently collude with this either overtly or covertly by asking them in some detail about such facts, thus reinforcing their fear that they are related to the loss. We all need to be aware of the impact of such questions and check out our own motivation in asking them.

Case history

Apparently suffering from infertility with no identified cause, Lyndsey, 35, was eventually able to tell me that she had been raped as a teenager and had never dared tell anyone. Her mother was very strict and said that she would be thrown out if she ever 'got into trouble'; her father continually undermined her verbally. She had decided not to tell her husband about the attack as it had been in the past but now was convinced that it was causing the infertility and was her fault. Over time, Lyndsey told me the story of the attack and we worked together on looking back at her as a teenager and putting responsibility where it lay, i.e. with the attacker. We were able to then move on to exploring Lyndsey's anger and sadness at the lack of warmth and acceptance displayed by her parents and by her mother in particular. Lyndsey is now contemplating telling her husband about the incident and resuming the infertility investigations.

The physical ache that many bereaved people feel is enhanced in women experiencing pregnancy loss who describe a physical void within. Women have told me of heightened feelings of being disconnected, isolated and depersonalized. In pregnancy loss there is a particular bodily sense of this in that it is actually something that was inside the body of the woman which has been lost or, in the case of infertility, where something that should be inside will not grow there.

The impact of this sense of a physical void was shown when Kohner & Henley (1992) relayed women's reactions to sex after having a stillbirth. Some women wanted to make love again in order for their bodies to no longer feel like a coffin while others could not bear the thought that another being would enter into the place where had last been inhabited by their baby. It is a unique experience in grieving.

Pregnancy loss can precipitate feelings of isolation from external groupings, or as one woman described it to Ann Oakley: '... being alone in a world of mothers' (Oakley *et al.*, 1990 p. 106). Other women who had miscarried told her that 'The impact of peers and siblings having children increased the sense of isolation. They no longer shared central experiences, and the embarrassment and awkwardness of others made them turn away' (p. 220).

Women who are already mothers when the crisis occurs can experience this exclusion as a feeling of alienation from their existing maternal role. Many of those around them expect such women to gain comfort from their existing mothering and this in turn makes them feel particularly odd and uncomfortable when they do not. I now make a point of telling women who are already mothers that I would not be surprised to hear that they have this reaction. Many women have told me with great relief that they have felt at best numb and at worst rejecting towards existing children. They want to mother the child that they have lost or have wanted to conceive, not the ones they already have.

Case history

Zubaida, 26, had two children aged 5 and 3 when she lost her third baby a few hours after it was born prematurely. She was very ill herself after delivery and remained in hospital for five days. On a home visit a couple of weeks later, something about how she was reacting with one of her children made me open up the question of her reaction to them. Zubaida was enormously relieved to know that she was not alone in feeling rejecting towards her live children after a loss. She had been feeling very guilty but nevertheless very antagonistic to them to the extent that she could hardly bear to have anything to do with them. After her session, she was able to explain this to her husband and family too and allowed herself the time she needed to 'be with' the child she longed to mother, before being able to 'return' to her live children.

Seeing mother and unborn child as separate (referred to earlier) can therefore be detrimental to the woman's emotional well-being. Listening to women's own accounts of pregnancy, birth and pregnancy loss, points to the need to find out (in counselling) what meaning the woman herself wants to place on her relationship with the baby that has been or is growing inside her, or that she would like to have growing there.

Oakley relayed the distress felt by many women at the detached language used in hospitals and by health professionals to describe their baby and their experience. Terms such as 'fetal remains', 'products of conception', 'fetal wastage' were particularly highlighted (Oakley *et al.*, 1990 p. 11). Interestingly, she also reported that a baby tended to be called a baby as long as all was well, e.g. at a routine scan. However, once problems arose, women reported that professionals suddenly 'renamed' the baby so that he or she became a 'fetus', an 'embryo' or even a '16-week pregnancy'. This detachment may be at least in part due to the professional's own need to depersonalize the baby as something 'other'.

The theme of 'reclaiming' the baby appears in writings and accounts from all areas of reproductive experience. Thus, birth mothers in adoption started coming forward once there was an external validation that they have needs too, particularly through the work of the Post Adoption Centre (Howe *et al.*, 1992). Several recent books (Neustatter, 1986; Davies, 1991; Leroy, 1990; Kohner & Henley, 1992) have acknowledged women's wish to talk about their feelings of loss for the baby in stillbirth, miscarriage and also abortion – feelings echoed through the self-help movements.

Unless, and until, women are afforded the opportunity and external validation to (slowly and if it feels the right thing to do) incorporate this into their grieving – then it may in turn distort the grieving process unhealthily. Hey *et al.* (1989) talked of the importance of women gradually learning to let go emotionally of the baby which is no longer physically inside them while retaining the memory as a positive part of themselves. Women need not only to internalize a positive image of their baby but also a positive image of that child with themselves as mother: this is true for both intended and unintended pregnancy loss. Thus I have helped women reconnect with and mourn their miscarried and aborted babies, and the babies they have given away for adoption.

Case history

Both Leila, 23, and Angela, 29, were stuck in their grieving because they had not felt able to ask anyone what had happened to their babies. Leila had had an abortion at 9 weeks pregnant, which she still felt to have been the right decision. Angela had miscarried at 11 weeks pregnant while on the toilet at home. Both were haunted by the thought of what had happened to their babies. Both had tentatively tried to ask, but their questions had been brushed aside. In counselling, we were able to acknowledge that the disposal of their babies had not been in a manner that they would have wanted – and the acknowledgement and mourning for that loss was then enough for them to be able to move on.

Women's experience of the process of the loss itself is also crucial to understand. The counsellor needs to be able to identify where the handling of the situation by those around the woman has made emotional recovery more difficult for her. When the woman can see that she was influenced by that process as well as influencing it herself then she can better move away from the potential for self-blame. Highlighting some of the processes which have regularly presented problems for women's recovery may also be useful in considering how the services themselves can become more therapeutically sound.

In the public arena of the medical world, infertility, miscarriage or stillbirth is likely to be treated primarily as a biological malfunction, a technical problem requiring a medical (physical) treatment solution. For the woman, however, it is a multidimensional experience and she needs to be allowed to negotiate and experience different routes without being swept along on the professional's time-scale and the institution's procedures. Of course, in the path to pregnancy loss, there are sometimes compelling medical reasons to move the woman along. Nevertheless, even within necessary medical procedures, there is often time to stop and check the emotional state of the woman and slow things down to allow her emotional state to keep pace more closely with her physical experience.

For example, where abortions are offered following the diagnosis of a fetal abnormality, doctors tend to arrange the abortion very quickly. When asked why, they typically reply that women and couples request it. Yet women seeking abortions on 'social grounds' also request a speedy service to which doctors do not seem as compelled to respond.

Grief-work patterns and my work experience indicate that it better aids the healing process if women and couples are allowed to spend a little longer in the 'anticipatory' grieving state. Doctors may therefore serve their patient's interests better by delaying the process. It may be important for them to consider whose needs are in fact being met by dealing with these abortions so quickly.

There may be times when women going through the process of loss feel so swamped with feelings of helplessness that they appear to want to be taken over and be dependent on someone who will offer them support, guidance and direction. Decision-making may be especially difficult for women if they revert to this childlike state. Such women may see themselves as at fault for having intense emotional reactions if those feelings are not acknowledged as normal by the person in whom they are investing so much trust.

Some women do not enter this highly dependent state, but may be too numb to counteract any assumptions that they have done so. For these women, the danger is of feeling taken over, and of losing control. As women, this may critically connect with feelings of having only illusory control over their lives anyway and this can mean that even relatively small losses of control are experienced as proportionately major losses. Again, professionals need to be aware of the effects of their actions and the need to allow women to maintain maximum control at all times.

Case history

Jasmin, 33, had been brought up in a household where her father's word was law. Jasmin had struggled to develop self-confidence since leaving home and going through university. She felt pleased with her efforts to date, held down a professional job and worked hard at making her marriage an equal partnership. She went to pieces several months into routine infertility investigations when her results had gone missing a second time and the doctor had been verbally dismissive of her assertive stance in asking for additional investigations and an earlier follow-up appointment. The doctor immediately referred her for counselling. Early on in our work, we recognized triggers of power and control issues for Jasmin in the hospital procedures and attitudes of the doctors and were then able to tackle them by Jasmin using counselling to work on that for herself and by me feeding back to the doctors about the unhelpfulness of their approach.

Woman's self-confidence is invariably low at such a time, even when they are reassured by medical advisers that they are entirely blameless. When no cause for infertility or fetal abnormality or miscarriage can be found or where the woman herself has decided to end the pregnancy (in abortion) or not take on the parenting (in adoption), the potential for self-blame and lowered self-esteem is even greater. At such times, women often impute critical meaning into non-critical remarks and become especially receptive to intended critical comment. Relating to those women who already tend to distort messages received to correspond with prior negative internal representation, may be additionally difficult. It can be useful for health professionals to understand this in order to assess their patient's reactions more accurately and to cope with any feelings of rejection that they may themselves experience at the apparent rebuff of their helping.

Relating to women with their male partner present also needs forethought. Professionals sometimes prefer to relate to the man in these situations, with the inherent danger that the woman feels invisible. This is exacerbated where the professional talks to the man as if he is the woman's father rather than partner, again heightening the woman's sense of lack of control.

For some women, this latter action can coincide with them feeling anger towards their male partner and his (often) seeming emotional frigidity. This anger can spill over in the time immediately surrounding the loss, or in the aftermath. It needs to be acknowledged and worked with constructively with either the woman alone or the couple. This can then encourage the man to openly connect with his 'weak' feelings of sadness and abandon his stance of being strong and in control in order to 'help' his partner. Men are also caught in gender roles around grief reactions, just as much as women. If their partner's anger is instead dismissed or rejected as an emotional overreaction on the part of the woman, a positive opportunity for work is lost.

Of course, not all women feel anger towards their male partners at this time. However, in my experience, women almost always express regret that their male partners are not able to show their feelings or too quickly get them under control again after showing them. Women feel (and fear) that their partners do not care about the loss as much as they do, that they have soon forgotten and a chasm between them starts to open up. Women also not infrequently express the regret that they are thereby denied the chance to sometimes be the strong one in the relationship and a comfort to their partners. They can thereby feel less legitimated in seeking comfort at those times when their own distress feels overwhelming. It's one of life's ironies that women are cast as the emotional nurturers and caretakers and yet men cite their role as needing to be strong for their wife as their barrier to connecting with deeper feelings.

The tasks in feminist counselling

We now consider ongoing tasks in counselling, further to those already identified. Just as in delineating a grief-work model, so is it possible to identify a 'linear' model of counselling – but with the same proviso that counsellor and client will without doubt not stick to the straight and narrow and the journey may be long and complex!

First and foremost, the counsellor needs to allow and encourage a woman client to tell her story, and the counsellor needs to listen. Interestingly, both Monach (1993) and Oakley *et al.* (1990) commented on the fact that respondents in their studies positively welcomed the chance to talk to an attentive listener. The counsellor needs to try and understand the meaning of what the woman is saying and help her use that meaning positively.

In my experience, women almost always want to explore their own experiences of being mothered. This is true of women in counselling and in other therapeutically helpful settings. In counselling, it often seems to be the case that the woman's experience of mothering has been particularly damaging. Thus women may have been denied 'good enough' mothering through the death of their mother, her desertion either physically or emotionally, or where she has been unable to combat the destructive effect of her male partner.

Women need the opportunity to reflect on that in a way which can be or can become creative. In the reflecting and remembering however, (sometimes for the first time in a conscious way), women can feel overwhelmed at times with critical feelings towards their own mothers. They may feel that they are thereby likely to be criticized themselves in view of their probably incomplete separation from those experiences. The potential to feel judged by the counsellor is great and the skill of the counsellor is in coping with that and eventually working towards the woman recognizing the needy mother and child of that early relationship so she can let go of the need to blame her real mother.

The counsellor needs to identify together with the woman client the psychological tasks that are associated with the problem encountered (e.g. infertility, coping with a stillbirth); the stage that she is at in dealing with it; and the degree of impairment that she has in coping.

This involves identifying with the woman what feelings and ideas are emotionally comforting to the client, which feel dangerous and frightening and which feel exciting and liberating. There will be times when they explore feelings of fear because they sense that there is something important to unlock behind them. Sometimes there will be an awareness that the client has 'moved on', indicated by perhaps a shared feeling of elation or peace – without either the counsellor or client necessarily being able to identify the route or the turning point.

The woman's social system will similarly need to be identified, including its positive reinforcing states and its negative ones. The impact of changes there will need to be determined.

Central to any understanding is the importance and meaning of control to the woman, and its meaning within the counselling relationship. This includes how the woman identifies her optimum state of 'being in control' and what could be achieved in this respect. Moreover, both she and the counsellor need to be aware of the acceptability of new states of control and coping mechanisms to existing relationships. Changes will have impact on other areas of the woman's life and on other relationships, and the counsellor needs to remain alert to this.

When the woman is able finally to internalize a more positive internal representation of herself she is then ready to move out of the counselling relationship with this new idea of herself.

Throughout the counselling process, the interaction between the representations that the counsellor and client ascribe to each other and the use made of them is critical. The development of a more positive sense of the client's self will, in part result, from this dialogue.

Within counselling situations in reproductive medicine, some or all of the following stages will hopefully be attained by the woman:

- adjusting to life without the baby that she lost or longed for
- letting go the identity that she was pursuing for herself – as mother, mother to a particular child or mother at a particular age
- reconnecting with herself, and, if appropriate, with her family, partner, friends, social network
- developing a changed role and identity for herself about which she can feel positively
- feeling in an optimum state of control.

Hey *et al.* (1989) suggested that women need certain key experiences from others to help them in achieving the necessary grieving stages. Thus they talk about the need for:

- *Confirmation* – that no woman is completely alone or abnormal in losing a baby nor in responding to it in the ways she does
- *Information* – about their bodies, (including miscarriage, ectopic pregnancy and so on); and about the structure and informing principles of the health services and of mourning
- *Affirmation* – that, individually or together, women can do something positive, either by understanding something that they previously had not, or by finally allowing themselves to grieve fully and freely, or by taking action for some kind of change. (This has been named 'Coming through and going on').

I would add two further crucial stages:

- Consensual validation of suffering – that there is something common to all women going through this type of grieving;
- Reinforced permission to stop grieving – that women may need to be told that it is alright to move into a stage of 'facing the reality of loss' and of 'going on', and that it makes them no less a woman as a result.

In trying to draw out such patterns, the feminist counsellor is incorporating a central tenet of feminism – the belief in the positive value of recognizing and naming experiences common to women. By deindividualizing experiences, as well as accepting that there will be unique differences within them, it is possible to reach through the loneliness and connect with it.

In also giving women the message that they can move on from grieving, feminist counsellors are incorporating an awareness of the mixed messages that women get about their coping abilities through stereotyped female images. Women may receive strong messages that they should construct their coping quickly – to 'hide' their temporary collapse and 'get over it'. This may include the message that they should not talk about the baby overmuch as this is somehow unhealthy.

There is usually an alternative message too: men are expected to be less upset than women and for a shorter time because they are supposed to be 'stronger' and have more important things to occupy themselves with in the public world. Women may find an expectation that they will be more upset than their male partners, but that this must follow equally strongly prescribed patterns to avoid any pathological label being attached to them. Thus, women are expected to resume basic tasks relatively quickly to give the outward appearance of coping; but they are not expected to get over the loss too quickly or completely in order to conform to the role of a 'proper, caring woman'. As Irving Leon has said '. . . to forget her loss would be a form of abandoning her own' (1990 p. 77).

It has, hopefully, been clear from what has already been said that I would distinguish between the need to offer therapy via counselling and the need to provide a therapeutic atmosphere within which some women will manage without counselling and other women will be better enabled to move into counselling.

Additional models of helping

Supportive listening

Many women make good use of supportive listening; of being allowed to tell their story as often and for as long as they want to, uninterrupted and without advice or judgements (no matter how well meaning). This can be provided by health and other professionals, or partners, family, friends, and other members of the social network.

Self-help groups

Self-help groups also offer members supportive listening although the woman usually needs to be emotionally free enough to be able to give attention to other group members in turn. Such groups can play a very important part in validating feelings and experiences and can also lead on to empowering members to seek to effect changes in institutional practices which have been commonly experienced as unhelpful.

Many of the changes that have taken place in hospitals have come about through pressure from self-help movements such as the Stillbirth & Neonatal Death Society (SANDS), the Miscarriage Association and Support After Termination for Fetal Abnormality (SATFA). These organizations predominantly comprise women and are testament to the power of coming together with common experiences, validating them by talking about them together and thereby feeling empowered to press for changes. This may often occur in the face of strong resistance from health professionals who regularly voice the argument that it is only neurotic women who join such organizations and make a fuss!

It has been written that: 'A death is a death, whether of a loved companion or of an unknown half-formed foetus; but the nuances of mourning and recovery should not be limited, however they may initially be shaped, by institutions either of bricks and mortar or of social norms' (Hey *et al.*, 1989 p. 148).

Institutional changes

Institutional changes, especially in health service delivery, should constantly be considered if they might improve the therapeutic atmosphere which women need to inhabit. These include changes in particular relationships that are established, even if only for brief times – such as the doctor/patient, nurse/patient or radiographer/patient relationship – as well as changes in wider institutional practices such as how to handle the disposal of the miscarried, aborted or stillborn baby.

In the hospital in which I work, there have been significant changes in the last few years to reflect parents' wishes and feedback from counsellors and others. There is now a 'Book of Remembrance' for all babies; an annual Remembrance Service; the opportunity for all babies or fetuses to be cremated or buried and for religious services to be held for them; a room on the ward redesigned and set aside for women who are or may be miscarrying, with streamlined medical procedures available for this contingency; a monthly drop-in clinic staffed by midwives, social workers and health visitors for women going through subsequent pregnancies after a stillbirth; booklets available for parents particular to their experience; and a bi-monthly information and support group evening for women and couples having difficulty in conceiving.

Changes in society

Changes within wider society are more difficult to bring about. Societal norms are largely outside of our control although changes at interpersonal and institutional levels can start to seep upwards, and public dialogue can certainly be prompted by more localized movements.

Conclusion

In this chapter, we have seen that the experiences of gender affect experiences of pregnancy, parenting and our interaction with reproductive medicine. In the development of the female psyche, women have a greater tendency to develop a sense of low self-esteem. They also may have a need to connect their identity and status with others (usually men and/or children), and have a drive to be nurturing of others in ways which may feel unsatisfying if expressed at the expense of their own needs.

I have gone on to consider how these experiences influence the ways in which women cope with crises arising in relation to their reproductive selves. I have outlined my belief that the most constructive ways of helping women cope with these are: to listen to them more carefully; to encourage them to speak more openly from within themselves; and to affirm the specificity of their experiences while trying to help them identify the commonalities with other women too. In keeping with this, the importance of other influences on women's lives, for example ethnic identity, sexuality, class, disability has been mentioned. Ways of increasing an understanding of their interconnectedness and separateness have been explored.

The importance of women's own experiences of being mothered as well as of their later life experiences has also been outlined. Indeed, the importance of professionals better understanding women's experiences is a constant theme. This is especially true in the current move within the medical and scientific world to see mothers and their unborn children as separate while women themselves stress the crucial significance of being allowed to define for themselves the nature of that relationship.

Different avenues for creating a more woman-centred way of managing reproductive health services have been outlined within the belief that individuals can influence at least some of the structures in which they participate even though they are also always partly a product of them. Such participation can be both through any psychic restructuring resulting from individual therapy and through the experiencing of other indirectly therapeutic situations.

Out of the immensely painful experience of pregnancy loss in general, women may even come to expand the very parameters of their femininity and masculinity. I worked with Bernadette for several years on and off. During this time, she was only able to see herself as wanting to be a mother and that drove her through numerous treatments, four miscarriages, and the death of a son and a daughter who each lived for only a few days. One day, she came to tell me that she no longer needed to see me. She was ready to move on with 'a necessary sadness' but also with a new strong sense of herself as a creative woman with living left to do. We cried together for all the babies that she had lost and for the children she would never help nurture to adulthood, and she then left telling me to tell the women clients I was still seeing that

> ... there's green grass out there and bright yellow and blue flowers that I haven't seen for years. All I've been able to see is grey, but I can see colour now ...'

N.B. My thanks go to those women whose stories are contained in this chapter in so many different ways and with whom I have had the privilege to work. Many thanks also go to friends and colleagues who have been so helpful in reading and commenting on earlier drafts, including Lesley Blackthorn, Iris Singer, Pat Spallone and, of course, Sue Jennings. Finally, thank you to my family, Julia, Jonathan and Phil for all their patience, love and cups of tea during the seemingly endless, and at times fraught, hours of writing.

N.B. Please note that any case examples used in this chapter are an amalgam of case histories, rather than specific histories, in order to preserve anonymity.

Chapter 4

Male Mysteries: Factors in Male Infertility

Sammy Lee

Introduction

For a number of reasons, many societies in the world are male dominated. Indeed, medical specialists, even in the field of obstetrics and gynaecology are predominantly male. Moreover, infertility specialists are almost always gynaecologists! Perhaps as a consequence of the predominance of men in this field, investigations and treatment of infertility have always been focused on the female problems of infertility. Historically men have been able to deny involvement in infertility and until very recently, little attention was paid to the man in most infertility clinics (which even now are often within gynaecology units in maternity buildings). Indeed, in Asiatic, African and Middle Eastern cultures today, even if the male is actually known to be contributing to the infertility problem, this fact may not be overtly discussed; and it's often the lot of the female partner to bear the brunt of the infertility guilt (see the case history below).

Furthermore, in these societies the possession of many male offspring is equally as important as the possession of land and cattle. It is interesting to note that in the Bible, a man committed to a 'barren' marriage is allowed to take on further wives – consider Abram, Sarai and Hagar. It is a theme that runs deeply throughout the millennia of history and prehistory; childless male heroes are constantly encouraged to take on a new partner. More often than not, when infertility is finally overcome, for example in the Bible, the child is a male.

But it is not just other cultures that favour male offspring. There are still several titled, aristocratic, landed English families that place great importance on the need for a male heir to maintain their lineage.

Generally it is important to bear in mind when counselling that cultural and ethnic backgrounds must be considered. People from different backgrounds are likely to harbour different outlooks – perhaps favouring male offspring even more than we do – and have differing lifestyles.

Case history 1
There are men who cannot accept the diagnosis of male subfertility, and this

is particularly common amongst Arab, Asian and Greek men. One such couple had just received a diagnosis of male sub-fertility. The specialist had suggested that there was almost no chance of success which had left the man in a terrible state. The interpreter suggested to me that the diagnosis had brought about a crisis as it had left no possibility for hope, thereby leaving the man very depressed. The interpreter explained that for Arab men, there was a type of pride invested in one's fertility; to denude a man of this 'spiritual' need was to leave him impotent, mentally as well as physically.

Cultural, ethnic and religious issues relating to male infertility

It is important to note several additional points relating to culture and male infertility. Much of humankind (strict Catholics and orthodox Jews for example) is not allowed to practice contraception. Many religions place great emphasis on fertility, within the sanctity of marriage. In traditional societies a barren couple experiences a loss of status. In particular, even if the man is the root of the problem, it is the female generally who stands to lose the greatest amount of status. In the Bible infertility is often described as God failing to bless a relationship. The phrase 'Go forth and multiply' (found, of course, in the Bible) is a tenet of many religions. Even within the broad aspect of Christianity, infertility is barely acknowledged. If you are good, you will marry and have children. An unspoken inference is that if you are barren, it is God's will, and probably you are being punished for some sin.

Hence many infertile couples believe that they are indeed being punished by their god for some unknown act of sin. This often leads to feelings of guilt among infertile couples. When dealing with this issue of guilt and punishment, I explore the idea of the client giving themselves permission to have children and try to affirm their right to do so. It is very important to dispel their fears and anxieties on this matter.

It is very important to check that the fertility treatment on offer does not conflict with the patients' ethical, cultural or religious beliefs.

In some religions, all *gametes* must be used, no seed may be wasted; the semen sample unused for IVF *must* be placed into the vagina; similarly, all embryos resulting from IVF must be used, and furthermore freezing is not acceptable. The Pope is in principle against 'assisted conception', which is viewed as a collection of unnatural practices. The Chinese traditionally rely on acupuncture or medical herbalism, whilst Africans, and many Asians rely on fortune-telling and Shamanism. It is important to remember that for many Africans and Arabs masturbation is taboo and humiliating. The Chinese are tremendously embarrassed about infertility, especially the women, and Asian women are likewise usually tightlipped on the subject.

Much has been written very recently about 'sex selection'. In Indian and Chinese society, male offspring are greatly desired and there are some who argue that in these societies it is the cost of a dowry and the cost of bringing up females that makes this desirable. In Indian society, for example, males are further desired because the male stays in the family home and will be the family heir and also lights the funeral pyre. This is particularly pertinent with regard to the next case history.

Case history 2

Mr G, an Indian man with azoospermia had declined donor insemination (DI). Several years later, after a serious illness, and now being infirm, Mr G was willing to entertain DI. He claimed to be resigned to his position of being unable to father a child himself and stated that he now wished to have DI treatment for his partner's sake, rationalizing that this was the only way they could now have a child. He offered both religious and cultural reasons for declining DI initially. No one will know about the treatment other than he and his wife. Interestingly, the prospective child was to look after him in his infirmity! There were additionally strong family pressures to produce off-spring.

Some hidden agendas

In the 1980s and 1990s more attention has slowly been paid to the male problems of infertility. But even with better understanding, greater enlightenment and clear opportunities for diagnosis, it is interesting to observe that in spite of the availability of advanced male sperm function testing, many specialists still pay little attention to this subspeciality. Reasons for this remain unknown. It is possible that because of our historical ignorance about male infertility, the *status quo* demands that we continue to ignore this aspect of infertility. Another possibility is that gynaecology and hence infertility are disciplines that centre on women and not on men. The male consequently is an unknown quantity for most of these specialists. My own experience in this area may throw some light on the matter. I am often referred men who have a low [sperm] count for further diagnosis. Often these men have *no* count, 'low' being used as a euphemism. It seems that both male and female gynaecologists find it difficult dealing with infertile or sub-fertile men. When talking about male infertility, we are highlighting a difficulty in providing diagnosis as well as a problem in explaining to men that they have sperm dysfunction.

How men feel about infertility

Men often feel very uncomfortable when placed under the spotlight in a clinical setting. Often the man appears to be detached, remote and uninterested in proceedings – even though he may in actual fact be full of anxiety. Invariably, and fortuitously the female partner also attends (in more than 90% of cases). It seems that the masculinity of the man is seen as being under threat. It is often quoted that the link between virility and fertility means that a diagnosis of infertility is a major blow to a man's belief in his own manhood; this is without doubt an important issue, but just how important remains unclear. Some men have episodes of impotence, and logically, it is probably these men whose virility needs affirmation, whilst the others may not feel their manhood to be under the same threat.

Putting aside the feelings relating to loss of potency, men also often experience a feeling of guilt and self-blame and a sense of uselessness begins to surface. Indeed, in many cultures, a man's ability to have offspring is linked to his social standing and potency in society. Confirmation of male factor infertility (such as with sperm dysfunction), brings all these emotions to a head in the man. Shock and panic are accessory emotions, and they may persist in sub-crisis for years. In women, emotions which may persist over several years are those of denial and loss; aspects of bereavement may last for many years. But for men, this feeling of bereavement does not seem to be so important, although, whether this is due to denial is still unclear. Rather, the male will often volunteer that the feeling of guilt and uselessness are the key long-term emotions. Anger is also prevalent in men although it will usually be denied at first. The anger is not always explicit, nor necessarily present at home, but is more easily displayed at work. Often the anger is released over issues unrelated to infertility, but over any irritating issue, particularly at work. A key word which is often unspoken is frustration. Because of the overwhelming tendency of men to deny their plight, there is often an irrevocable commitment to isolation. This self-imposed isolation makes men particularly difficult to deal with both from a medical point of view as well as a counselling aspect. Loss of self-esteem is also undoubtedly common and is by contrast always readily acknowledged; the man may deny anger and deny feelings of loss of virility/potency, but he will almost always be willing to disclose a loss of self-esteem. However, in my experience, it is still very difficult to explore such feelings with men.

'Types' of male reaction

It occurs to me that this is the ideal point in this chapter to explore the types of men I have come across in my work. There are essentially three types and the list is an over-simplification and is therefore by no means comprehensive, serving only to give a general outline: the quiet arms-folded type; the apparent extrovert; and the explosive type.

Case history 3

This involves the **quiet, arms folded type** who, when a diagnosis of poor sperms is made, will not initially participate. He is reluctant to talk and refuses to engage; often the partner makes the running. He is apparently strong and silent, but in fact stuck in absolute isolation and complete denial.

Mr and Mrs F were both aged over 40. The couple were undergoing IVF treatment. A feature of the case was the absence of the husband throughout the treatment cycle. The nursing sister made a point of mentioning to me that the husband appeared an odd man – very quiet, seemingly shy and who showed little interest in giving any support to his wife. He was always polite, but would not engage in conversation and left the clinic at the earliest possibility. On the day of egg collection, he would produce his sample and leave immediately afterwards returning only to take his partner home. He clearly loved his wife, but it was also clear that he was somehow greatly inhibited in being able to offer her the emotional support she clearly needed. Several attempts at IVF were unsuccessful. This type of personality is very common.

N.B. *The remainder of this case history is used in the section describing possibilities for dealing with male clients.*

Case history 4

This involves the apparently **extrovert type**, who quickly accepts diagnosis and then readily accepts the donor option. A fast resolution, but are there hidden dangers?

Mr C was azoospermic and had elected with his partner to have DI treatment. During counselling, he was relaxed and quite willing to explore his feelings regarding his condition. He had clearly come to terms with his diagnosis. He felt no anger, no frustration and did not feel he was being punished. He reported that he had obviously at first asked 'why me?' and had cried a little, but had very quickly resolved the issues. He assured me he was OK and was looking forward to the treatment and to holding and playing with his prospective child. He was in fact in a hurry to get going.

N.B. I do not know the outcome for this couple, but I am aware that, oddly, some successful couples elect for termination of pregnancy after they have had *successful* treatment with DI. I personally wonder if this type might be more prone to such an outcome?

Case history 5

This involves the **explosive type** who finds it hard to accept the situation. Potency and virility are an important issues. The man will desperately seek to avoid and therefore shift blame, and is often very angry.

Mr A is a very westernized Pakistani man. However, Mrs A was dressed in traditional garb and had little to say, while he did all the talking. He made it clear he did not like seeing junior members of staff. He showed great anger at having to masturbate to produce samples for analysis. He was also angry about his wife always being the focus of attention at the clinic. He stated that he was to blame, so why did they not focus on him? Mr A was also superstitious about fertility, and seemed to believe that he was under a curse. The couple had consulted a seer and sought traditional remedies for their infertility, but these had been no more successful than western methods.

To summarize for all these types, there are a number of issues which should be considered. There are not necessarily any number of consistent themes, since different types of people will perceive different issues as vital. There is often a link seen between fertility and manhood. Often men in these cases are introverts, with a few extrovert exceptions: anger is overt only in rare cases, where the male partner is spoiling for a fight and the anger almost always being transferred. It is important to note that even an introvert under extreme provocation can act as an extrovert or even as an angry explosive type.

The diagnosis of male sub-fertility is a big blow to a man's self-esteem. In some men, even in cases of azoospermia, there is complete denial. Often, they will all ask 'why me?'. It is almost as if the answer to this question will in some way salve the pain. They will often complain that other less deserving people have children, and it seems a gross injustice that they cannot. Inevitably there are also issues over the apportionment of blame. There exists also the issue of 'divine retribution'. It is common for the female partner to express relief at the shifting of burden when the spotlight falls on their male partner. The summation of all these feelings, especially within the medical setting is often a growing feeling of total uselessness in the man. There seems so little that may be done for male infertility: any treatment options seem to centre almost entirely on the blameless partner, the female. This results in the man feeling marginalized. When looking at cultural differences, there is an added emotional charge – for example Middle Eastern men often cannot accept that they are the cause of the infertility (*see Case history 1*).

Dealing with men suffering infertility

What can be done for these men?

I feel it is important to explore men's feelings of anguish in these situations in detail. There are no real answers to the 'why me?' and the 'what have I done to deserve it?' questions, but in my experience it has been useful to affirm the absurdity and apparent injustice of life, to acknowledge the unfairness of the situation. It may be useful to challenge the client's feelings of guilt and uselessness. It may be helpful to explore ways of bolstering their self-esteem and marshalling their own potential inner resources.

It is rarely an option for men to explore potential resources with their male friends. When they have tried to share their problems in this area, the response from male friends is usually to make a joke of it or to trivialize it; everyone always has an apocryphal tale to tell. A common response is to offer to help out with the wife, and sometimes there is embarrassed silence, then it is swept under the carpet and the matter becomes taboo.

As a consequence, men often report that they feel very hurt. They have a sense that the whole world knows about their plight and is laughing at them. They often express resentment and bitterness that they are 'jaffas', or that they have been 'firing blanks', and many find it ironic that they have spent years worrying about contraception. There is little that I have ever found of use to say, when men report these feelings of hurt. It seems enough just to listen sympathetically. Sometimes I have found it useful, when counselling the strong silent type, to ask them about their experience of talking with their male friends as a means of engaging them.

Many men in this situation share a type of depression, and seem to experience a quiet desperation. It is not easy being a 'genetic cul-de-sac' i.e. a person who is unable to pass on her or her own genes directly. I often ask these depressed clients how they view the future: do they see themselves being old, childless and bitter? (One wife actually piped up that it was her husband's life ambition!). It is certainly useful to determine how their fantasies of the future manifest themselves.

In many men a 'heroic' type of self-sacrifice occurs. Some volunteer immediately for DI and seemingly have all the right things to say (see Case history 4). This reaction does not mean that shock, disbelief and frustration are not present, but somehow they seek to resolve their anxieties too quickly.

Dealing with ambivalence

Ambivalence is also an important issue, for both men and women as can be seen from the following case history.

Case history 6

Mr and Mrs S have been attending the clinic for over three years now. There is a long history of low sperm count. The female partner is ovulatory and has a normal pelvis. In spite of their problems, they are an heroic couple in the way they struggle on. Mrs S has disclosed childhood abuse and Mr S is a builder and obviously carries out a great deal of manual work, undertaking heavy lifting to such an extent that he recently spent £3000 on orthopaedic surgery for his damaged back. Mr S is constantly talking about having treatment for infertility but it never happens (or has not for over 30 months now!). He is constantly talking of marrying his partner, but this also never happens even though he always seems genuine enough when he talks about it. The couple have considered fostering, but at the end of the day would really like a child of their own. Mr S is a small wiry man, who is one of those quietly spoken, very private people and shows very little anger. He understands that poor sperms play a role in childlessness, yet does not seem overly bothered by this fact.

I am certain that the absence of definitive action in this couple's case lies in ambivalence and we are still waiting to see how this couple's story will end.

In the context of male infertility, we are examining an area where men have hidden agendas and, importantly, we should bear in mind that it is not just physical factors that may affect a person's fertility. Perhaps there is a fear of growing up, establishing stable relationships incurring responsibility. There may be history of abuse in childhood. There is the real likelihood that for so-called unexplained infertility and some cases of specific male infertility, that ambivalence may be a major issue. Here it is possible that intervention with counselling or related therapy might be as useful as conventional infertility treatments, as is shown in the following case:

Case history 7

This couple, Mr & Mrs T were very intense. They felt they had been messed about by a well known Harley Street clinic and when I first encountered them they were very irate and fed up. Both smoked and drank heavily. They ran several businesses which kept them both extremely busy. It was not hard to understand why they were having such difficulty. Many sessions of counselling followed, involving a great deal of exploration concerning their lifestyle, and about their attitudes towards parenthood. This resulted in challenging their lifestyle and expectations, and in an agreement to undertake to define and pursue some different life goals. Slowly, their attitude to life and their lifestyle changed. N.B. *This couple now have their first child.*

Dealing with impotence and sexual failure

It is also important to consider circumstances where a couple fails to achieve sexual intercourse. For such couples sex has become meaningless, and they will often disclose that sex has 'become a grind' and therefore, because it does not produce the desired child, it has become a chore – hence they abstain from sexual relations altogether. In my experience long-term impotence is rare, though periodic impotence seems to be a side-effect of male infertility, usually arising at the worst point in a man's experience – for instance, when he is told that nothing more can be done, or that the only way forward is to consider DI.

With male infertility, up to 25% of couples may intermittently be in this strange state of celibacy outside treatment, particularly where the men feel that virility is linked to the ability to father a child. Here some psychosexual counselling may be most valuable, the main goal being to reassign sex within life's many priorities and putting the reproduction aspect into its true perspective. Often the couple may also be 'in a rut'. Exploration of family life often reveals a certain boring routine and the loss of spontaneity and sparkle. Goal-setting by way of 'doing something different' – perhaps re-establishing the idea of simply cuddling, or of going out either to the cinema or to a restaurant may all be useful tasks in dealing with general impotence. However, deep-seated cases of impotence require outside referral.

Accepting childlessness

Treatment is not always the right course of action. Sometimes acceptance can be a very powerful emotion. Being able to acknowledge and face up to fears and problems may help some couples to make decisions which allow them to control their own destinies. Treatment is not always essential, as shown in the following case history.

Case history 8

It is not uncommon to be sent patients who are desperate in their uncertainty. They want someone to tell them what to do. A particular couple had been treated once with GIFT and it had not been successful. The main problem appeared to be a very low sperm count in conjunction with low motility. The couple wanted to know what to do. Together we explored the couple's desires and motives and found that fear was a major issue. If they chose not to have treatment, would they regret it later on in life? The couple considered the effects of stress and its adverse effect on their lives and after counselling, the couple decided not to pursue treatment. N.B. *I received a letter from the couple, about one year later. They had succeeded spontaneously.*

Finally, the following case history may be a useful way of summarizing the various elements of this section on what might be done when counselling infertile men:

Case history 9
(This is a continuation of case history 3 used to illustrate the quiet type of personality with regard to male infertility)

Mr and Mrs F elected to have several sessions of counselling and a contract for six sessions was made. During the ensuing sessions, we explored Mr F's feelings regarding treatment. Mr F felt terribly isolated, he never spoke to anyone about their infertility, he worked hard. The treatment was really for his wife. He was happy to fund it and participate because it was what she wanted. For himself, he would have been happy to accept the diagnosis of infertility and quietly get on with his life. He felt guilty and useless. He did not see impotence nor virility as an issue. Having established Mr F's feelings, further exploration took place regarding his understanding of his wife's feelings and attitudes (it seemed that they were unable to talk about these issues together at home). During this exploration, Mr F disclosed some of his fears. He wanted a child very much, but was desperately afraid of failure. He certainly felt that he was being punished for something. When considering goal-setting. Mr F was asked whether he thought that his fears might be making him freeze out the world and more importantly his partner. He agreed to think about this and how he might effect some changes. Throughout the remaining sessions, Mr F became much more attentive to his wife and seemed much more relaxed in the remainder of the sessions. In the last session, Mr F made a further disclosure about his childhood, which was very relevant to his feelings regarding punishment and fear. It seemed to provide him with some form of release or emotion catharsis. N.B. *I am happy to report that Mr and Mrs F finally succeeded with IVF and now have a baby boy.*

Dealing with donor insemination: the male aspect

Before moving on to the discussion and conclusion of this chapter, we must digress and look at implications counselling for donor insemination. When counselling men who are considering, or who have chosen to have DI, there are a number of issues which must be explored.

One should bear in mind that with DI, once again, treatment focuses on the woman despite the problem lying with the man. So, even with DI, the man is marginalized, feels useless and is in many ways isolated. As well as dealing with the implications of DI, it is also an opportunity for the man to explore his feelings regarding his plight. These feelings have been discussed extensively already. It is also pertinent to explore the man's feelings regarding DI itself. Some men arrive easily at a decision to employ DI, but most men agonize over it, and some men are highly resistant to the idea, but eventually acquiesce. In my experience DI is often initiated as an option by the female partner. It is rare for the man to have to persuade his partner to take up DI treatment. There are also situations when the female partner may ask for DI treatment to be kept secret from their partner.

The vast majority of men have grave reservations about DI, although they may accept to undergo the treatment. However, despite the reservations, it is clear that when the decision is made, it is always made in an optimistic manner and is often viewed as a gift for the partner. This is probably a good point to consider the implications. It is important to consider their own feelings about DI and the prospective child. They have to consider their possible changes in financial, social and psychological circumstances. They must consider their own families, and how they will feel about DI, or indeed, if the respective families will be told. Couples must consider whether they will keep the DI a secret. If they choose this option, they must consider the likely complications and problems. In my experience, up to 90% of all couples considering DI will wish to keep the treatment a secret (limited to close family only, often to the man and wife only).

They must also consider the needs of the prospective, unborn child. The welfare of the child is of paramount importance (for a detailed discussion, see Chapter 15). Unusually, here counsellors are expected to take action if they feel that the prospective child is in any danger (presumably from abuse?). Under such circumstances, one assumes the couple might be barred from treatment should the doubts prove to be substantiated. It is also worth pointing out that a couple must consider that treatment may not necessarily succeed. This is one area where counselling is strongly advocated in the code of practice regarding the Human Fertilisation and Embryology Act of 1991. Finally, we should bear in mind that the use of donor semen, and indeed the whole problem of male infertility itself, in certain circumstances, can lead to severe emotional difficulties. The stresses and strains of treatment may lead to failed marriages or even the termination of pregnancy following successful treatment outcome. The careful use and availability of skilled counselling should ensure that such sad outcomes will be minimized.

Discussion

Male infertility is a field that is still in its infancy. Counselling in male infertility is in a similar state. However medical and scientific advances offer much hope for the future. It is to be hoped that any such advance, when it comes, will help to alleviate some of the pain that surrounds the seeming 'life sentence' of male infertility.

A diagnosis of infertility is a fundamentally shattering event, comparable to a major life crisis. The emotional issues that arise are similar to those of bereavement (although this is not the only model), often following → surprise → denial → anger → isolation → grief → acceptance. The triangle of guilt–fear–anger should also be uppermost in the counsellor's mind. Barbara Mostyn has suggested that for some clients these emotions feed each other and form a vicious circle. The provision of counselling is vital therefore, if we are to avoid further isolating and abandoning these men. As the men begin to adjust to their diagnosis they need urgent attention, not just with regard to research, but also in terms of dealing with their actual emotional responses.

Acceptance of being a so-called genetic *cul-de-sac* takes time, support and understanding, and we need to explore how best to deal with men's emotions in this area. With DI, it seems that no man is able to embrace this option readily. It is also important to acknowledge that even modern treatment of male infertility centres on surgery for the fertile female partner. This lack of tangible treatment for the man himself leads to further isolation, loss of self-esteem and a feeling of uselessness. We therefore urgently need to investigate the needs of men regarding their marginalization. We also need to address the fact that men attend insufficiently to their own needs, in my view being all too frequently ready to shoulder blame. We must further explore the male experience of infertility. In terms of the science, it seems that progress in understanding male infertility will help by providing men, who have a strong need for information, with resources to understand their physiological plight.

A model for counselling

At this point, it might be useful to summarize my model for counselling when dealing with male infertility. It is influenced by Egan's three-stage model and the London Hospital Medicine College Diploma Course (see Appendix 4) and is by no means complete (nor ever will be).

Exploration

The client must be 'engaged': this involves establishing a trusting and safe environment for the client. Once an empathic relationship has been established (often because the female partner almost always attends, and it is the female partner who initially makes the running) the exploration process may begin. The client's diagnosis, his feelings about it, his fears, his hopes and other emotions may be explored. A major skill in this process centres on the use of metaphor. Even the most silent man will 'engage' when he is allowed to use his own metaphors; and may thus offer up even some of his innermost feelings. The use of visualization can also be a vital tool. When a man is in despair, he may often be brought out of it by asking him to visualize his feelings or using images as a means of externalizing inner issues. Having thus attached the emotions to a 'real' or seen object, the 'light at the end of the tunnel' may materialize.

Insight

Through the process of exploration and challenge, insight may be achieved, and once insight has been established there is the possibility of moving on. This model is non-directive and client-centred, thus when insight is achieved and goal-setting becomes a possibility, the process of goal-setting is never imposed.

Action-goal-setting

We explore the range of possibilities and the client decides which goal or goals he and his partner will aim for. By examining the issues, confronting their emotions and dealing with them through action, clients will be better placed to impose their own will on the direction of their lives. In this setting, one of the most important issues is that they are enabled to make well-informed decisions on their treatment. The model is based on Egan's three-stage model of exploration–new insight–action, with the power of metaphors and visualization as additional vital ingredients. As we begin to understand more, and with greater personal experience of counselling, this model is bound to evolve.

Conclusion

A public acknowledgement of the existence of male infertility and the ignorance surrounding it may lead to more openness about it and therefore less public stigma about male infertility. Perhaps more access to counselling will also help to alleviate the stigma, anxieties and the isolation associated with it. We need to further explore the intensity and pain caused by such a diagnosis, and to explore the need of support; is it useful to know that men in this position are not alone?; is it useful speaking with others in the same plight?; how much time is needed to adjust, and to cope with male infertility. We need to explore a man's need to be father; and how men view fatherhood. Finally, and by no means least, we need to explore the role of overall stress in male infertility counselling and how its reduction will help.

If we are able to attend to some of the research outlined above we should be able to provide effective access to counselling for men and we will be able to provide better support and therapeutic intervention for them. It is to be hoped that the social stigma of male infertility will continue to be eroded and that ultimately, we will be able to overcome the isolation that accompany a diagnosis of male infertility.

Chapter 5
Working With Partners: Counselling the Couple and Collaborating in the Team

Paul Pengelly

Introduction

Most infertility treatment is undergone by partners in male–female couples, from a desire to bring children into their relationships. This chapter explores the significance of partnership and gender, both for counselling and for working relations between practitioners in the treatment team.

In a heterosexual couple, the man and woman between them embody the total biological reproductive system; at the same time, they also form a psychosocial system which is the matrix for their personal and social identities as adults. Just as their sexual relationship carries both physical and emotional aspects of their partnership, so the way they manifest their biological fertility – or fail to, or choose not to – will have profound significance not only for themselves but for their wider family and social relationships. It follows that, even though medical intervention may be focused on the body of one partner only, practitioners should be aware of the likely psychological implications for both partners, individually and as a couple.

These ideas will be familiar to practitioners who adopt a holistic, or integrated, approach to medicine generally, and to infertility treatment in particular (Inglis & Denton, 1992). So, too, is the principle that counselling may be needed – whether from clinical staff in the course of their work, or more specifically from a designated counsellor – to help patients make informed decisions and cope with distress and anxiety (HFEA, 1991).

What may not be so familiar is the idea of the couple relationship itself as a focus for counselling. I shall argue that this offers an approach which can be both effective and economical of professional resources. I shall then show how this 'couple approach' in patient counselling can also reveal some principles for partnership in the counsellor's working relations with colleagues within the multidisciplinary treatment team. These arguments are based on research and training work in the field of infertility counselling, drawing also on earlier research into inter-professional work with couples (Woodhouse & Pengelly, 1991) and the theory and practice of marital psychotherapy developed at the Tavistock Marital Studies Institute (Ruszczynski, 1993).

Counselling with couples

The research project on which this chapter is based began by studying a sample of couples who were about to start IVF treatment in relation to: their experience of infertility and its attendant medical interventions; their use of counselling in the treatment centre (at the Royal Free Hospital, London); and the relevance of a couple approach to counselling.

My colleagues and I found that couples tended to organize their partnerships in very specific ways to cope with the crisis of infertility. The relationship itself was often their main resource during the practical and emotional stress of investigation and treatment. When the stress exceeded their immediate capacity to cope, counselling which focused on their interaction with one another could help them restore and improve the functioning of this resource system. This process was empowering for couples, since it enabled them to use their own combined capacities better, not only in coping with stress but also in choosing how they would use what the treatment centre could offer – and this included the counselling itself. We also found, however, that this potential in the couple relationship was not always apparent from the way partners presented themselves to the treatment centre.

The sections which follow summarize our findings on how these infertile couples experienced their predicament, how they organized their partnerships to deal with the emotional stress of infertility, by means of internal and external defences against anxiety, and how counselling which addressed these couple issues could be effective.

Couples' experience of infertility

The threat of losing their fertility goes right to the heart of a couple who are failing to conceive a baby. It can be felt as destroying their entire *raison d'être* as a couple – their belief in their value to one another as creative partners – as well as threatening each individual's profoundest sense of his or her personal destiny and purpose in adult life. Fears of threatened loss and failure were vivid and painful for most of the couples in the research project. At the same time, they had to deal with the conflict between these negative fearful feelings and the more positive hopeful feelings which they were struggling to keep alive. Knowing rationally that the medical technology on which they were placing their hopes had a low success rate, they nevertheless went on hoping against hope in order to sustain the quest for a baby. These pressures could put them under enormous emotional stress, both individually and within their partnerships.

Many of the couples had been pursuing their quest for long periods of up to ten years. As well as the repeated testing and the previous treatment attempts that were part of the quest itself, the women's reproductive histories included miscarriages, terminations, tubal surgery, ectopic pregnancies and sterilizations. Men as well as women spoke of the emotional pain and anxiety surrounding all these kinds of events, both before and also during their quest for assisted conception. Both also complained that no counselling had been available at earlier stages.

Internal defences: the psychological 'division of labour'

To focus on the couple, and on both partners' feelings, is not of course to imply that women's and men's experiences are the same. It is precisely in the sexual and reproductive area that their physiological and related psychological differences are most salient.

In our separate research interviews with male and female partners, we indeed heard marked differences between their emotional experiences and their psychological strategies in most of the couples. The women felt the imperative desire for a baby more strongly. More than half of them also knew the impediment to successful conception lay in their own bodies, and all experienced infertility as a devastating attack on their female identity. They felt guilty, and those whose infertility was unexplained were just as liable to blame themselves as those who had a diagnosis. They also expected and feared the blame of others, especially their partners; some were afraid their partners would leave them if a baby was not forthcoming.

Most of the women indicated that they had not expressed the full force of these painful feelings openly to their partners; some felt their partners understood enough to be supportive, some doubted that they could ever understand, while others simply did not imagine that such things could be discussed between partners at all. This lack of open communication seemed all the more difficult to bear because very few women had anyone else they could confide in; out of shame, sometimes mixed with envy, most had become isolated from their families and friends.

They often seemed to speak as if this predicament was inevitable for them as women – just as inevitable as the fact that they, not their menfolk, had to undergo the physically painful and invasive procedures of IVF treatment. Looking at men's and women's accounts together, however, we concluded that the seeming 'passivity' of the woman was often part of an active collaboration between the two partners in each couple, based on a largely inarticulate belief that this was the way to deal with the inordinate stress they both felt. To understand this collaborative dynamic we need to explore the men's perspective too.

On the whole, the men did not feel so personally devastated by infertility as their partners. Those in whom a 'male factor' problem had been diagnosed (only a handful) did feel undermined in their masculine function of begetting children, and feared that their partners would reject them – one had offered his wife a divorce immediately after the diagnosis. More typically, however, a man's first response to questions about feelings would be to refer to his partner's emotional distress. Most began their replies with 'She', hardly with any 'I'; a small group began with 'We', and will be considered in the next section. These men saw themselves as performing a specific and separate function in their relationships, by organizing, managing and keeping the quest going on their partners' behalf.

Some men, when asked again about their own particular feelings, could reveal their personal anguish over, for example, the crisis of a partner's ectopic pregnancy, or their own frustrated longing for children. Many men admitted to hating the ordeal of having to produce their samples of sperm by masturbating in the only men's toilet on the unit. As they invariably emphasized, however, this was 'nothing compared to what she's had to go through', and in general men discounted their own feelings as not worth dwelling on.

The one emotion that many men did feel free to express was anger at doctors, hospitals and treatment centres for the way they felt they and, especially, their partners had been treated. This was something the women seldom expressed on their own account, and the men only did so in the relatively separate and confidential setting of the research interviews. Indeed, many of them exempted the hospital itself from any blame, as if wishing to preserve it as 'good'. It seemed here that the paramount need was to protect the couple's investment of hope in the current treatment centre, which meant suppressing any frustrated or angry feelings, except privately in relation to the past.

Protection, in fact, seemed a prime concern for both men and women in their behaviour towards each other as well as the hospital. Male and female partners would regularly speak of their wish to shield each other from distress and humiliation. Their respective efforts to achieve this took very different forms – the women by taking emotional pain on themselves, the men by sympathizing and searching for solutions. Sometimes the two partners in the couple seemed unaware of each other's silent protectiveness; sometimes they were quite aware, and grateful for it, but confided separately to their interviewers that it did not in fact remove the essential pain.

We can now see the psychological 'division of labour' in which men and women were collaborating in most of the couples in the sample. They seemed to share a set of assumptions about male and female roles

– separate but, as they hoped, complementary – which is widespread in our culture (Wirtberg, 1992, describes an identical pattern among infertile couples in a rural area of Sweden).

At a deeper psychological level, this gender-based division of labour between partners could be seen as protective not only of the other but also, and primarily, of the self. Men were liable to become more anxious than women about experiencing overwhelming emotion; and women were liable to become more anxious than men about ever managing to find a solution. Each therefore (not necessarily consciously) delegated the task he or she was most anxious about to the other, and (more consciously) tried to sustain the other in carrying it.

It seemed to us that for many couples the division of labour had so far been sufficient to afford them mutual support. This was more likely to be so the more partners could openly recognize and appreciate what they were relying on each other to carry, and thus value their inter-dependence as a partnership.

At the time we interviewed the men and women, however, they were experiencing the heightened stress of being on the brink of the treatment programme. We could see how, for some couples, this was eroding their capacity to communicate to the point where their respective concerns could be neither voiced nor heard between them. They were therefore feeling more cut off from each other just at the time when they most needed each other's support.

Internal defences: 'perfect harmony'

Whilst a division of labour was the predominant pattern, a small number of couples appeared to have organized their partnerships in another way (perhaps following another, more modern, set of assumptions). Psychologically, their strategy for managing the stress of infertility was for the two partners to be emotionally at one at all times. This emotional unison, moreover, depended on their experiencing only positive feelings; there was no thought of blaming each other, no question of either partner despairing. For them, it seemed, a shared anxiety about having any difference between them (which itself might be felt as destructive) outweighed all other anxieties.

These were the couples in which the men partners began with 'We', when asked about their feelings. Some had become experts on their partners' fertility problems – there were no 'male factor' cases amongst this group – and they suffered empathically everything that their partners suffered in the course of investigation and treatment. Both partners seemed to be following an unwritten rule that their separate identities as woman and man should be submerged in the interests of their joint survival as one entity.

Like the division of labour, this psychological strategy for avoiding anxiety seemed to have functioned well enough for the couples who adopted it. Since they could have no disagreements with each other, however, it was not surprising that they were among the most extreme in their blaming of doctors and hospitals (expressed by the men) and their hostility towards their families (expressed by both the women and the men).

External defences: the 'united front'

Virtually all the couples, whichever internal defence system they showed in their own relationships, appeared to feel that they would only be acceptable to the hospital if they presented themselves outwardly as united and worthy of becoming parents. For some this was linked with a belief that their bodies would only conceive if they were in the right, 'worthy', state of mind, which they studied hard to achieve. But the effort to maintain an external appearance of unity could lay further stress on the couple, and further restrict their capacity to manage their often turbulent feelings.

To present a united front meant always hiding negative feelings, whether of desperation, anxiety or anger, which were believed to be unacceptable. The 'perfect harmony' couples, who already suppressed any such feelings internally, also concealed their external hostility (which had been confided to us in the research interviews) in their face-to-face dealings with the hospital. In the 'division of labour' couples, men concealed their anger, women their pain, and both concealed any stress between them. Virtually all the couples seemed ready to comply with whatever was required of them at the treatment centre (not least the invitation to take part in our research, which hardly any refused). The external 'positive united front' thus tended to mask both the existence of stress and the way partners were using their relationships to try and manage it.

The couple focus in counselling

In many treatment centres (as seen in the second part of this chapter) the result of such masking may be that counselling is not thought of until a clinician is faced with a patient in acute distress – usually the woman partner on her own – i.e. when the couple's defence system has broken down. At the Royal Free Hospital, however, it was routine for all couples to see the counsellor, together, during their first visit on being called up from the waiting list. This was not a counselling session; but in introducing herself and explaining her role the counsellor was able to make the offer of counselling in person, and couples could explore informally with her whether they might find it useful. Nearly two-thirds of the sample accepted the offer.

Most of these couples took only one further session, in which the partners could clarify medical information and think through the implications of success or failure and how they would manage these together. They also voiced some anxieties – often apparently for the first time in each other's hearing. These included the strain of secrecy, the woman's envy of fertile siblings and friends, the man's feeling of being subservient to the woman's preoccupation with getting pregnant, and how this could affect their sex life.

These couples seemed to be functioning relatively well at this point. They could get some relief from the opportunity of talking things over, affirming that their infertility was a shared problem, and hearing that the anxieties they expressed were normal in their situation. They were evidently helped to keep their joint internal defences (of whichever kind) flexible, and to modify their external defences through experiencing the counsellor as the 'human face' of the treatment centre – with whom some worrying feelings could, after all, be revealed and discussed. Some touched on deeper, more painful feelings, but indicated that they did not need to discuss these at present.

A smaller number of couples took up two or three sessions. The imminent approach of treatment seemed to be forcing them to face some ambivalent feelings, usually in one partner, which they had not been able to work through together. These centred mainly around two kinds of issue: first, the struggle by men or women who already had children by previous relationships to understand and accommodate their new partner's desire for children now; second, the conflict between children and career in career-centred women who also had misgivings about becoming the dependent one in the partnership.

With the counsellor's help, the ambivalent partners in these couples were enabled to voice the more negative side of their feelings more fully than before. This brought relief and new understanding between the partners (except for one couple whose relationship was evidently in such difficulty that they broke off treatment). For most of this group, therefore, counselling appeared to provide a safe enough space for them to share specific anxieties, which they had been suppressing for fear of threatening their cohesion as couples. This reduced the pressure on their joint defence systems, which they were enabled to re-establish in a modified form, based on greater mutual understanding.

Only three couples took up a more extended series of sessions (between four and ten). Their quests for children, too, had been extended over many years, and this was their first opportunity for counselling. Their anxieties, all stemming from unexpressed negative feelings, seemed similar to those of other couples but had become so unmanageable between them that they felt immobilized. In each case the partners were helped to make links between their current predicament and painful issues in their earlier lives which they had been counting on each other, or a baby, to resolve. With this understanding , they were able to renew their commitment to IVF as their shared choice, but without feeling the survival of their partnerships depended on it.

Empowering the couple

In fact, virtually all the couples who took up counselling were enabled to increase their sense of having choices, and resources, as they went through the treatment process. In particular, they were helped to enhance or recover some of the resourcefulness of their own partnerships through using the counselling process, at different levels of intensity, to explore negative feelings which they had been afraid of. This also meant that a minimal amount of counselling time could be more effective because it was directed towards restoring the clients' own main coping mechanisms.

For most couples, in fact, counselling did not oppose their joint psychological defence system, but rather increased its capacity to accommodate a wider and more realistic range of emotional communication between the partners. The defences were still needed, not only to manage the stress of treatment but also to keep anxiety about the final loss of fertility at bay while hope remained. That ultimate anxiety could sometimes be acknowledged but, understandably, couples were not ready to do the emotional work of coming to terms with it at this stage.

Collaborating in the team

If partnership is recognized and can be worked with as a resource for infertile couples, what about partnership in the infertility treatment team? This question was addressed in a research workshop designed to supplement the in-depth study at the Royal Free Hospital with a broader sample of counselling practice. The workshop was attended by five counsellors (all women) from different infertility treatment centres, and met weekly for three months. At each session, one member would present for study either a counselling case or a description of her role and the working relationships in her own setting, and the issues that arose there; each member also completed a questionnaire covering two areas – her counselling work overall, and her view of her team's attitudes towards counselling.

The referral system

These two areas of interest turned to be closely linked with each other, most obviously through the practice of referral. All seven cases presented in the workshop had begun with clients being referred to the counsellor, mostly by doctors and in one case by the nurse-coordinator.

The questionnaires confirmed that referral by clinical staff was the general pattern in all these treatment centres. It was exceptional for patients to seek out the counsellor direct, though they were in theory free to do so.

This was the exact opposite of the system of access to counselling at the Royal Free, where couples were able to determine their own use of the counselling offered. Also very different was the pattern of who became the counselling client. At the Royal Free it was the couple, but with the workshop counsellors it was often the female partner only, reflecting the different way in which the referral system worked.

There were two main types of situation which led to referral. The first was an overt display of distress or indecision by the patients – usually by the woman partner while seeing a clinician on her own. The second was any prospect of treatment involving donor gametes or surrogacy, which invariably led to referral of the couple as a matter of policy; in some centres counselling in such cases was known as 'mandatory', which in practice seemed to mean not only that the centre was obliged to offer it but also that couples were expected to attend, and sometimes that the counsellor was expected to report back to the doctor that they had done so.

In the first type of referral, the woman partner, if referred 'in distress' on her own, often continued to be seen on her own by the counsellor. Even if both partners were referred, the woman often attended all or most sessions alone, and the counsellor usually accepted this even though he or she might regret it. The high proportion of 'women only' in counselling bore out the questionnaire finding that both their clinical colleagues and the counsellors themselves automatically tended to think of the woman as essentially the patient in the infertility treatment setting.

The absence of the couple

Another pattern that emerged was that even when both partners did attend (including all of the 'mandatory' type of referral) their relationship as a couple was not addressed – we only heard of one instance where the counsellor did this. That seemed all the more remarkable, since all these trained counsellors worked skilfully with their clients' painful feelings, and could help them understand how these might be linked with other painful issues in their family relationships, past and present. This particular partnership, however, seemed to be the one relationship that could not be focused on. Sometimes the woman client would confide her anxieties about it in an individual session – for example that her partner did not understand her feelings, or would not want to talk about his. But there was a pervasive assumption that these difficulties were impossible to work through, either in the partnership or in the counselling itself (which the woman was sure her partner would not attend).

Overall, the picture that emerged from the workshop material was of two systems which reinforced each other's assumptions. On the one hand were the couples who could not communicate with each other about emotional pain, and who tacitly agreed that the woman partner should carry it and receive counselling help. On the other hand was the treatment team, including the counsellor, who also saw the woman as essentially the patient (or, in the original sense of that word, the sufferer).

The division of labour in couple and team

This did not, however, leave the men without any role. From the counselling material, in fact, it appeared that these couples had made the same psychological 'division of labour' as we found in most of our research interviews at the Royal Free. Once again, the women seemed to experience the need for a baby as more central to their identity, but felt trapped and dehumanized by the clinical procedures and often feared they would be blamed and rejected by their partners (even when the infertility was unexplained); thus the problem, and the helplessness, were vested in them. The men, on the other hand, as before assumed the role of seeing their partners through the problem by organizing, managing and protecting, and by trying to remain determinedly positive. Any painful feelings they may have had went unrecognized; there were signs that some of them also felt threatened and humiliated, but they seldom expressed or explored this in the counselling.

Here it should be emphasized that in the workshop we were hearing about couples referred for counselling, for most of whom the infertility experience had become too stressful for them to manage unaided. At the Royal Free, where we had access to a more general sample, a degree of 'division of labour' seemed quite functional for many couples, as long as they were able to stay in touch with each other's different stand-points yet appreciate their interdependence.

In the workshop cases, too, there could still be a functional value in the division of labour at some points. For one or two couples, for example, it looked as if it was the man's more detached position that enabled him finally to say the unsayable 'enough is enough' and call a halt to treatment, after repeated failures; though it was the woman who undertook the main work of coming to terms with this, at least so far as attending counselling sessions was concerned.

More often, however, the detachment of the man and woman was clearly dysfunctional for these couples, in their interface with the treatment centres.

Case history: splitting the difference

The couple's infertility was unexplained, and the husband was not accompanying his wife to counselling sessions; instead, he went to tell the (male) doctor that he thought she had an anatomical problem in having intercourse. She was duly examined, but the feature he described was found to be so slight as to be negligible. This examination took place at the time when the wife was supposed to be having her weekly counselling session, but the counsellor only heard about it the following week when she enquired why the wife had missed the appointment.

It was at this point that the counsellor brought the case to the workshop, commenting that she thought the husband's behaviour might be his way of dealing with his own anxiety at being unable to impregnate his wife. Agreeing with that, we also saw in this case how the division of labour could become a 'total splitting' – and not only between wife and husband, but at the same time between counsellor and doctor.

The counsellor then changed strategy, insisted on the husband coming to a joint counselling session and enlisted a male counsellor to join her. For part of the session he engaged the husband in thinking about his involvement in the treatment process, including the very practical point that giving up his heavy drinking could well improve the quality of his sperm. Then the woman counsellor (who was also an art therapist) invited both partners to paint a picture together. She brought their remarkable 'couple painting' to the workshop: the wife had filled the middle of the huge sheet of paper with wild, dark shapes, some swirling, some jagged, while the husband had carefully made an elaborate border, two or three layers deep, all the way round the outside.

The counsellor helped them explore the meaning of this particular 'division of labour', how they had in fact collaborated in depicting it, and the functional value it could have for them. This was our one instance of a counsellor focusing on the couple relationship; sadly, the workshop ended without another opportunity to follow it up, but two further points can be made. First, it was clear that the two counsellors also operated a 'division of labour', which now modelled a functional interdependence instead of the dysfunctional splitting which previously occurred between counsellor and doctor. Second, though this splitting affected both the clients and the professionals, it was by no means clear that any one partner or practitioner was solely responsible. Once the doctor who examined the wife realized that the husband's complaint about her was unfounded, he was glad to discuss the problem with the counsellor; the husband, too, was more readily drawn into the counselling than the wife had feared. And, when further joint sessions were proposed, the wife became anxious about whether she could still have her individual sessions.

The recognition of counselling

We should therefore bear in mind the unconsciously collaborative nature of this kind of splitting between, for example, the doctor and counsellor role, and the tendency for fantasies to proliferate across it

(Wilson & Wilson, 1985), when considering what the counsellors said about the way counselling was regarded in their treatment centres. Most felt counselling was given low priority, or seen as a last resort rather than as a positive part of the service offered by the centre. Similarly, most counsellors saw themselves as less than fully integrated in their teams. This was partly related to the fact that they were all part-time in this work, whereas the rest of the team often worked together full-time. In three of the five treatment centres, the counsellor had no colleague in the same role, and not all counsellors were included as a matter of course in team meetings.

In the daily practice of the treatment centres there were other indicators of how far counselling was or was not integrated. Each centre had its own way of giving patients information about the treatment programme at the outset. There was always a verbal explanation, usually given by the doctor in charge, which was supposed to cover counselling among all the other aspects. In some centres there was also written information; the counselling content of this could be minimal – for example, only the inclusion of the counsellor's name on the staff list – though at one centre the information pack contained a whole sheet devoted to counselling. At none of the centres did the reception arrangements provide for all new patients to meet the counsellor in person for information about counselling, as they did at the Royal Free Hospital.

The counsellor in the professional culture

Counselling and assessment

A particularly sensitive and uncertain question for all the counsellors was whether it was part of their function to help assess couples' suitability to be offered treatment; for example, in terms of their emotional stability and potential to care for a child. The statutory HFEA Code of Practice (HFEA, 1991) states that such assessment is the responsibility of the whole multidisciplinary team, and must include consideration of the welfare of any resulting child. But it remains silent about what specific part the counsellor might play in this. Some counsellors felt strongly that to take any part in assessment was incompatible with their confidential helping role; others thought it was feasible, provided the tasks were clearly separated.

The Code does emphasize that assessment must be distinguished from counselling *per se*. In some of the workshop cases, however, it sounded as if it was the doctor's second thoughts about the couple's suitability which had led to the referral for counselling. This was implied rather than specified, but these counsellors felt they had been given a mixed message and were left confused about their task, with clients who (like those at the Royal Free) could not easily discuss their own anxiety about how acceptable they were.

From the counsellors' side, there was also the question of how to deal with any misgivings of their own about couples' suitability, which might arise in the course of counselling. Most said their approach would be to seek discussion in the team meeting, indicating their concern without disclosing confidential material; in this way they would try to ensure that the whole team took responsibility for recognizing doubts about the case rather than leave it to the counsellor.

The disposal of professional anxiety

To achieve shared responsibility for such decision-making, however, seemed no easy matter. Not only were counsellors unsure of their acceptance in the team, they also reported a general sense of being left to carry anxieties which other members of the team did not want to deal with. Although one or two spoke of some interest among their clinical colleagues in the emotional impact of infertility, and its treatment, most said they encountered resistance to any serious consideration of this. Patients referred in distress were sometimes labelled 'difficult', but from the counsellor's point of view the difficulty appeared to lie in her colleagues' inability to manage their own anxiety when faced with distressed patients or ethical dilemmas. It was said to be generally unacceptable for staff to speak of anxiety in themselves, or any disturbing feelings arising from their work; many doctors especially were perceived as taking a 'no-nonsense' approach, and some reportedly stigmatized any staff anxiety as 'neurotic'.

Such attitudes were seen as powerfully influencing the working culture of treatment centres, in which doctors were naturally the dominant profession and counsellors felt especially weak. Against that background, counsellors sometimes felt it was too difficult to uphold their counselling objectives when these appeared to conflict with medical treatment objectives: for example, when treatment schedules seemed too inflexible to allow time for adequate attention to clients' emotional needs in counselling; or when treatment was apparently being pursued, unstoppably, beyond the clients' emotional capacity to cope. Here too, as with questions of assessment, the counsellors felt constrained by the need for confidentiality; if they were to argue a case for delaying or ceasing treatment, they were bound to do this without disclosing relevant information which was known to them but not to the doctors.

'Mirroring'

These were some of the forces which seemed to structure the internal working relationships in treatment teams so that they could all too easily (and quite unwittingly) replicate or mirror the 'splitting' interaction observed in some of the couples. This well-documented process (see, for example, Mattinson, 1992, and Britton, 1981) regularly occurs in groups of professionals who avoid addressing and understanding their task-related anxieties together.

Such unconscious mirroring tends to follow the most obvious pathways. The natural and, in itself, functional division of labour was that the (mostly female) counsellors were concerned with emotional pain, the (mostly male) doctors were concerned with organizing hopeful solutions; these were their proper respective primary tasks. But the belief which sometimes took hold of counsellors, that they were powerless to influence or communicate their concerns to the 'unfeeling' doctors, suggests that the two disciplines could also re-enact the same splitting of roles as the patient couples; and with the same loss of interdependent functioning. This was made all the more likely by the obvious differentials between counsellors and doctors in terms of authority, status and gender. As Will & Baird (1984) put it, 'these real professional vulnerabilities provide lines of least resistance along which mirroring may occur.'

Conclusion: re-empowering the team

Just as the division of labour in the couples could develop into a dysfunctional split when the stress of infertility exceeded their capacity to cope, so this parallel process among the practitioners could occur when they too were seeking to ward off a feared overload of anxiety, from working with anxious patients in a highly sensitive field. It sometimes seemed, for example, that the referral of a distressed patient for counselling was the occasion for the clinician's anxiety simply to be passed over to the counsellor to deal with (an invitation often duly accepted by the counsellor), rather than an opportunity for the two colleagues to communicate and think about it.

For that to happen, however, the infertility treatment team needs structures which would allow for more open dialogue between practitioner colleagues, from their different roles, different status and different points of view. Counsellors, who are trained to provide a safe and containing space in which people can express and understand their anxieties, ought to be in a strategic position to promote such structures, but they first need to examine the part they themselves play in professional dysfunction: to re-empower their colleagues, and their client couples, they need to re-empower themselves.

There was already some evidence of re-empowerment in the workshop numbers. By the time the workshop ended, sufficient awareness had developed to enable the counsellors to question whether they were really as powerless as they sometimes felt. One was actively involved in redrafting her centre's printed information on counselling; others became more determined to seek similar opportunities to influence policy and practice, and to review the part they played in team meetings. Two, who were not clinicians by background, made a point of witnessing IVF treatment for themselves, for the first time. They observed, in close juxtaposition, both the invasive experience undergone by the women patients and what was demanded of the clinicians in carrying out such procedures swiftly and accurately. Their appreciation of both patient and clinical perspectives seemed to offer part of the basis for new kinds of communication between colleagues.

Chapter 6
A Family-Systems Approach to Infertility Counselling

Robert Bor and Isobel Scher

Introduction

Infertility is defined medically, but problems arising from it may be thought of in the family-systems approach to therapy as problems of loss and secrecy about loss.

Human reproduction is at one level a private, individual matter; while at another, it has implications for couples, their relationships with others and for social functioning. The birth of a child is a punctuation point in the family life-cycle that has a ripple effect throughout the wider kin network. Women become mothers, brothers become uncles, parents become grandparents, and so on. Although the birth of a child leads to numerous changes in relationships, it also affirms our capacity to do what generations before have done: to protect, feed, care for, nurture and teach their young.

Reproduction, child-bearing, childbirth and child-rearing are such central human processes and events that they can be described as natural. In this context, a deviation from the desire or capacity to reproduce is viewed, at best, as unusual and, at worst, a disaster of nature. Research has traditionally focused on the plight of the family adjusting to the birth of a child, and to developmental issues in families (Berk & Shapiro, 1984). By way of contrast, less has been written about the psychological effect on couples who experience fertility problems. A family-systems approach recognizes the personal and interpersonal psychological processes associated with human reproduction.

The family-systems approach to counselling is always contextual, taking into account socially constructed views of the problem, couple and family dynamics, and the relationship between the couple and health-care providers. The counsellor in this situation must first establish for which of the partners infertility is most a problem, and also the nature of the problem for each. The effect of the problem on the family and the extended family should then be addressed, as should the influence of the family on the problem. The meaning given to having children should also be discussed, both as a couple and within a family, as well as for each individual. Consideration is given to a couple's fear of loss, or consequent loss, and this should form a central part of the counselling process.

All of these issues are addressed in family-systems counselling against a backdrop of developmental themes – for the individual, couple and family; historical events in the family, across generations; past experience of coping with loss; and lastly the evolving relationship between the couple and the health-care team. The family-systems approach is derived from a conceptual framework about psychological problems and the therapeutic process, and guidelines have emerged for conducting such counselling sessions.

The approach does not prescribe how people should relate to one another or what decisions people ought to make. The term family-systems may imply working towards a traditional, patriarchal family structure. However, the approach described in this chapter in fact takes a more neutral view about relationships; but also recognizes the social and political forces (including gender issues) which act to influence relationships.

The first part of this chapter sets out some of the psychological problems that arise from infertility which affect families. This is followed by a description of the family-systems approach in infertility counselling.

Beliefs about parenting

The desire to start a family can seldom be explained by any one factor. It may be a combination of conforming to social expectations, redressing balance in a family structure where other siblings do not themselves have children, an antidote to loneliness in a marriage, the need for an heir, or more hands to help with household and other work, amongst others. Child-bearing and the start of a family are often emotional experiences and parents may expect to be taken over by 'magical thinking' and be consumed by pleasure and happiness.

The reality is that a child will force the parents to define or redefine their role in the family, and with one another. Parents may have to decide who will be the most responsible for the day-to-day care of the child. The traditional pattern of a mother caring for her child, freeing her husband to work, is increasingly being challenged. Not only are there changes in the workplace and patterns of employment, but there is some recognition that the biological family is not the only source of parenting. Extended family networks, fostering and adoption arrangements, and even children brought up by same-sex couples are possibly alternate forms of parenting. Counselling should address the couple's beliefs about the extent to which they view parenting as being driven by biological and social associations between themselves and the child.

This can help them in reaching decisions about treatment and options regarding adoption, among other consequences of infertility.

Background

A large proportion of women in Western societies who have planned to start a family will come into contact with a range of health-care providers at different stages in the course of pre- and post-natal care. For those who experience fertility-related problems, their first contact with health-care professionals may be at a time of personal stress or crisis, as these problems are not usually anticipated in advance. Psychological issues for these women and their partners may need to be explored through counselling. Infertility counselling can help people to make informed decisions, to adjust to new and sometimes unwelcome circumstances, and to solve personal problems. Some consequences of infertility may require special attention in counselling. These include issues arising from *in vitro* fertilization, artificial insemination by donor (DI), surrogacy, and fostering and adoption. Couples who either choose not to have children, or for whom child-bearing may not be an option (such as in same-sex relationships), may also benefit from counselling.

While the provision of psychological support in infertility settings is important, some women and their partners may thus be disadvantaged. Most approaches in counselling and psychotherapy favour working with individual clients. Infertility has implications not only for the individual, but also for the couple and family. Yet counselling for couples and families requires the acquisition of different psychotherapeutic skills, which may entail a shift in the conceptual framework regarding psychological problems, how they evolve, are maintained and how they can be resolved through counselling (Watzlawick, Weakland & Fisch, 1974).

Unlike traditional counselling approaches, which usually focus on the pathology and history of the individual client, a family-systems approach addresses the needs of individuals, couples and families, and may also include members of the health-care team. Even without formal training in marital and family therapy, counsellors used to working with individuals can use the approach to broaden their understanding of the client's problem and the counselling process. It is not within the scope of this chapter to provide a detailed description of the approach and readers may wish to consult other texts on family-systems counselling (Jones, 1993; McDaniel, Hepworth and Doherty, 1992).

While emotional and psychological issues associated with infertility may prompt people to seek support through counselling, family-systems counsellors acknowledge the interrelatedness of biological and psychological processes. Counsellors work closely with their medical, nursing, technical and administrative colleagues, and try to avoid dichotomous mind/body arguments. We recognize, for example, that the failure of reproductive technologies to help a couple have a baby can result in the couple feeling hopeless and depressed. Similarly, the pressure experienced by a couple to have intercourse 'on command' over a few days during treatment for infertility, can result in sexual problems and impotence in some male partners.

Addressing beliefs about medical problems

The prevailing social context of health and illness mediates personal responses to medical problems and, ultimately, how people cope with them. Both the meaning ascribed to the medical condition as well as beliefs about how the person 'contracted' or 'acquired' the problem may need to be explored in counselling sessions. In many societies, for example, a couple are not viewed as adults until they have children. Because of the high premium placed on having children, infertility can lead to secrecy, shame, severe depression and even suicide. The length of time since fertility-related problems are first noticed is a mediating factor in what meaning people derive from the medical problem. A woman who has not conceived after three months may be tempted to view her difficulties as transient, whereas a woman attending an infertility treatment centre for two years may have all but given up hope.

Meaning is also derived from views about biological processes. Genetic factors rather than social forces may determine whether a couple is able to bond with their child. For example, some parents may feel that they do not have right to discipline a child who has been adopted because 'the child's really someone else's child'. This can, in turn, lead to a self-fulfilling prophecy in which a child later feels that he does not really belong to his adoptive parents and may start to rebel against them or constantly challenge their authority. Ideas about what it means to be a 'real' parent can therefore lead to psychological problems for both parents and children.

Meaning attached to the 'cause' of the problem and how it is treated is equally important. Feelings of guilt, shame and blame are often associated with causation of medical problems: 'If only I wasn't on the pill for all those years . . .'; 'How can we possibly adopt! Maybe we'll be getting damaged goods'; 'How can you expect me to feel close to my daughter? After all, my great contribution to making her was to jerk off into a bottle in a toilet in a grey-painted clinic!'. There is almost always a therapeutic issue arising from the meaning of the medical problem, its social consequences, and the changing definitions of relationships that may need to be addressed in counselling sessions.

Boundaries and 'boundary ambiguity'

Both reproduction and infertility can challenge family structures, roles and relationships. Boundaries regularly undergo change within the family, and between the family and social systems. Changes to relationships and the structure of the family can give rise to 'boundary ambiguity' (Burns, 1987).

Preparation for parenthood begins before couples become actual parents; a fantasy child may be psychologically present in the family long before conception has even taken place. Raphael (1983, p. 231) suggests that 'the image of the relationship and the baby may represent conscious memories, but also unconscious fantasies [which] may also be powerful factors in leading to the beginning of the mother-infant relationship'. The couple may start to view themselves as a triad, giving rise to boundary ambiguity, which is characterized by the psychological presence but physical absence of a family member. Infertility extends the period of ambiguity, particularly during treatment. Parenthood and grandparenthood are in limbo and, in a multigenerational context, this can have distressing consequences. A child may be a gift to one's own parents, the means to mending damaged relationships in a family, or an opportunity to re-balance the family ledger whereby grandchildren can be shown the love and attention denied to their own parents (Burns, 1987).

Secrecy

In the field of human reproduction, many psychological problems experienced by people stem from the dissemination of information about a medical condition and its consequences. A family-systems counselling approach gives a high level of priority to interpersonal dynamics stemming from secrecy, confidentiality and privacy (Karpel, 1980). Problems stemming from secrets have implications for social boundaries, roles and relationships. For some couples, the social shame of infertility may result in their not disclosing information to relatives and close friends. Consequently, they may be denied the support of those relatives and close friends.

Some solutions to the problem of infertility may also be hidden from relatives as there remains suspicion and stigma of families where children are conceived with donated gametes (Schaffer and Diamond, 1993). Where a child is created by a procedure which disrupts the genetic link, the couple may have to confront issues about what it means to be cut off from one's biological connections. This may also affect the future parent-child relationship, Fostering and adoption may give rise to similar problems as there is a premise that 'the child's experience of biological-familial continuity and connection is a basic and fundamental ingredient of his sense of self' (Colon 1978, p. 289). Symptoms of psychological distress in some children, such as shoplifting and disruptive behaviour in the classroom, may reflect unresolved issues about secrets pertaining to their pedigree. Children born to parents who have experienced fertility-related problems are more likely to be overprotected by their parents. This suggests that the legacy of infertility may later have implications for the child's ability to successfully negotiate the process of leaving home at a later stage in his development (Burns, 1990).

Health-care staff are not immune to the effects of secrets. Where a couple have chosen not to tell others about the problem of infertility, they may come to rely on professional carers for support. Members of the health-care team may themselves feel burdened with private information. The counsellor should be aware of and recognize the limits of his or her responsibility, which may help to prevent inappropriate feelings of responsibility within the family.

Dealing with loss and anticipatory loss

The experience of loss may first bring people to counselling (Mandelberg, 1986). Yet, the anticipation or threat of loss is itself as challenging and painful as actual loss (Rolland, 1990) and should be addressed through counselling at an early stage of treatment, and not only when actual loss leads to the withdrawal of the medical system and a referral for counselling.

Losses may include unrealized plans and ambitions, loss of continuity in the family, loss of the assumption of parenthood, as well as loss of hope. Loss is frequently punctuated by a transition from the status of potential parenthood to non-parenthood (Matthews and Matthews, 1986). One effect on couples of the increasing range of available technologies to assist with biological parenthood, as well as the alternatives, such as adoption, has been for the plight of the involuntarily childless to be ignored. Yet, almost without exception, everyone attending an infertility treatment centre is likely to confront issues pertaining to loss (Jennings, 1991), even if these include the loss of not being able to have a child in the 'normal' way; that is, without medical intervention.

Sexual responses as well as the biological function of marriage or partnership may also be brought into the spotlight, as may the couple's expectation that they will have control over their personal and reproductive world. It is not surprising, therefore, that research consistently demonstrates that marital relationships can be severely stressed both by infertility and its treatment (Humphrey and Humphrey, 1987; Shaw, Johnston and Shaw, 1988; Weinshel 1990). At each stage of investigation and treatment, the couple are faced with new decisions which have implications for the viability of their relationship.

Matthews and Matthews (1986) have observed that the way in which the couple and their respective families deal with pressures and challenges to their reality is mediated by several factors. These include: the duration and outcome of their infertility; the extent to which the couple have a shared construct about how best to deal with the problem, or whether issues such as blame and responsibility have skewed this, and the reactions and responses of family members to them. To this can be added the central role that health-care providers play in influencing the couple's response to anticipated or actual loss. Some health-care providers may unrealistically convey too much hope to the couple about the potential outcome of treatment. Staff who themselves experience difficulty dealing with loss or who are excessively stressed by their work are more likely to do this. As a consequence, the couple may be distracted from facing up to the possibility that treatment might fail.

In some cases, beliefs about blame, responsibility and guilt may serve to 'deflect' the couple from the overwhelming emotional pain of infertility, miscarriage or the loss of a child. The pain may be in relation to 'separation anxiety, existential aloneness, denial, sadness, disappointment, anger, resentment, guilt, exhaustion and desperation' (Rolland, 1990 p. 30). The feelings may be both intense and ambivalent: there may be a desire to be closely and deeply connected with a family member; and at the same time, a need to escape from all the emotional pain and therefore a longing to feel disconnected from some people and the problem. Furthermore, some of these painful feelings may have to be endured in secret and in isolation because the couple may have chosen not to tell anyone about the problem. Coping with the uncertainty of treatment for infertility or pregnancy may be as difficult for the couple as the certainty brought about by bad news.

The consequences of loss can be discussed in counselling, as can thoughts about how the loss can be resolved. This may lead to discussion of ideas about grief and mourning, and the concept of time in psychological healing. Counselling about anticipatory loss can start with hypothetical and future-oriented questions (e.g.: 'What effect might it have on your relationship if you were unable to have children?'). The use of questions in counselling is discussed later in this chapter. The threat of loss or the experience of actual loss places people at risk of psychological problems. People can 'have difficulty imagining their future because of its potential loss . . . they can lose the systemic flexibility that allows the future to hold new meanings' (Penn, 1985, p. 305). An important task for the counsellor is to push the couple or family-system forwards in order that they do not become stuck at a particular point in their development or around a particular event. This may entail creating a meaning for the loss, helping sustain a measure of hope that will help the client or couple to carry on, and helping them to maintain their competency in dealing with the loss. Where the couple have chosen to separate, the counsellor may also be required to help them to end their relationship. The section below describes how some of these theoretical ideas can be applied in therapeutic practice.

Basic tenets of a family-systems counselling approach

There is a range of therapeutic approaches in counselling. Whichever route one takes in counselling, a 'map' is necessary to help conceptualize problems and their possible resolution. Theory is important in the practice of counselling, as under-developed or vague theoretical ideas are a recipe for confusion in counselling sessions and for both confusing and abusing the client. The authors of this chapter define systemic counselling as follows:

> it is an interaction in a therapeutic context, focusing primarily on a conversation about relationships, beliefs and behaviour, through which the client's apparent 'problem' is framed and reframed in a fitting or useful way, and in which new solutions are generated and the problem takes on a whole new meaning. This can lead to different views about the problem, or different behaviours in relation to the problem, thereby leading to its resolution.

Theory and experience should guide the counsellor in conducting sessions with clients. The ten basic tenets of a family-systems approach are described below:

(1) Focus on the family and relationships

The family (both biological and social) is a person's primary social system. Problems about reproduction may arise in the context of family relationships and can be resolved within them. The family does not need to be present in sessions for the counsellor to explore the impact of the problem on relationships with others.

(2) Respect people's own beliefs and practices

The objective reality of infertility affects people in different ways, and counsellors should avoid imposing their ideas or solutions on others. Counsellors endeavour to retain a degree of neutrality with respect to people's ideas and practices, although this may be moderated by practices that have legal implications. One task of the counsellor is to seek to understand a person's social and cultural context, irrespective of the person's gender and sexual orientation, race or disability, and help that person to generate solutions to problems that fit with them and their context.

(3) Behaviour and problems occur in a context

They should be examined and understood in the milieu in which they arise. The basic axioms of communication (Watzlawick, Beavin and Jackson, 1967) are central in this regard. These are: one cannot *not* communicate; *every* communication tells us something about a relationship; and communication always includes ideas about content (*what* is being said) and process (*how* it is said and what this conveys).

(4) Changes in an individual will affect his or her relationships

If something happens to an individual it will have an impact on other people and may affect how they behave towards them. The birth of a child, for example, may disrupt the dyad of the marriage relationship. The father may feel excluded from the close mother-infant relationship and himself be slow to bond with the infant. His wife may resent his being distant from them and feel that he has withdrawn from their relationship. In turn, she may become seem depressed to her family and friends.

(5) Problems associated with reproduction may have both psychological and medical consequences

The medical system typically views problems as residing in an individual. In reproductive medicine, which by definition, is usually a problem that confronts a couple, this may lead to one person feeling blamed. Irrespective of the number of people present in the counselling session, the ideas and concerns of people from *at least* three different (but overlapping) systems can be addressed: (a) the client system (usually a couple); (b) the family system (usually those related to or close to the client(s), and (c) the medical and health care systems (doctors, nurses and related specialists, and sometimes reception staff, other counsellors and laboratory personnel, among others).

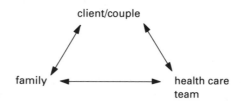

The triangle depicted opposite, of which the counsellor is a part, is the minimum unit or relationship network which the counsellor addresses in sessions. While these three sub-systems closely interact, ideas and beliefs emanating from additional sub-systems may need to be discussed. These include the close friends and work colleagues as well as the extended family of each client as well as the needs and considerations of the unborn child.

(6) Consideration of the sociomedical context of human reproduction

Counselling cannot be separated from events and advances in biology, medicine and medical technology, nor from social, ethical and political forces. If, for example, a clinic is unable to offer a particular treatment to their clients, this will have implications for their care. The counsellor may then have to deal with the anger and frustration of patients who might feel that they are not being offered a full range of possible treatments.

Laboratory tests and medical treatments for clients who experience infertility or who wish to terminate a pregnancy are costly and a sizeable proportion will be forced to pay for their care. There is, therefore, the possible additional consideration of clients' financial resources, and how these directly affect the choices available to them. One consequence of having limited financial resources is that clients might feel resentful and angry. These feelings may be directed at health-care staff and need to be discussed in the course of counselling.

(7) Relationships between people are punctuated by beliefs and behaviours

New ideas and beliefs can lead to different behaviours, and *vice versa*. Behaviour, thought and emotion are interdependent. Counsellors can intervene with clients with respect to either their behaviour or their ideas and beliefs. Family-systems counsellors tend to focus their interventions on ideas and beliefs.

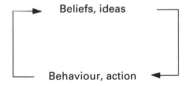

Beliefs, ideas

Behaviour, action

(8) Concerns associated with human reproduction do not inevitably lead to psychological problems

An emphasis on professional psychological care in relation to infertility may inadvertently cause some people to believe that they have a psychological problem (Edelmann and Connolly, 1987). A family-systems approach recognizes that problems may arise for some people and at different stages and at different times.

(9) Problems may occur when reality is denied

A woman who is unable to conceive, for example, despite years of specialist medical investigations and methods for assisted conception, may be denying reality when she travels overseas for a series of expensive 'miracle' treatments.

(10) Enhance people's competencies and coping abilities

This is in contrast to an 'error-deficit' approach to counselling in which people are sometimes led to feel blamed for a problem or are viewed as 'damaged' or 'pathological'. A couple who seek a medical opinion about infertility from several different specialists may be described as 'denying their problem'. By way of contrast, a family-systems therapist might reframe this as their not wanting to relinquish their hope of having a child. This could lead to an extensive discussion about their feelings of hope and hopelessness, and what it might mean to them if these feelings were to change. Where indicated, clients can be helped to be more assertive in dealing with the medical system and having their needs met.

A family-systems approach to counselling is usually purposeful and problem-focused. In this respect, it may differ from explorative psychotherapy. The actual process of counselling is described next.

Family-systems theory and the process of counselling

Assessment

Defining the problem is a key task in systemic counselling as the counsellor avoids bringing to the session preconceptions of what the problem (if any) might be. All forms of diagnosis and counselling involve asking questions that result in disclosure of the relevant information to the counsellor. Questions form an integral part of the process of assessment, which in turn is inseparable from the process of counselling. The process of assessment is not merely a procedure for labelling, for this by itself may be destructive. Rather it is seen as an ongoing process of observing, examining and clarifying a stated problem within its whole context. The aim is to formulate appropriate methods of dealing with that problem. During each counselling session, systemic counsellors are simultaneously engaged in three key procedures or activities: hypothesizing; the circular interview, and neutrality and curiosity.

Hypothesizing

A team of Italian psychiatrists, led by Dr Mara Selvini-Palazzoli, introduced the circular interview as a means for conducting a systemic investigation of family relationships and psychological problems (Selvini-Palazzoli *et al.*, 1980). In order to guide the counsellor in this problem-defining task, he or she needs to develop a hypothesis, or calculated guess, about the problem and what it may mean. Hypotheses are composite ideas about a person's relationship patterns with respect to a symptom or problem. The Milan team, who first described the use of systemic hypotheses in counselling, were not concerned about the truths of the counsellor's explanations or ideas, but rather the usefulness of their formulations. All relevant information about relationships and the medical problem is used in the formulation of a hypothesis. An example of a hypothesis is as follows:

Case history

Mrs J has been attending the clinic for treatment for infertility for two years. So far, treatment has not resulted in her becoming pregnant. She has become increasingly depressed over the last few weeks. Her husband has indicated that they should stop coming to the clinic and accept that they probably will not be able to have a child, though the couple have not openly discussed this. Mrs J, who is an only child, seems ambivalent about whether to give up treatment. On the one hand, she appears to agree with her husband, but on the other hand, she feels that she would be disappointing her parents who look forward to the day when they become grandparents. Her doctor has not discussed with her further options for treatment, but has asked Mrs J if she would like to speak to the clinic counsellor. To date, there has not been open discussion between the couple, and between the couple and clinic staff, about whether treatment should be discontinued. The decision about further medical care also involves addressing the important psychological issues of hope and despair. It seems that there is anxiety talking about this because of the implications of loss of hope for this couple. The task of raising this with the client has been 'delegated' to the clinic counsellor, in the belief that the counsellor's main role is to help people to cope with 'bad news'.

Hypotheses reflect the counsellor's view of reality rather than what is 'really' occurring. They are revised within sessions, as new information comes to light, and between sessions. The construction of a hypothesis involves making use of all available information to create a therapeutic reality. The hypothesis should be circular and relational, which means that all information gathered in the session relevant to a symptom should be used to create a new view or understanding of the problem. It is through the process of questioning, which is described below, that the ideas in the hypothesis will be put to the test.

The circular interview

The counsellor's interview with the patient is an important source of information: 'a clinical interview affords far more opportunities to act therapeutically than most people realize' (Tomm, 1987 p. 3). Circularity, as opposed to linear cause–effect reasoning, is a hallmark of the systemic counsellor. The counsellor conducts the session using feedback from the client or couple about relationships and interactive patterns (Selvini-Palazzoli *et al.*, 1980). In the traditional medical model, psychological problems may be seen to be caused by biological changes or repressed events. Irrespective of the source or the cause of the problem, the medical model focuses on the individual who is seen as the locus of the problem. Investigations proceed along a linear course, linking past events to psychological symptoms. One effect is that someone or something is blamed for a problem.

When the technique of circular questioning is used, the process of the interview itself will reflect circular and systemic thinking. Thus, the underlying philosophy and methods used to conduct the process of diagnosis and treatment are congruent. Questions are the main catalyst for client change and healing and they provide clients with opportunities to make further choices in their lives. There is a wide range of questions that can be used in counselling. Linear questions, sometimes termed 'closed questions', usually require a 'yes' or 'no' reply from the client and are helpful if factual information is required by the counsellor. 'Circular questions' apply to the range of interventive or therapeutic questions that are used in addition to linear questions in systemic counselling. Some examples of questions are set out below:

Question	Example
Linear question *(closed question)*	Have you previously had an abortion?
Future-oriented question	How do you see your relationship if you were unable to have children? [or] When do you think that the pain of not being able to have kids will most show?
Relationship question	Which of your parents gets more upset when they think that Jenny may never have children?
Difference question	Is it easier for you to live with the uncertainty (and in hope) of not knowing if there are problems with the fetus, or the knowledge (and maybe the distress) of any possible problems or abnormalities?
Circular question	If I asked Pete what first attracted him to you, what do you think he would say?

Hypothetical question   Sue and Mary, if you were a heterosexual couple, at what stage in your relationship do you think you would be considering having children? What might be happening in the relationship around that time?

Using the process of circular questioning (Selvini-Palazzoli *et al.*, 1980) the counsellor is able to track very closely not only relationship patterns in the present, but any changes at the time the problem first appeared. The basic tenet is always to ask questions that address a difference or define a relationship. Clinical experience confirms that the use of questions as a means of conducting the counselling interview is especially pertinent to dealing with personal issues which are of a sensitive nature.

Posing questions also provides the clients with the opportunity to view themselves in the context of relationships and in an interacting system. Hypothetical or future-oriented questions are particularly effective in helping people to talk about difficult or painful realities. There is no such thing as a 'wrong' question, although certain questions will be more useful than others; everything the counsellor 'does or says, or chooses not to do or not to say, can be thought of as an intervention that could be therapeutic, non-therapeutic or counter-therapeutic' (Tomm, 1987, p. 5). The questions that the counsellor asks help to construct a therapeutic reality. This reality in turn enables the counsellor to formulate a particular intervention; or this new reality may become an intervention in itself.

Neutrality, empathy and curiosity

Systemic counselling, as previously described, is not founded on a normative view of problems and relationships. Most counselling approaches stress the importance of the professional's neutrality in relation to decisions and experiences of their clients. Systemic counselling is no exception to this rule. This distinguishes professional counselling from advice-giving and support. On the one hand, the counsellor strives to retain a level of neutrality with regard to some of the client's dilemmas and problems. This has to be balanced with careful consideration of the legal and ethical implications of any actions, as well as empathy, which is a hallmark of counselling.

Empathy may be conveyed in two different ways in systemic counselling. Listening to clients, respecting their views and attempting to understand their predicament or problem more fully is one description of empathy. The counsellor is also being empathic when he or she moves at the rate or pace that the client dictates. If the counsellor introduces ideas to clients before they are ready to accept them, the counsellor is imposing his or her views and potentially making assumptions about clients. It has been suggested that a counsellor's warm and empathic style facilitates problem-solving. Undoubtedly, the counsellor's interpersonal style is important if the counselling relationship is to develop. However, empathy and listening alone are unlikely to fully satisfy the client's expressed need for change. Empathy is also conveyed to the client when the counsellor is curious about the experience and ideas of the client. Asking questions and avoiding making assumptions about the meaning of what the clients says or does in the session, helps the counsellor to guard against becoming prescriptive or judgemental.

Defining the problem in counselling

A clear definition of 'the problem' is required by the systemic counsellor working in a medical system, or with people with medical problems. This is an integral part of counselling and provides an opportunity to refine the initial hypothesis and will directly affect the outcome of counselling. For counsellors to understand the definition of the problem, they may require answers to certain key questions. The first of these is to identify the context in which the problem is defined and for whom it is most a problem. There are four main contexts in which problems arise:

Defining the context of the problem

(1) The problem of the client is related to his or her family system. *Example*: the client's parents, who are deeply religious, see their daughter's infertility as a just punishment for her having had an abortion as a teenager.
(2) The problem presented is related to friends or other social support systems of the client. *Example*: a couple have observed that many of their friends are settling down in relationships and are having children. They now feel under pressure from them to start a family as a way of conforming to and maintaining these relationships.
(3) The problem presented is related to other therapeutic systems with which the client maintains contact. *Example*: another counsellor, who has previously worked with the client, feels that it is morally wrong for a lesbian to have a child. The client terminated the relationship with the counsellor because she felt that her lifestyle was being judged. She now wonders whether that counsellor may have been right and she and her partner decide to seek counselling in an infertility clinic to hear another view.
(4) The problem presented is related to the system within which the counsellor works. *Example*: a consultant in an infertility treatment centre refers a couple to the counsellor because he is concerned

about the deleterious effects of treatment on their relationship. Although the couple did not have a very good relationship at the start of treatment, the consultant feels that treatment has aggravated their difficulties. He indicates to the counsellor that they should be given marriage counselling to 'help them to stay together'.

A systemic counsellor working in this field need not presume either the presence or the nature of a problem until it is defined or confirmed by the client or a system of which he or she is a part. These systems include the client's personal and social milieu, the professional health and social-care systems, or the wider social and political system. The way in which clients view their problem will in part be a response to how others view it. Similarly, an only child growing up in a family where he or she was conceived through IVF, may feel over-protected by his parents. When a boy for example reaches a stage when he sees his friends becoming more independent, he may become disruptive at school as a way of drawing attention to himself and rebelling in a less emotionally charged setting.

In summary, the overriding aims of systemic counselling are;

(1) To engage the client and others in counselling, and to provide a supportive context in which sensitive and emotive issues can be openly discussed.
(2) To identify whether there is a problem and, where appropriate, to define the problem and identify for whom the problem is most a problem.
(3) To help people to make informed decisions.
(4) To prevent individuals, couples, families and other systems from becoming psychologically 'stuck' around problems pertaining to human reproduction, and therefore to help people to continue to grow and develop emotionally in the context of all of their relationships.
(5) To identify and discuss each person's greatest fear or concern, to work towards the resolution of problems and to reduce personal stress and anxiety to manageable proportions.
(6) To help people to talk openly about change and loss for themselves and other members of the family.
(7) To describe to each client a relational context for their problem and thereby reframe the problem.
(8) To normalize and affirm the experience and feelings of each family member, as well as those of professional colleagues.

Use of the genogram

This section describes how some of the aims of counselling sessions can be achieved. Many systemic counsellors draw a 'genogram' or family tree with the client in the first session as a way to identify members of the family, and to begin to explore the implications of problems in a multigenerational context. A genogram provides a graphic representation of family history and relationships, and can also include information about emotional closeness and distance between people and across generations. This is not only a powerful method of engaging someone in counselling, but it can also be considered a therapeutic intervention as the problem can be viewed in a wider context from the outset. Eliciting a family history can prompt conversation about change, loss, patterns of support and secrecy. The process of constructing the family genogram with an individual, couple or family can arouse interest in people's past and present, and open up discussion about future possibilities (McGoldrick and Gerson, 1985). This is illustrated in the following case below.

Case history

Mrs S was asked by the school counsellor to come and discuss her daughter's progress at school. Jane (aged 6) had recently fallen behind in her school work and had become socially isolated from friends. During their discussion, Mrs S also revealed that Jane had started bedwetting and it was becoming increasingly difficult to prepare her for school in the morning. The counsellor asked about how Mrs S and her husband were coping with these problems and whether they had any ideas about their possible cause. She also drew a genogram of the family.

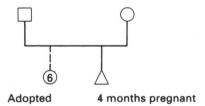

Adopted   4 months pregnant

Fig. 6.3

Mrs S told the counsellor that she was four months pregnant following IVF. In addition, she revealed that because she was unable to conceive in the past, they had adopted Jane. They had not told their daughter that she was adopted, nor that her mother was pregnant. Mrs S and the counsellor spent some time exploring ideas about Jane's sense of belonging in the family, and the fear that she may be displaced by the arrival of a 'real' son or daughter in the family. With Mrs S' permission, the school counsellor contacted the counsellor working in the infertility clinic and they discussed now best to help the family with issues about disclosure and family relationships.

The use of the genogram in this counselling case helped the client and counsellor to open up discussion about family relationships, secrecy and psychological symptoms.

Exploring the relationship context of the client's problem

Drawing a family tree is a helpful way to view the client's family. Systemic counsellors also focus on the interfaces of the client's significant relationships. For example, one might explore how the current problem affects relationships, and the anticipated effect it may have if the problem were to persist; or the problem were to deteriorate; or the problem were to be solved. Some of these points are illustrated below, using a range of different questions, in the excerpt from a counselling session:

> *Counsellor* Mr F, what concerns, if any, might you have for your relationship with your wife and your unborn child if the doctors suggested that your wife try to conceive through DI?
>
> *Mr F* I don't like the idea of her having another man's sperm inside her. I would think that it's someone else's baby.
>
> *Counsellor* So how do you think that would affect your relationship with your wife and the child?
>
> *Mr F* I'm not sure that I would want to sleep with my wife again. And maybe I wouldn't bond with the baby.
>
> *Counsellor* What do you think would be your wife's response to what you have just said?
>
> *Mr F* I doubt she would agree with me. But then it's easy for her – it's half *her* baby.
>
> *Counsellor* And if you chose not to go through with DI and you didn't have a child, how might you view your relationship with your wife?
>
> *Mrs F* Can I say something here? I've already told him it's okay if we don't have a kid. It's more him that wants one anyway. It's like he wants a boy to teach to play soccer. But I've told him you don't choose the sex of your baby. What if it's a girl?
>
> *Counsellor* For whom in the family would it be most difficult if you chose not to have a child?
>
> *Mr F* My father. He keeps nagging me and saying that time is getting on. He wants grandchildren.
>
> *Counsellor* Does he know the difficulties you have had starting a family?
>
> *Mr F* I couldn't tell him I haven't got enough sperm. He'd think of me as less of a man. And maybe he'd blame himself for that. Worse still, he'd probably tell me to leave Carol and try having a family with another woman.
>
> *Counsellor* What might you do if you were given that advice?
>
> *Mr F* That may be the beginning of the end of my relationship with my father. I wouldn't have him interfere with my relationship with Carol. Nothing is more important to me.
>
> *Mrs F* I've never heard you say that until now! It's taken all this time to hear that, and then it's got to be in a room with a shrink!
>
> *Counsellor* What does that mean to you, Mrs F, now that you've heard your husband say that?

> Mrs F   I guess our relationship is more 'OK' than I'd ever allow myself to believe.
>
> Counsellor   And what might that mean to you?
>
> Mrs F   We'll survive this problem: there's hope.

In this case, at least six levels of the problem can be conceptualized and explored with the couple: the husband's low sperm count and his association with his masculinity (including his relationship with himself and his father), the couple's inability to have a child together (the marriage relationship and their view of themselves as a family), the potential solution of DI (the relationship between the couple, the donor and the child); expectations of and pressures on the couple from others (the couple's relationship with each family of origin); the expectations of the child conceived and each of the client's views and expectations of counselling and the (male) counsellor (the triangular relationship in the counselling room).

Conclusion

The family-systems approach is more than a school of counselling; it represents a way of conceptualizing about problems and therapeutic work. The theory of counselling people with fertility problems described in this chapter, as well as the associated therapeutic skills, can readily be adapted and used by counsellors who choose to practise other counselling approaches.

While reproductive health-care has become increasingly medicalized, there is also a trend, through counselling, towards improving the psychological and social well-being of people affected by fertility problems. The family-systems approach recognizes that infertility is not only the problem of the person who is medically described as infertile. Furthermore, while infertility may be the presenting problem in counselling, there may be the psychological problem of loss which needs to be addressed. Counselling has application both where emotional factors may be contributing factors of infertility (Bresnick & Taymor, 1979) as well as helping people to cope with the psychological stress of the impact of infertility (Bresnick, 1981).

Although birth and death are the most basic human events, their timing is not always predictable or certain. The task in counselling is to clarify the meaning of infertility and consequent childlessness not only for the couple, but also for the family and extended family. Issues in the health-care team should be accorded equal importance and should be included in the counselling context.

Chapter 7
The Fertile Ground: The Role of Art Therapy in the Fertility Clinic

Jean Campbell

Introduction

The primary function of art therapy in the work of an infertility clinic is to offer a way for people to work creatively with the unconscious (or less conscious) aspects of their involvement with fertility, sub-fertility and its treatments. It may be integrated into verbal counselling in order to facilitate communication, or used in its own right as a direct therapeutic aid.

This chapter is concerned with the importance of art therapy in the treatment of infertility, whether unexplained or medically diagnosed. It is based on extensive work with individuals, couples and groups at a 'high-tech' fertility clinic at the Royal London Hospital. Art therapy also contributes to the training of medical students and fertility counsellors.

Background: what is art therapy?

Art therapy involves the use of spontaneous art activity to bring about change, for the better, in a given human condition. Creative work such as painting, drawing or modelling is used to communicate and express feelings, thoughts and ideas. Both the act of spontaneous image-making, and the work which is produced are considered to have meaning for their creator. The therapist helps clients to understand the images and how they relate to the issues which have brought them into therapy. In the context of infertility, art is used as a visual language. It allows people to give shape to complex ideas, thoughts and feelings, which are often grounded in pre-verbal experience or are simply beyond words and therefore too difficult to articulate verbally at first.

The physical attributes of the art media can be used to reflect real and imagined sensations and experiences; for example, paint can be used to explore positive and negative feelings about body fluids, or feelings of loss of control, while clay can be used to model body forms.

Images produced by clients and trainees alike often reveal varying degrees of conflict. The conflict, more often than not, is about trying to hold on to a positive, healthy sense of self while coping with physical

113

conditions and treatments which are about body dysfunction. Women in particular have been able to create intimate images which explore feelings about their bodies, locating what, for some, becomes the focus of their emotional distress.

From a broader perspective, issues of power and control are also relevant to women's gynaecological experiences. Art can be used to reaffirm a positive self-image and a sense of personal power.

Art therapy demands active involvement, and can be both physically and emotionally stimulating. It can help with the treatment and management of stress. It provides safe ways to express and explore intense feelings such as anger, frustration and despair. Couples, in particular, have been able to utilize image-making to improve communication and understanding between them.

While the spoken word may be forgotten, the permanence of the images of art therapy means that they can be referred to easily when needed. These images also provide a permanent record of the counselling from which other professionals can learn. They also afford insights into the complex interrelation of emotional, spiritual and physical issues. There is much to be gained from giving medical students, for example, an opportunity to 'see' images of emotional states which may underlie physical conditions; for example a purple vagina-like shape against a green background with a head grimacing in pain at its centre showed one woman's feeling of helplessness and despair about her endometriosis.

In line with the ethos of the clinic, a more holistic therapeutic involvement with clients is promoted. This means taking into account the whole person – mind, body and spirit in relation to their medical problems. Clients are supported whilst they gain insight into emotional conflicts which affect their ability to make appropriate treatment choices, or to cope with distress.

An even more obvious reason for using art therapy in fertility work is that it channels creativity to address that most creative aspect of life, namely, procreation. As one client put it, 'being unable to have a baby strikes at the heart of my sense of myself as a creative being'.

It is no coincidence that much of the language and symbolism used around artistic and visual creativity is also used in relation to fertility: for example, 'bearing original fruit', 'conceiving an idea', 'nurturing and giving birth to a concept'. There are obvious parallels between creating art and creating babies: both involve the transformation of matter or raw materials to produce something which is unique. Thus, artists also speak of feeling as though they are being taken over by a powerful force when they let go, unleash or give in to this indefinable energy reminiscent of conception, orgasm and also birth.

There are other strong links between art and fertility. Most cultures have a legacy of fertility imagery, both pre-historic and contemporary.

Fertility images are still used in many cultures to mediate with deified powers that be. Regardless of how advanced and effective fertility treatment becomes, people need outlets to communicate their more spiritual connections with the forces of creativity. Often, during counselling sessions, clients will speak of their fertility by using timeless symbolic imagery. One female client spoke of herself being like barren land, waiting for the dam to burst and flood her so that she would become fertile and able, like mother earth, to bestow her gifts on those around her.

In counselling, such imagery is held in the minds of the client and the counsellor, but art therapy provides an opportunity to give concrete shape to such imagery, to explore their own 'fertile ground'.

What happens in art therapy

The underlying principles and processes of art therapy give a framework by which to understand and structure the work. Art therapy is mediated through dynamics generated within what has been described as the 'triangular relationship' (Inscape, 1990). In an acknowledged therapeutic setting, the elements of this triangle are the client/artist, the image or artwork, and the therapist.

In a typical session, the client is invited to work with the materials provided and do, for example, a drawing, painting or sculpture. The work can emerge completely spontaneously, with the client allowing the image to come – the so-called non-directive approach; or the therapist may suggest a theme based on an issue relevant to what brings the client into art therapy – the directive approach (Campbell, 1993). In both modes, the artist or client works without a predetermined idea of the finished product. Time is usually set aside for reflection and discussion on the thoughts, feelings and sensations which come from making and looking at the image.

As the quality of trust builds up in the relationship, the client becomes more expressive, images flow with greater ease; a personal visual language is created of colour, line, texture, abstract or figurative forms. This will have a degree of symbolic content. Diana Halliday, a pioneer of art therapy in this country, calls this process 'art from within'.

There is no judgement of good or bad art; the *meaning* is of primary importance, rather than aesthetic judgements on the art itself, to those involved in the making of it. Both therapist and client work together towards understanding what the artwork reveals of the inner, less conscious aspects of the client's emotions in relation to the issues that bring her (or him) into therapy.

The art therapist is required to 'hold' the integrity of the work, an attitude akin to the 'unconditional acceptance' adopted by Rogerian counsellors. (Rogers, 1996). This bias of the therapist dictates how images are worked with the meaning ascribed to them and the structure of the session.

Theoretical ground

The development of art therapy in the UK and in the USA has been extensively chronicled (Waller, 1984 and 1991). Two interwoven roots have been identified: developments in art education and development in psychotherapy theory and practice. From the influence of progressive ideas in art education and the 'Child Art' movement that sprang up between the wars came the notion that 'art was a means of developing a seeing, thinking, feeling and creative human being' (Waller, 1991).

While such ideas support the intrinsic benefits of artistic self-expression, the psychotherapeutic strand uses art like a therapeutic key or analytic tool. Margaret Naumberg, a Freudian analyst and founder member of art therapy in the USA, 'saw the object as both integrative and healing, and also an aspect of the transference relationship between the therapist and the patient' (Waller, 1991).

With emphasis on the power of the creative act, the role of the therapist is mainly that of facilitator. He or she provides space, time, materials, acceptance and understanding. With the emphasis on art as psychotherapy, a 'psychodynamic' understanding of human development and function provides the art therapist with a framework by which to interpret all aspects of the client's engagement with the work. This includes symbolic or hidden meaning in the images, and also the client's interactions with the therapist.

Art therapy encompasses a wide range of therapeutic practice, from in-depth art-psychotherapy at one end, to 'helping approaches' which utilize the techniques of art therapy to varying degrees, at the other. Many practitioners use the tenets of the main psychodynamic schools of thought as a framework to guide and understand interactions in their sessions.

Early Freudian theory, especially with its map of levels of consciousness, acknowledgement of unconscious motivation, psychosexual development and dysfunction, is a keystone to psychodynamic practice. As Naumberg writes:

> The process of art therapy is based on the recognition that man's most fundamental thoughts and feelings, derived from the unconscious, reach expression in images rather than words ... The techniques of art therapy are based on the knowledge that every individual, whether trained or untrained in art, has a latent capacity to project his inner conflict into visual form.   (Naumberg, 1966)

A Kleinian approach considers a person's artwork as an echo of relationships with 'internal objects' or 'inner images or ideas' we hold of our parents as children (Weir, 1987). Through art therapy, the client is able to re-engage with the inner task of maturation, to work through the conflict (he or) she was unable to resolve before and come to a more workable balance between the demands of the inner life and the external world.

Art therapists may also be influenced by the work of Carl Jung. His identification of personality types, the dynamics of conflict between opposing internal forces (archetypes), and the pervasive power of the collective unconscious can also give focus to art therapy. 'Jungian principles and techniques give a sense of direction and meaning as an exploratory model, and offer ways of mobilizing inner psychic resources through the transcendent function of symbol making' (Nowell-Hall, 1987).

Yet another approach is the humanistic one, which regards people as more socially reactive, self-determining beings, less at the mercy of uncontrollable drives generated via early formative relationships. Emphasis here is on using spontaneous image-making, not on plumbing the depths of the unconscious, but to clarify how people see current relationships or issues in order to envision possibilities for change.

Though the influence of psychotherapy theory and practice is very important, the 'art' in art therapy is grounded in appreciation of the healing power of visual creativity. As part of their training, art therapists are introduced to writings on creativity by artists and psychoanalysts such as Milner (1950); Ehrensweig (1984) and Winnicott (1971). Milner (1950) in *On Not Being Able to Paint* applies her psychoanalytic mind to explore her own quest for visual creativity.

The kind of spontaneous image-making which is fostered in art therapy is akin to play. In his chapter, 'Creativity and its origins', Winnicott (1971) broadens our perception to view play as a demonstration of a creative attitude. The objects which are created do not take centre-stage, rather it is the act of creation which attests to the person's state of being in the world. Through creativity, people can gain a sense that they can affect what is 'out there', as opposed to feeling that they are totally at the mercy of the powers that be.

> It is creative apperception more than anything else that makes the individual feel that life is worth living. Contrasted with this is a relationship to external reality which is one of compliance, the world and its details being recognized but only as something to be fitted in with or demanding adaptation. (Winnicott, p. 65)

It follows then that utilizing peoples' creative capacities at times of emotional distress is not about distraction but, rather, a way of reclaiming a capacity which most of us used naturally in childhood to make sense of and manage the vicissitudes of life. Likewise, introducing visual creativity to counselling training sessions heightens students' self-awareness and broadens the scope of learning. Both clients and students learn through taking 'visual risks'. Without knowing the final outcome, images are produced based on personal thoughts and feelings. Verbal risk-taking may follow on from this act. Carl Rogers (1970) expands on this theme:

> ... the mainsprings of creativity appear to be the same tendency which we discover so deeply as the curative force in psychotherapy – man's tendency to actualize himself, to become his potentialities ... This tendency may become deeply buried under layer after layer of encrusted psychological defence; it may be hidden under elaborate facades that deny its existence; it is my belief however, based on my experience, that it exists in every individual and awaits only the proper conditions to be released and expressed.   (p. 140)

Such theoretical ideas on the relevance of creativity to therapeutic work both inspire and guide the development of art therapy in the fertility clinic. The actual nuts and bolts of art therapy practice however have been shaped by direct work with clients.

How much and what ground to cover: practice issues

Though most art therapists work within the field of psychiatry, more recently there has been growth in the number of practitioners in physical medicine, for example in AIDS units and medical centres treating cancer. (It is also worth noting that the first employed art therapist worked at a chest clinic). To my knowledge, however, the Rowan clinic is the only fertility treatment centre in the UK to employ an art therapist.

In seeking to develop art therapy practice aligned to a counselling service within a fertility clinic setting, my priority is that the clients should find such work relevant and useful. To this end, a number of basic guidelines have proved useful. First of all, it is important not to 'psychopathologize' infertility (Jennings, 1992). By that, I mean that, though people can experience, and show, very distressed emotional and mental states, these states are a reflection of individual life-histories, social circumstances and well as treatment experiences; and the psychopathology not inherent to infertility itself.

The photographic image of the moment of conception, when the egg is surrounded by sperms frantically trying to penetrate it, provides an apt visual analogy for the way fertility can activate a wealth of interrelated issues. Infertility may be the nucleus of the client's problem, but it is the activation of unresolved feelings which can cause turmoil. These may relate to sex, sexuality, parenting experiences, bereavement and loss, relationships, gender, power and control. Images relating to all the issues mentioned above have come up in clients' art work.

Knowing how far or what level to work at, is equally important. As art therapy can sometimes give quicker access to unconscious life than pure verbal work, the work needs to be carefully paced and focused so that it does not 'disable' the client. Art therapy, after all, is offered for the clients to use in order to help them understand and manage themselves more effectively. But the parameters and limitations of the work must be defined not only by the needs of the client but also with reference to the primary task of the unit. The following example of brief work illustrates this point.

Case history

Anne and her partner attended one session of the art therapy group. The group was given the theme of 'my ideal family' to work on. Anne became very distressed by her picture. Drawn faintly in brown and grey pastels, a grey winged figure hovered above a baby's cot. Anne did not want to talk about it in the group. As the couple had found group work difficult and because they had marital problems that were only indirectly related to fertility, we (the counselling team) recommended marital counselling with Relate. Anne accepted the offer of five individual weekly art therapy sessions, to be followed by a couple session.

Anne had a diagnosis of secondary infertility – she had a teenage daughter from a previous marriage. Her gynaecological history revealed a minefield of distressing events including many miscarriages. She was frightened of having another miscarriage, and felt worthless. We agreed to focus the work on her miscarriage experience and her self-image in general. Anne came to four individual sessions and also attended the couple session. A life chart drawn in the first session chronicled significant life events, including the pattern of her miscarriages. This 'blueprint' provided themes that were then expanded. In one picture, Anne was keen to get the colour of an aborted fetus just right.

At first Anne was very anxious and spoke incessantly while she worked. She was encouraged to work in silence for longer periods and to express more of her feelings about the events shown in her work. She drew a self-image of her torso, with a scream coming up from her belly. Her hand cuts off the scream leaving her with a lump in her throat. This image of unexpressed despair brought up other areas of repressed grief. A tirade of ambivalent feelings about her mother threatened to overwhelm us. It was crucial that Anne was helped to make connections with her present situation. It is at this point that we come full circle back to the haunting image from that first group session. Two siblings had died and mysteriously disappeared during her childhood. Anne had not been allowed to go to the hospital. Her next picture – of her fertility – was of a field of spring flowers with a blue door in front of it. When I asked her what the door represents, Anne slipped into her usual defensive mode; a stream of complaints about the doctors who 'fail to treat me right'. We tried another route. I asked her what part of her gets aborted with the fetus when she has a miscarriage. She replied 'my unworthiness. I carry a bad gene like my mother'. The session finished with Anne writing a goodbye note to her last aborted fetus. Her final gesture was to take away all her pictures except the first.

I was very challenged by the work with Anne. Her referrer (a senior nurse) had astutely picked up that her abrasive and difficult behaviour in the clinic masked her acute anxiety and vulnerability. Via spontaneous image-making, Anne was able to gain some insight about her distress. Since childhood, she had fostered a fantasy about her mother 'killing-off babies'. She identified with her mother and saw her repeated miscarriages as an echo of her mother's behaviour. Giving shape to such ideas which sit at the core of inner self-distress is like the 'naming' of which Michael Jacobs speaks: 'Naming tries to help people find their shadows and to name them, a process which the counsellor assists but does not dictate.' (Jacobs, 1986, p. 24).

Anne's present distress, including her sub-fertility, was clearly connected with her childhood experiences both real and imagined. The breadth and depth of such experiences indicated the possible need for a lifetime of therapy, but that was not what the client wanted. Rolling up her pictures and removing them from the clinic was a clear message that she had gone as far as she wanted to.

Knowing how far to venture into peoples' psychic world is a particular challenge posed by using art therapy in the clinic. It cannot be desirable to incapacitate people emotionally in a situation in which they are already physically vulnerable. Anne was very clear about how far she wanted to go. Other clients, however, particularly those who are struggling for emotional stability, find it difficult to defend their personal ground, so it is very important to find a level to work which feels right for both art therapist and client.

Though it is not possible to ignore elements of transference in the work, in art therapy for infertility I try not to foster the kind of 'in-depth' transference relationship which is the foundation of full art psychotherapy. When working with a transference relationship in art therapy, the artwork is viewed as a visual reference to particular feelings which the client has for the therapist. These feelings are usually a replay of relationships which the client had with significant figures from her past.

The regression and dependence inherent to this approach puts people in touch with the 'child' part of themselves. Although this may be an important part of inner preparation for parenthood, in a fertility treatment setting, it is the 'adult' and potential parent that needs to be supported and reaffirmed. Also, people having fertility treatment are already in heavily dependent relationships with the clinical personnel. They have to cope with very invasive treatment where even the fundamental act of procreation is taken over by medical staff; so I take care not to 'invade' them psychologically or artistically.

I am also mindful of the fact that the play aspect of spontaneous art activity invokes childhood memories for many people. Artwork brings to mind child-parent or child-teacher relationships. However, the kind of relationship which seems to work best for art therapy in this context is more akin to the 'therapeutic alliance' which Dryden (1991) speaks of. We agree to work together, to learn what image-making tells us about the concerns of the client. I avoid interpreting the meaning of the work, and concentrate instead on helping the client to come up with their own ideas.

There are times when transference material can be worked with in more depth, for example, in individual art therapy sessions, when the client has already had therapy experience and in groupwork.

That said, however, it does not mean aspects of people's inner life cannot be worked with in art therapy. I would suggest that having an understanding of people which takes into account the connections between their life histories and their inner life and motivations, is vital to art therapy practice in fertility work. Without such a psychodynamic understanding, it would be hard to keep the often powerful and some-times disturbing images produced in perspective. I have found super-vision by an analytic art therapist necessary and very useful.

Confidentiality

There are specific issues related to confidentiality where art therapy is concerned. We have to take responsibility for looking after not only what is disclosed verbally, but also concrete representations of an equally intimate nature. Clients are concerned to know what will happen to their pictures and who will see them. With these concerns in mind, I always ask clients' permission if I need to show their work to others. For example, artwork can be a powerful visual aid when giving talks to other medical professionals, especially medical students. Art-work is treated with respect, and stored carefully. Fertility clients are anxious what is revealed in their work should not be used against them. This is a valid concern, given that the HFEA does suggest cases where people can be assessed for parenting suitability.

During a talk to obstetricians on the emotional effects of infertility, I once mentioned that a client who developed a psychotic illness after treatment had painted a picture of her depression some months earlier. At the time, she had refused further counselling. One doctor's response was to ask whether the client's picture indicated that she needed a psychiatric assessment. However while art therapy is used as a diag-nostic medium in some institutions, in fertility work I feel this would be inappropriate. Apart from the fact that there are too many ethical issues involved, it raises the question of whose needs the art therapy is there to serve.

Working with images in counselling

Image-making is introduced to clients when there are clear signs that they may benefit from working through spontaneous artwork; for example, when the client has difficulty with words (too many or too few); or when clients bring up issues of body or self-image. Another unique asset that image-making brings to counselling is that it can symbolically contain or hold verbally based work. The following case history illustrates this point.

Case history

The client was a young woman and mother who desperately wanted to have another child. Her second child had died a cot death. The client was in a state of frozen grief, walking and speaking as though she was only 'half there'. It soon became clear that she had not come to talk about fertility treatment; what was uppermost were unexpressed feelings about the child she had lost. Sorrowfully, she spoke of the love she had not been able to give and her guilt about what had happened. She acknowledged her need for more in-depth bereavement counselling, and to delay further fertility treatment.

Towards the end of the session I felt the situation called for some kind of symbolic gesture to both contain the moment and mark a turning point for this grieving mother. I asked her if there was anything she wanted to give to the baby who had died, and invited her to draw whatever it was. She drew a deep red heart, cut it out and made an envelope for it. She planned to find a special place in her room to keep it. This painting represented a transitional stage in her grief-work; taking back part of herself which had died with the baby.

Asking a client to draw an image about something that is difficult to find words for gives focus to the session; the image acts as a bridge and can help the client to become more articulate. The following is an illustration.

Case history

A young woman was in a dilemma as to whether or not she wanted to have another child or to end her relationship. She was at a loss for words to describe how she felt. I suggested she did a drawing about it. The image was of an egg shape drawn as a black ring with a pink, swirling, flower-like centre with a yellow nucleus. The black ring was her partner and the relationship, while the pink section she described as representing the improvements taking place. The yellow centre represented hope for even better changes. The outer ring for her seemed the most dominant factor: it encapsulated the ambivalence of the protective prison in which she felt secure yet stifled. She was unaware that the image looked like the cross-section of an egg – a perfect symbol of the nucleus of her concern.

When clients are very anxious or struck by 'verbal diarrhoea' drawing or painting can help both client and counsellor to get to the heart of the matter. A client, for example, who later disclosed her history of eating disorders, spent two sessions pouring out an endless diatribe describing painful and personal events. My experience of contact with this client was as though I was drowning in a mess. By introducing drawing we could identify more clearly the components of her distress. Also, by suggesting she worked in silence for a while, we were able to create a space for both of us in which to stand our ground.

When verbal-based counselling or therapeutic work becomes stuck or sterile, images can renew engagement with this work by both parties. It may be that the client and the counsellor feel at a loss with the complexities and multilayered nature of an issue. In which case, space to work visually and non-verbally can help to identify what is possible within the counselling, and what may need other therapeutic intervention.

Image-making can be introduced during any phase of the counselling process: to give visual shape to how the client perceives their problem; to facilitate more in-depth exploration as trust develops in the relationship; as well as towards envisaging future changes.

Clients can be invited to draw a 'life-line' – a visual history of personal development which highlights significant life events. This simple exercise allows the clients an opportunity to take stock of their lives. Repeated motifs and use of colour may indicate connections between events.

Bodywork with images

Many counsellors would agree that body language is part of the information which is 'processed' in counselling. Usually, it is a matter of the counsellor noting pieces of non-verbal communication including postures. The client may be asked to talk about body sensations, or sometimes, the counsellor may even suggest that the client alter their posture and breathing pattern in order to allow themselves to experience the feelings from which they may be cutting themselves off. It is possible to add another dimension to this work: there are instances where clients can benefit from drawing and painting how they experience their bodies. The very act of creation can release body tension.

Giving concrete shape and form to what is felt inside can also promote insight. This can be particularly useful when part of the identified problem stems from the client's difficulties in owning or expressing feelings. In one moving session, the husband of one of the members of an art therapy-based group, modelled in clay a small baby lying on its back, clutching a bottle. Tears filled his eyes as he spoke of what childlessness meant to him.

The dripping of red paint on a large group painting triggered suppressed memories of a miscarriage for another client.

Bodywork with women

It is not uncommon for women fertility clients to have a very poor self-image. Feelings of sexual guilt, past events or abuse can obscure a woman's understanding of her clinical problem. Also, the need to keep hope and a positive attitude to medical treatment, prevents many women from addressing their anger, distress and resentment about the invasive nature of the treatment.

Some women, often with long histories of infertility and treatment, do paintings which show 'bad' or rotting parts inside their bodies. One woman, who attended an art therapy based group for couples and individuals with a wide range of fertility-related issues, produced a very powerful image in response to the theme of 'an inner self-portrait'.

Case history

To begin with, she was asked to lie down on a large piece of paper. Her partner drew an outline of her body. She was then asked to show how she felt inside herself: a kind of mind-body-and-spirit portrait. This exercise seemed particularly relevant for this client, as she was often preoccupied with fears about her body.

Using paints and crayons, she showed how she felt inside. Black and red shapes represented malignant growths in her groin, red highlighted hot throbbing legs. A mixture of red, black and brown blobs and zigzag lines in her chest and belly region rose up to her throat. Her toe and finger nails were painted. She wore a bow in her hair, the eyes were closed. She did not draw a mouth.

During the discussion time she spoke about the choking sensations in her throat, holding her throat to emphasize the discomfort. She described them as coming from feelings inside her which she could not talk about. It was pointed out to her that she had not drawn her mouth (clearly connected with her inability to give expression to those distressing feelings). She was then asked to draw a mouth on her figure. She drew a large open mouth and then proceeded to literally 'draw up the badness' (red, black and brown blobs and squiggles) from the throat area, and out of her mouth. This spewing discharge marked a cathartic moment, punctuated by a deep sigh from her. A moment of silence descended on the group.

A more detailed account of how artwork was used in this couple's first counselling session is given below. Another woman painted a large image of a womb. Two thirds of the picture, in black, red and brown, was taken up with a fetus/breast shape. The rest of the space had blobs of dark shapes appearing to fall away from the main image.

The artist became quite distressed when she realized what she had painted. She was later able to go on and work with her image. Diagnosed as having unexplained infertility, she had gone ahead with another attempt at assisted conception before she had dealt enough with the grief from a miscarriage. Treatment failure had left her with an even heavier burden of grief.

Sometimes women need to work on their own, but there are also advantages to couple and group-based work.

Couple work

The main purpose of introducing art therapy to couple counselling in this setting is to provide a non-verbal outlet and means of communication between the couple. Their reasons for coming and goals for the work need to be aired at the start of the session. Infertility and treatment regimes can put relationships under a lot of strain. Guilt, anger, sexual frustration and blame are never easy to deal with. Yet, when they are brought out into the open, stress is often reduced and the couple's coping capacity increased.

Art therapy is of benefit to couples in relationships where talking about feelings is difficult for one or both partners. The images which they create open a path through their difficulties.

Couples can work individually or together. Partners can be invited to comment on each other's work. Images can be used to clarify what belongs to the individual and what is shared, as well as to form a bridge of communication between them. Some of what is felt can be seen; giving almost literal meaning to the use of the phrase 'Now I see how you feel', or 'I see what you mean'. Couples are given an opportunity to play together, to use their imagination to create new possibilities, mess about, discover or rediscover new aspects of each other's personalities and capabilities.

Such experiences, as they involve the couple being together in a different way, can sometimes provide the right kind of trigger for a reappraisal of their relationship.

A couple who had been trying for a baby for three years requested art therapy sessions:

We felt we'd done a lot of talking around the issue of fertility and that it was time to allow our feelings to express themselves in a different, perhaps more direct way. We discovered that the work we did during the sessions threw up a lot of emotions – anger, confusion, grief – that we had buried away deep inside ourselves.

We also discovered some very positive feelings within us. We realized that we do create together, that we do possess a great deal of creative energy between us. The most powerful image to come out of the sessions was one of the home that we create together. This was a very confirming message about our relationship.

Like others, this couple used spontaneous artwork to reaffirm their commitment to each other: they exposed their true feelings through images.

One exercise that I sometimes use with couples is to ask them to make a vessel together in clay. The results are often surprising. Such work helps to fortify the couple against treatment disappointment; an appropriate focus for supportive counselling, given the low success rates of many fertility treatments.

Sometimes, through the artwork, male partners can allow themselves to show loss and distress. As in the case of the couple described below invariably it is the woman who is in floods of tears during counselling. Male partners will indicate that they are only there to support the woman. With a visual language to facilitate 'the language of emotion' a fuller picture emerges. Some women express relief when they see some of what their partners feel about what is happening to them.

Spontaneously produced images can be very revealing. As an onlooker I can often see a lot more of what is going on in the work than the couple can. Knowing what to draw their attention to and when is crucial to the work. Too deep an intrusion at the wrong time, motivated by my own needs rather than what the situation requires, can lead couples to close ranks.

There is no way of predicting what a client may 'get in touch with' via spontaneous artwork. The same applies when working more directive way with given themes. What may seem a well thought out idea may provoke images that prove difficult to handle.

We had reached half-way through a series of six sessions with a couple who were struggling with whether or not to halt trying for a baby – the woman had a history of recurrent miscarriages. It seemed a good idea to invite the woman to work on a full-size body image, as a number of references had been made to negative feelings about her body. A powerful and disturbing image emerged. It showed ambivalence about her sexual self – around the whore/virgin conflict. She spoke of feeling exposed; an aspect of herself was shown to her partner before she had had the space to come to term with it.

It could of course be argued that images emerge because they are ready to, i.e. the moment is 'ripe'. However it does not always follow that it is also the right moment to talk about them. The right moment for the image and the right moment for words may not coincide and the art therapist needs to be ever-watchful.

At other times however, a painting may be all that can be shared. In one session with an African woman whose spoken English was very poor, painting gave her a more effective way to communicate her despair about treatment failure. She painted for 10 minutes using two colours, black and red. She applied the black first in furtive strokes but moved on to using red with angry, firm strokes. As she moved from black to red paint her mood of depression shifted to anger about her desperate situation.

Case history: Mrs and Mr W

This is an example of how artwork was used during a first couple session: The couple were referred for counselling by a senior nurse at the fertility clinic. They had a five-year history of unexplained infertility. Two treatment attempts had failed. They were ambivalent about making their third and final attempt. Mrs W had developed anxiety attacks shortly after the last treatment. Within moments of entering the counselling room Mrs W was in tears. She spoke of having panic attacks, breathlessness, sleeplessness, preoccupation with images of death and of having near hallucinatory experiences. Mr W, though clearly concerned, seemed embarrassed by his partner's visible distress. I asked them to draw, on the same piece of paper, their individual preoccupations, shared concerns were to be depicted in the space between them.

A pictorial summary of their current situation was produced, drawn with wax pastels. Mrs W's images were pale and fragile, showing different aspects of herself: without hands; with two 'thought bubbles' – one containing a baby, the other a grave with a cross; as one of two people conversing, the man with his brain, the woman without.

Mr W used more colours and a firmer quality of line. He drew a small but revealing figure of himself with a grin seemingly frozen on his face, but with a rope knotted in his stomach. He also drew a cartoon Loch Ness monster grinning, with a hat on its head. A line was drawn down the middle of the paper with the image of a baby on the top. Mrs W described this as 'a barrier' between them.

We identified a number of issues for further exploration, possibly as tasks to work on:

(1) Improving communication between them – in particular enabling Mr W to speak more freely.
(2) Exploring the links between Mrs W's' death preoccupations and panic attacks and how they related to her fertility.

As they liked using art materials, I suggested they attended some trial sessions of the art therapy-based counselling group, followed up by a couple session. They were happy with this suggestion.

My reasons for inviting this couple to use image-making in their first session was based partly on an intuitive feeling that they would be able to engage with this approach to the counselling. I also noted the harsh division of emotional expression between them; Mrs W was in floods of tears while her husband blocked off his emotions. My hope was that Mr W would be able to share some of what he was feeling and thereby relieve Mrs W of some of the expressive burden. With the drawing as reference, they were able to say a lot about themselves, the problems in their relationship, and how infertility and treatment affected them.

Art therapy-based counselling group

As well as individual and couple sessions, patients were also offered the chance to join an art therapy-based counselling group for a period.

Individuals and couples were self-referred or referred by other counsellors or clinical staff. They had differing diagnosis of infertility but were united by the common experience that they all had problems coping with and wanted to do something about their situation.

Format and structure

Group members were advised not to meet socially while they attended the group. This was for a number of reasons: firstly in order to distinguish the group as a working, therapeutic entity, different from the patients' support group; and secondly, to maintain confidentiality. Such boundaries helped people to feel safe in the group. We also decided to close the group on a six-week basis to new members. This facilitated the development of trust which enabled intimate disclosures to be made. The group met for between one-and-a-half and two hours. The session was divided into two parts – image-making, and time to talk about what had been done. A range of groupings were used; in pairs, couples together, groups of three or four, or individually.

Again, artwork was based on a combination of given themes, or people's own ideas. In both instances, members of the group were encouraged to just allow an image to emerge rather than plan the final outcome.

We often used the same themes as those for individual and couple work including body image, sexuality, fertility, body stress maps and life histories.

In response to this theme one male partner drew a landscape of a field of corn with a barren patch in the middle. The foreground of the picture is of a river running under the field. Black – what he describes as 'dead' – fish lay on the bed of the river. When he came to talk about his work, he associated the fish with his 'useless' sperms. 'Why me' he cried out. The group was moved by this display of emotion from this usually very softly spoken man. They, in turn, were able to acknowledge their own grief about infertility.

The range of work groupings mentioned above were also used when it came to talking about the images and the making of them. Subgroupings were always used with care as there are always instances when talking in pairs can undermine a group: for example, when distressing details are disclosed within the pair but not shared in the larger group.

The value of an art therapy group

For the right client, there are specific advantages to be gained from such a group. Societal taboos, familial pressures, along with feelings of inadequacy or simple shyness, can leave those who have difficulty conceiving, feeling isolated and unsupported.

The group in question helped people to talk, and learn from those in similar situations to themselves. There was no pressure to talk, but people's curiosity about the images soon drew questions even from the shyest of members. Using image-making offers an easily accessible way for people to bond with the group. Members felt an affinity with what they saw in each other's work.

People have differing levels of artistic skills, but in art therapy as the emphasis is on the meaning of the work for its creator; members of the group soon learn to respect each other's work; respect for the work makes people feel accepted.

As people began to take more creative risks in the group, verbal confidence grew. Couples in particular, benefited by learning from each other the benefits of articulating feelings. Men also have the chance to benefit from seeing other men expressing tender and distressing feelings.

The group became a source of support for people through the different phases of their treatment. Members would share their coping strategies. It also provided a forum for people to learn to deal with their envy and resentment when someone became pregnant. Destructive feelings were worked through visually and then talked about.

Not all the work was problem-based. At times, there was also a need to enjoy being creative for its own sake. It was possible to see people's energy levels and spirits raised as they messed about, playing with the materials. The whole group would create work which celebrated life.

Art therapy and the training of fertility counselling students

The Rowan clinic is the venue for a diploma course in fertility counselling. Students come from a range of professional clinical and therapeutic backgrounds, including nurses, doctors and counsellors. Art therapy contributes to their training in two ways: students attend a personal development group structured around image-making; and it is also an opportunity for experiential learning of how art therapy techniques can enhance the counselling process.

The format of the training sessions is more or less the same as that described for the patients' group.

Personal development

It is difficult to distinguish between the images done by fertility patients and professionals who work with, or are in training to work with them. This observation is a reminder that fertility issues affect us all – if only because we were all conceived and born.

The high incidence of infertility in the general population also means that even in a small student population there are likely to be people who have distressing personal or familial histories in relation to fertility.

It can only be of benefit to those seeking fertility treatment that their counsellors are as fully aware as possible of their own connections with all aspects of fertility. Without this awareness it is all too easy to block out the painful, complex and intimate material which their clients bring to the counselling.

Through image-making students have the chance to bring to light some of their less conscious feelings, views and experiences around fertility. Students who have shared their own experience of infertility through their artwork have enriched their colleagues' understanding in a unique way.

A group is also used at times to alleviate the intensity of the course. Spontaneous drawing and painting helps them digest and process other theoretical and experiential input.

Because working with images quickly establishes a high level of trust in groups, students, once they become engaged with the group, show a remarkable capacity for self-exploration and risk-taking. Care has to be taken not to turn it into a therapy/treatment group. An exercise, for example, on a visual history of their own fertility produces a wealth of personal imagery. It can bring into perspective feelings and attitudes which the student was unaware of. Memories of past, sometimes suppressed, experiences can come into consciousness. When this occurs it is important that the student feels comfortable with how much he or she says about the issue. Excessive curiosity about another person's images is often an indication that whatever is contained in the image relates directly to the person who is most curious about it.

Experiential learning

The by-product of active involvement with a visual creative therapy is that it gives the students first-hand experience of how they can enrich their counselling practice with art therapy techniques. Even if the students would not feel able to use art therapy techniques themselves, they acquire enough knowledge to make appropriate referrals.

It is the same for fourth-year medical students who attend one to two art therapy sessions during their obstetrics and gynaecology training block. For one session they are asked to do a small drawing on the theme of fertility and infertility. The images are grouped together to form a large patchwork in the centre of the room. The images which are produced give focus to our discussion. In particular we see how repeated, or visually striking figures, colours and symbols reflect the students' views, feelings and ideas about the subject.

Another theme is a spontaneous painting or drawing on their first experience of delivering a baby. On average about 12 students attend the session, and contribute to many hours of moving, informative and stimulating discussions. For some students, this exercise provides a much-needed opportunity to process one of the most traumatic events in the their training.

Conclusion

Art therapy and its techniques is not suitable for all clients who come for fertility counselling. At times, despite clear indications that a client could benefit from expressing themselves non-verbally, they choose not to work in this way. When, however, couples and individuals have been able to draw, model or paint spontaneous images about what is troubling them, more often than not they gained from the experience.

Fertility counselling covers a broad spectrum of issues to do with people's, emotional, ethical, social, spiritual as well as physical involvement with infertility, treatment and treatment outcome. The flow of words and tears in counselling does make a difference to how people are able to cope.

In the counselling room of the fertility clinic, people struggle to find words or other suitable ways to express their pain, hope and frustration. This is particularly true when what is stirred within them relates to unconscious or preconscious experience. It is here that art therapy comes into its own for a lot can be said via the language of image-making. Spontaneous art activity allows people to work between their inner and outer selves. Words tend to flow more easily after clients have created their drawings.

Art therapy both supports and enriches the role of counselling in the clinic. Essentially, I think it acts as a kind of counterpoint to the physical treatment concerns of the clinic, and through this the overall health of the clients is supported. They are aware that there is space, within the same establishment which attempts to treat their physical dysfunction, for input which supports them as whole beings. Women in particular have used image-making to explore body and self-image. Via the therapeutic work clients are helped to make more suitable choices and put the rest of their lives in perspective. This work is based on the understanding that people have a natural creative ability to give visual shape to what concerns them. Clients from differing races and classes are able to enrich their counselling experience in this way.

The depth and breadth of art therapy work created by professionals in training to work with fertility clients, shows the value of this creative input. Once the fear of ridicule or exposure is addressed, the right climate for creative activity is established. In this setting, students are able to extend knowledge of themselves and others more rapidly than would be possible in a purely talking-based group. From both clients and professionals in training a wealth of images are created which shed a particular kind of light on how we all understand the human experience of procreation, creation and infertility. Many of the powerful, tender and sometimes beautiful images which are produced remain etched in the mind's eye long after words have been forgotten.

Art therapy in fertility counselling gives couples and individuals a creative and imaginative way to work with their experience of fertility and infertility. Whether it is used as a brief input in a mainly talking-based session, or as the main focus of communication, image-making can both focus and refine the therapeutic encounter. Thoughts, feelings and ideas which can be too difficult to talk about, or just beyond words, can be given shape via the 'visual language' of line, colour, texture and form as we have seen. Both client and therapist work together to understand how the artwork (the making of it and the actual painting or sculpture) sheds light on the issues which concern the client.

The depth of work depends on the needs of the client. For some it is a matter of one or two drawings to help to clarify needs and implications of treatment. Where 'therapeutic counselling' (HFEA, 1993) is in indicated however, art therapy makes a distinctive and effective contribution. It can be seen as a kind of mirror which helps the client to readjust an often distorted image of themselves as flawed, infertile beings. For some clients, drawing images about the ways in which they feel flawed has been the first stage in a process of self-healing.

It is not only distress and confusion which can be thus expressed; images of hopes, desires and those which connect people with powerful, archaic ideas of fertility have also been enlightening. To some extent, the very act of visual creativity reaffirms peoples' capacity to be creative in a wider sense.

The value of art therapy to fertility work is summed up for me by these words from a client:

It's like you put it out there, [a spontaneous painting about what she is going through] it looks back at you, you can have a good look at it, and then it doesn't feel so bad.

Chapter 8
Birthmasks: Ritualization and Metaphor in Fertility Counselling

Sue Emmy Jennings

14   Now Reuben went in the days of wheat harvest and found mandrakes in the field, and brought them to his mother Leah. Then Rachel said to Leah, 'Please give me some of your son's mandrakes.'
15   But she said to her, 'Is it a small matter that you have taken away my husband? Would you take away my son's mandrakes also?' And Rachel said, 'Therefore he will lie with you tonight for your son's mandrakes.'
16   When Jacob came out of the field in the evening, Leah went out to meet him and said, 'You must come in to me, for I have surely hired you with my son's mandrakes.' And he lay with her that night.
17   And God listened to Leah, and she conceived and bore Jacob a fifth son.

Genesis 30:7

Introduction

This chapter is concerned with a cultural and creative context of counselling people with fertility problems. Infertility clinics are busy places where people from a great range of ethnic diversity attend. Just as Djahanbakhch *et al.* suggest (see Chapter 12) that counselling roles need to be understood in relation to Eastern and Western cultures, we can go further and look at the 'culture of medicine' itself in relation to the need for ritual in all forms of healing, and especially in reproductive medicine. Western people can rediscover their own 'rituals of repro-duction' through the counselling process. As well as discussing the importance of the ritual of counselling, this chapter emphasizes the importance of the metaphoric and creative content of counselling, which can be enhanced by artistic and dramatic methods, and dramatherapy in particular.

What is dramatherapy

Dramatherapy is the therapeutic use of drama and theatre: a human, creative process whereby we give dramatic form to thoughts and feel-ings.

We engage in dramatic interactions throughout life, from a few weeks old, when infants imitate the sound and expressions of people close to them, and then move from imitation to innovation with the expectation that those people will imitate us. Our earliest symbol, often called the 'transitional object' (Winnicott, 1971) becomes a dramatized 'other'; we name the toy or the blanket and talk to it and then answer on its behalf As children our play is organized within the dramatic conventions of make-believe and we increasingly distinguish between everyday reality of the concrete world and dramatic reality of the imagined world. Because we can use our dramatic imagination, we are able to hypo-thesize, to imagine how life might be, or how we would like it to be.

Dramatherapists make use of normal dramatic human development in order to intervene therapeutically where appropriate. This develop-ment usually follows three stages which are complete before the age of six: The first stage is 'embodiment' where everything is experienced through the human body, through the senses and the ways in which we are held. The second stage is 'projection' where expression is projected into toys and media outside of the human body. The third is the 'role' stage where ideas of playing characters, human and otherwise, become the dominant mode of exploration in play, (Jennings, 1990). These three stages of embodiment, projection and role (EPR) develop in a context of dramatic rituals which are a part of family and social identity. Dramatic development and rituals are shaped aesthetically in theatre performances which not only entertain but are able to articulate themes that otherwise would be inexpressible. The three main modes of dramatherapy process and practice are: dramatherapy as develop-ment; dramatherapy as ritual; dramatherapy as performance (Jennings, 1994)

Dramatherapy is particularly pertinent for people who are having problems with their fertility. It enables them to give form through masks or models to their feelings about infertility; it provides a structure with limits where painful questions can be explored through metaphor and symbol; and it gives a ritual pattern within a cultural context that enables people to work through issues and move on. Above all, it is based on the human developmental dramatic cycle and the relationship between everyday reality and dramatic reality.

Dramatherapy is able to assist us to articulate areas of ourselves that need to be given dramatic form, especially in relation to distorted per-ceptions of ourselves and others. For example the text of Shakespeare's *King Lear* (see below) can help us understand the power of the feelings of someone who feels that she is barren because she has been cursed.

Rites of passage

The Dutch anthropologist Van Gennep identified the rituals that accompanied all major life-stages such as birth, coming-of-age, marriage, death, and called them 'rites of passage' (Van Gennep, 1960). Rites of passage always have three distinct stages, usually known as 'separation, transition, and reincorporation'. The person undergoing the rite is first separated from their customary grouping; then goes through a transitional period of learning, and is finally reincorporated in their new social status. A Western church wedding ceremony illustrates the point: the bride is ritually accompanied by her father to the church and is 'handed over' (separation). There is then a period of question and answer and statement of belief, accompanied by ritual music (transition). The bride, together with the groom, then leave the church in their new status as a couple (reincorporation). These three stages accompany all rites of passage in all cultures. They mark our passage through life as we move from one status and role into another, and are usually accompanied by ritual music and dance, special clothes and decorations, celebratory food, the giving of gifts, and various symbols of birth, fertility or death.

If we are ill, we can also see a similar medical rite of these three stages as we are separated from our home into hospital, go through a period of treatment wearing ritual gowns, and are reincorporated as we leave hospital as a well person. We even acquire new names temporarily: while we are ill we are called 'patient' and if we take time to recover we may be called 'convalescent'. There may be issues around whether we agree with the doctor that we are better and the ritual may be fraught with conflict if there is not agreement that a person is ready to leave.

Counselling, too, can be seen to reflect these three stages as the person (or couple, or family) is separated from their usual group; goes through a period of counselling (whether it is one session or many), and is then reincorporated into their lifestyle, having changed in some way. Of course, for the person who attends several sessions, they may have a difficulty with reincorporation after each counselling visit.

The counselling is ritualized by the space (the counselling room), naming (client and counsellor), and by the absence of food-sharing and gift-giving (unless it is actual payment for the counselling in the private sector – but see Case history 2 below). However, there is some uncertainty as to whether counselling is a ritual or a treatment, which may imply that a person is either medically ill or psychologically disturbed. Can counselling be separated from psychotherapy in relation to rites of passage? According to Silman (Chapter 12), this potential confusion between psychotherapy and counselling is exacerbated by the HFEA requirement that a fertility counsellor should provide 'therapeutic counselling', as well as support counselling and implications counselling. Silman suggests that therapeutic counselling should in fact be termed psychotherapy and should only be applied where there is a 'disorder of the psyche' and appropriate referral then made. He is more concerned that people have the opportunity to explore their desires and the necessary compromises that are needed in achieving those desires. I would like to propose a framework for a rite of passage for infertility counselling which provides signposts for both counsellor and client, and clarifies outcome and resolution. This rite should accompany medical investigation and treatment.

Fertility counselling as a rite of passage

In considering the actual process of individuals through their treatments and counselling, I have considered various literature and play texts in relation to themes of barrenness and fecundity. It is interesting how many ancient myths and stories, Shakespeare plays and religious writings have three stages of development which move from the abundant or fertile, to the barren and empty, and then to reunion and reconciliation.

In *King Lear*, for example, we have the early images of the fertile land that is about to be divided between Lear's three daughters: then the stark cursing of Goneril's fertility by her father which leads into the barren heath scenes and Lear's madness; then, after the peak of his madness (which is full of sexual imagery) there is a reunion, compromise and acceptance.

> *Lear*   It may be so, my lord.
>   He kneels
>
> Hear, Nature, hear! Dear goddess, hear!
> Suspend thy purpose if thou didst intend
> To make this creature fruitful.
> Into her womb convey sterility,
> Dry up in her organs of increase,
> And from her derogate body never spring
> A babe to honour her. If she must teem,
> Create her child of spleen, that it may live
> And be a thwart disnatured torment to her.
> Let it stamp wrinkles in her brow of youth,
> With cadent tears fret channels in her cheeks,
> Turn all her mother's pains and benefits
> To laughter and contempt, that she may feel
> How sharper than a serpent's tooth it is
> To have a thankless child! Away, away!
>
>   Shakespeare, *King Lear*, I.iv.273–280

The fertility counselling process

When people are unable to have children and treatments are not possible, the process of fertility counselling as a rite of passage incorporates the following stages:

Stage 1: fertile desires; Stage 2: barrenness; Stage 3: reconciliation.

Fertile desires

This stage is where people explore their longing and wish for a child, and the means of trying to achieve their wish.

Barrenness

This is the stage where people express their distress about their infertility and acknowledge that they are unable to bear a child.

Reconciliation

This is the stage where people come to terms with their infertility and consider other life-choices.

Stage 1 in fact covers both 'support' as well as 'implications' counselling. It is the whole exploration of the scenario of longed-for parenthood in relation to people's lives, past and present. People are helped to articulate their feelings about fertility and to weigh up all the issues concerning possible fertility, and treatments.

Stage 2 is a very painful time, when people have to confront the fact that they will not have a child – by any means. It is the barren landscape, where people feel without hope and deprived of life ever being fulfilled. People feel angry, sad, guilty, blamed, shamed, let-down, hopeless, depressed, and find different ways of expressing these feelings. It is a grieving stage for 'the child they are unable to have' (Jennings, 1990).

Stage 3 is only possible when people have been able to express the feelings associated with grieving and are able to reconsider the possibility of life without children, or at least without their own biological children. It is important that sufficient time is allowed for reconciliation work. This stage can also lead into a reappraisal of the original desire i.e. 'what else in my life do I desire, since I am unable to have a baby?'

When people are actually proceeding with treatment for their infertility problems, then the process becomes more complicated: Stage 2 will now include either treatment success, or treatment failure; and Stage 3 will include either celebration or reconciliation.

If treatment clearly followed these 3 stages it would be simpler. What in fact happens is that after a first treatment failure, people often go back to stage 1 again, buoyed up by renewed hope that 'this time it will happen', and in many cases they lurch between stages 1 and 2 for months and even years, while the rest of their world falls away. Unless people are celebrating a successful treatment they need to be able to deal with 'interim failure' even if they choose to embark on further treatment.

If the ritual three stages are used as a framework for all infertility counselling, then clients will feel safer in a structure that carries them through the treatment journey, rather than bounces them back and forth.

Metaphors of fertility and infertility

Metaphor is often used in counselling as a prompt for exploration: a client may use a metaphor or a counsellor may offer one. For example:

Client   I am all at sea and don't know where I am . . . *or*
Counsellor   It sounds as if you are quite swamped by what's going on.

I find that the extended exploration of metaphors can bring about major shifts in people's feelings and understanding. For example, I usually reply within the metaphor if the client uses one, for example:

Client   My life is just empty and nothing will grow.
Counsellor   Can you describe this empty garden?

This dialogue might then lead into the creation of a 'secret garden' in sand play and bring in issues such as who had the key and what did the key unlock.

Case history: 1

Mr and Mrs Smith had been referred for implications counselling (see Introduction and Chapter 1) before any decisions were made about treatment.

Mr Smith was found to have very few sperm, and those he did have had a low motility. His wife was ovulating regularly and her blood tests were all normal. They realized that if they wanted to have children, then they would need to have donor sperm for DI (donor insemination). They came back to the clinic and Mr Smith said that he wanted his brother to donate sperm so that there was a genetic link. Known donorship is not banned but is not recommended (HFEA Guidelines, 1991) since it can cause further complications.

Session 1:

When the couple arrived, they were extremely tense, almost to the point of hostility, and I had to spend time clarifying the role of the counsellor: that I was not there to judge the situation but to assist them reflect on the implications of the decisions they were about to make. Mr Smith kept interrupting me and said that they had already discussed everything, and shouted, 'So can we just get on with it'. I responded as if he had meant 'get on with the counselling' and I summarized the areas for us to talk about:

(1) The positive and negative implications of his brother being the known genetic father of any child in relation to a) Mr Smith, b) Mrs Smith, c) his brother, d) his sister-in-law, e) their children aged 10 and 14, f) the parents of the brothers, g) other extended family, h) the intended unborn child, i) any future children.

(2) The feelings of the brother & sister-in-law, individually and as a couple, about Mr Smith not being able to biologically father children.

(3) Their thoughts about what they would feel if any treatment did not result in a child.

This signposting is very important to ensure clarity of focus and understanding for the clients. It is an important 'landing stage' in the therapist/client communication, and helps to ground people's feelings and create a feeling of security concerning the limits of the enterprise.

It is also important to set priorities within this signposting. I suggested that we addressed the issues in reverse order and that in relation to (1) it could be helpful if the brother and his wife would also attend for a session. I was surprised that they both looked extremely relieved and readily agreed to a plan of four sessions where we would reflect on each of the themes. I proposed that the next session would focus on the possibility that the treatment might not work, and that the following session would look at his and his wife's feelings about his lack of sperm and how they were both dealing with the issue as a couple. The final two sessions would look at the implications of the other people involved, one with the brother and his wife, and one for them to attend on their own. It was stated clearly that if further sessions were thought to be helpful, then these could be negotiated.

Session 2

It was important for me to hear the couple talk me through their own wishes for a child, and also for them to listen to each other. Mrs Smith was not a very articulate person and needed time and space to proceed at her own pace. She was very softly spoken and did not say very much until after her husband had said what he wanted to say. He said that he had not thought about children until he had actually got married, but had always assumed that he would have children. The idea that he was not fertile had been a tremendous shock and one that he could not readily talk about.

His parents did not know there was anything wrong and he had mentioned it in total secrecy to his brother who had thought it rather a joke to be able to assist his sister-in-law to have a baby. Mrs Smith said that this had been very difficult for her; she was shy and her brother-in-law had always teased her and made sexually explicit comments, even though she knew they were jokey. Mr Smith said that one of the reasons he loved his wife so much was that she was unlike his rather loud and crude family. It was said quite spontaneously and was obviously something that she had not heard before. The effect on her was quite electrifying as she sat, with a faint pink tinge in her cheeks, obviously valuing the affirmation.

It is important to note that it would have been very easy to allow this session to generalize into 'couple therapy' rather than counselling that is specifically targeted towards the complex issues surrounding fertility. If the staff feel that more extensive therapy is needed, then we usually refer either within our own clinic or to another agency for 'marital or psychosexual or couple', 'counselling, psychotherapy or guidance', with a choice of orientation: arts, therapeutic, systemic, or psychotherapeutic counselling. However, with this couple, I felt that there was an issue in relation to the fertility issue concerning both the families as a whole which guided my next intervention.

Session 2 continued

I then proposed that we worked on the theme of 'people like me' and 'people not like me' – an introductory exercise (influenced by Kelly's *Repertory Grid* and Grainger, 1990).

(i)   each person writes down any adjectives that they would use about themselves;

(ii) each person writes down adjectives that they would not use about themselves;

(iii) each person lists other people, including family, that they would use the group (i) words to describe;

(iv) each person lists other people, including family, that they would use the group (ii) words to describe.

There is no value judgement attached to this; it is merely a vehicle to clarify perceptions of 'self and other'.

Mr and Mrs Smith wrote with zest as well as humour and we compared notes after they had finished. They had written about each other in categories (ii) and (iv), whereas most of their own families came under (i) and (iii), together with friends that they had had before they met. They were then able to talk about how difficult they found each other's family: she found his noisy and rude and he found hers disapproving and silent. She had not been able to tell her own mother yet that there was a problem with having children. They both decided that they had a lot to talk about, and I set some homework for them to draw their own family tree and to share it with each other.

Session 3:

They arrived for this session looking more relaxed, and said that they had decided that they did not think that using the brother's sperm was a good idea. Before even considering the implications of this decision, they had decided from their own discussion that it would create additional problems for them as a couple.

One way of exploring feelings about infertility is to create a 'landscape of the body' and on this occasion I decided to do the 'tree of life' exercise where

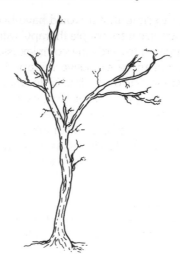

Fig. 8.1 The stunted tree.

a person imagines themselves as a tree. They then have to decide what sort of tree. Is it seasonal? Does it have flowers? Is it fruit-bearing? Does the fruit ripen? Is any fruit wasted or never ripens? (see Jennings & Minde 1993). They drew their trees (see Figures 8.1 and 8.2) with crayons and felt pens, and then looked at the feelings in their bodies which were triggered by the picture.

Mr Smith said that his stunted tree was in a barren landscape where nothing could grow: maybe it was after the ice-age or maybe after a war. Mrs Smith said that her rosebush in bud was in a garden: it was like perpetual spring, but nothing could flourish and blossom.

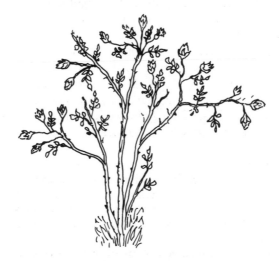

Fig. 8.2 The rose bush in bud.

Mr Smith looked very upset and began to cry silently. His wife, initially, looked very shocked and said that she had never known him to cry before, not even when his grandfather had died. She became very tender and they left the session very close, with an agreement to 'do something together in the country or garden' before the next session.

There was obviously a lot of scope for further work here, and I found it difficult to keep the fertility focus, which, after all, was the agreed contract. We had renegotiated the sessions since they were not using the brother's sperm, and they would spend the final two sessions with themselves looking at the various implications of having anonymously donated sperm. Of course the various people involved in all the 'implications' were very different once the decision had been made to use anonymous DI. There is always the question of 'who gets told' and many people want to start in complete secrecy. Of course, for this couple, the brother had already been told, and Mr Smith wondered whether he would keep the secret.

Session 4:
The couple explored various issues around distance and containment: for example, being able to tell certain family members that there could be problems, but that they were having a series of tests. We actually practised through various vignettes, (in which I also participated) being able to tell people in such a way that it did not invite further questions. They also rehearsed being able to be clear with people that it was confidential and not just to be passed on to everyone else. They felt this would give them time to think everything through, but, at the same time, Mrs Smith was optimistic that she would have some support from her own mother. There was a feeling of one-step-at-a-time now, rather than having to rush into things; and they both said that they had gone for a very long walk in the countryside and then decided to cultivate their garden!

Session 5:
In the final session, we looked again at the two pictures and within the gardening metaphors explored the possibilities of change. For example: 'the rosebush could be allowed to flourish' and then 'the gardener would need to be less protective'; 'perhaps the barren trees might be in the garden too'; and maybe 'become a strong tree for climbing'. 'But there must be enough room in the garden' said Mrs Smith firmly. They created a joint model with plasticine of a variation on the trees in the garden, allowing them to be closer to each other, but not too close. Even in this brief intervention, I felt that there had been an understanding and also a maturation within the couple's relationship. They had support counselling during the DI attempts; and at the second try Mrs Smith became pregnant and carried without problem to full term (Jennings, 1993).

This case history illustrates how the use of metaphor and imagery made it possible for this couple to modify their desires and make decisions about the most appropriate way to handle their infertility issues. Stages

1 and 2 were necessary for considering their desires as well as looking at the barrenness. In this case, the couple came back to tell me about the pregnancy, and, then again, after they had had the baby. There was a feeling of celebration of their new parental status.

The 'Trickster and the 'Naughty Bits'

Counsellors and therapists working in infertility clinics are very aware of the effect that infertility has on people's sexuality. Men may lose their potency after being told of a sperm problem; women may start to only allow sex on their most fertile day; and the couple themselves may find that their sexual relationship becomes focused only on procreation, and that their mutual desire and recreation get sidetracked.

Again, I have found literature helpful to me in my work; for example, I may think of characters such as Autolycus in *The Winter's Tale*, the Fool in *King Lear* or Mercutio in *Romeo and Juliet*. All these characters, in different ways, are 'trickster' type characters – as contrasted with heroes – and they usually upset the *status quo*. Their language is very sexual and full of innuendo; they usually live at society's margins, for example characters like Pan, Puck and Enki (Brinton-Perera, 1981), and can be both cruel and anarchic, as well as fun. In the above case history example, we can see that Mrs Smith's brother-in-law was something of a 'trickster' character and she found his sexual allusions very uncomfortable; but in response to his potential intrusion the couple soon found a way to be more relaxed and humorous. I find that the introduction of the trickster character can be helpful for people to rediscover the fun in their sexual relationship, and even make it possible to talk about 'the naughty bits'.

Case history: 2

Mr T and Ms S were referred for reconciliation work after medical investigations found that there was no possibility of their having assisted conception. Ms S had very severe tubal damage as well as suffering from endometriosis, and Mr T, too, had a sperm problem. They were devastated at the diagnosis, though I could detect that there was some relief at the fact that *both* of them had physical problems. As a mixed-race couple, they brought to the session strong cultural expectations in relation to their fertility. Mr T thought that as the man he should be able to inseminate his partner, and Ms S felt keenly that it was her role to be the carrier of his child.

Session 1

In the first meeting they were still in shock, and counselling was necessary to contain and allow for all the pent-up feelings surrounding the hopelessness of them becoming parents. We looked at the potential support structures within their own families, which turned out to be minimal, since there was family dissent that they were living together anyway. Well into this session they began to talk a little about their families and how they had met in the first place.

It is important to note that, since they had used 'flashback', this meant that I could introduce the overall context of their relationship, and allow them to express their 'desires' as well as their devastation that these could not be realized.

We had agreed a contract of four sessions and that we would look at the beginning of the story of their infertility as well as looking at the possibilities of different outcomes for the feelings of failure they were both experiencing now.

Session 2

In session 2 they both arrived looking pale but less frozen than they had in the previous meeting. They said that they had cried a lot together and that they had been able to care for each other. They went on to say that this caring was very much the basis of their relationship; they had met at college, had tended to be isolated, and enjoyed each other's company enormously. They did things together and it seemed a natural progression to set up home together. He was an only child, and she was one of five daughters who felt that she had an ambivalent role in her family (she was the second youngest child, the youngest being a boy). Her overriding feeling at the moment was that she was being punished for leaving home and living with a man from a different culture. He also felt very guilty as the only child, and he felt that his mother expected him to return home after college whereas in fact he had set up his own home instead. They were both teachers; he taught older pupils science and she taught middle school pupils dance and music.

I asked them about their early life together, and they readily described what a full life they had; they went out a lot to art galleries, theatres and concerts, and enjoyed each other's company. They also said they enjoyed sex and said it was a lot of fun. They then realized, with shock, how much of their shared activities they had stopped doing in the build-up to baby-making – including 'fun-sex'. They had stopped going out and also rarely did 'nice things', to use their phrase, when they were at home together. I suggested that they 'sculpted' their life, using any of the small objects – people, animals and so on – that are part of the dramatherapist's resources. She placed two monkeys close together with a tree, lion cubs and a cart-horse, and scattered some coloured beads around. He placed an elephant with a gazelle, a sheep, a goat, a lamb and a tiger, with two bright red buttons.

Ms S said: 'The two monkeys are us because we were funny and very physical and felt playful. The lion cubs are also the way we used to play together: even when college work got tough and we had exams, we could release all the tension by being funny or playful. The tree is the tree in my parents' garden and is a symbol for me of the fertility of the family and how I have let them down.' 'The cart-horse is you', she said as she looked at her partner, 'you are very steady and reliable. The beads are the colour that I must have in my life – which, of course, isn't there any more.' She began to look distressed.

Mr T: 'The gazelle is you: you are delicate but strong and you move like this. The elephant is me: I am large and clumsy, but I am very faithful. I think I am the sheep and you are the lamb or maybe the goat . . .' he paused, looking a little confused. I intervened. 'Is it anything to do with being hung for a sheep as a lamb, or maybe separating the sheep from the goats?' He continued, 'It is all about punishment; that's what the tiger is' and, looking at his partner's picture, 'and you have lions too, but they are little and playful. Can lions lie down with lambs? The two red buttons are us feeling very fulfilled.'

In this instance, the couple were very articulate and all I did was to *prompt* through the metaphor. There are multiple meanings here which the sculpting was able to contain effectively.

I asked them whether the picture for now would be very different from the one they had just made. Ms S was still looking upset and Mr W said that he ought to be the cart-horse and comfort her. They said that the playful elements were missing and that they both felt the infertility was a punishment because they had made their own decisions. Ms S was then able to say how guilty she felt at not being the boy, as the fifth daughter, and how abandoned she felt when the longed-for boy did arrive. He guiltily said that the tiger was his mother who would 'eat him up'. I moved the scenario on, trying to look at what they could put back into their current lives that had been there before. We reflected on the 'trickster' element in their sculpts – monkeys, lion cubs, a goat – and red buttons? They were given the task of talking about it together and come to the next session with some ideas. I suggested that they might like to use creative media to explore their ideas; techniques like 'the wheel of feelings', 'family role chart', 'the shape and colour of my life', (See also Chapter 6).

The issue for the counsellor here is not to get into their family dynamics, but to focus on their reconciliation to 'life without children'. This couple already anyway had many strategies that they could utilize for their own healing.

Session 3
They arrived with rolled up pieces of paper and said that they had done a lot of work at home. They talked me through the various pictures, and they had also created some diagrams of 'then' and 'now' with lists, using coloured felt pens. She had integrated the bright colour with the greyness, and he had drawn a wheel with different segments in which he wrote different feelings and said that they had kept spinning out of control. They had adapted their own structures for doing work together, which included the following elements, all of which can be developed in role-play and enactment, as well as with the use of masks:

The wheel of feelings
People draw a large wheel like a cartwheel and use it to contain feelings that are experienced as chaotic, out of control, and so on.

The shape and colour of my life
This can be used to express the 'here-and-now' before looking at possible changes.

Family role chart
This is used to look at family relationships and to consider potential change.

Then and now lists
Positive and negative factors in past and present events are written down and colour-coded: this helps people to focus on actual changes they would like to make.

Mr T and Ms S felt that they knew now what they needed to do to create a more satisfactory life for themselves. They still felt distressed, of course, and needed time to cry and get angry, but they realized two very important things: first, that they had a lot of creative strategies for expressing their grief; and second, that there were many things in their life that they enjoyed and needed to rediscover.

I set another task for them and that was to go and see the musical *Into the Woods* which is based on fairy tales and nursery characters and especially on the baker's wife who longed for a child. We restated the contract of four sessions and confirmed that the next meeting would be our last.

Session 4
They arrived with a big box and proceeded to talk about the musical which had been enthralling for both of them. They said it was a strange mix because, yes, it did emphasize their infertility, but it had been such a creative experience that they had both come away feeling very playful.

They had had a long discussion about going to see their respective families and seeing whether it was possible to tell them what had happened. We spent some time looking at this and how, without a family of their own, it was important to make new links with their own families. The ideas for this had come out of the family role charts. We made sure that the expectations were not totally unrealistic. We created some simple role-play to look at possible responses from the family, i.e. the worst response, the best response and the likely response, with the three of us taking on various roles and me being 'coached' by them in the part that was needed.

They ended up by saying that their sex lives had returned to normal and that they could enjoy the fun of sex as a way of being together, rather than just in desperation to have a baby. Finally, they opened the box, and in it was a cake that he had baked – apparently he always used to do a lot of cooking, but had stopped when he heard about his sperm count! They wanted me to share the cake as a celebration and had bought napkins, a knife and paper plates.

Perhaps traditional counsellors and therapists would challenge my participation in this ritual, but I felt it was absolutely in keeping with a coherent approach – the making and breaking of food, as a celebratory ritual. It was a very healthy signpost for their future life together.

Two years later, I had a telephone call to say that they had adopted a mixed-race little girl and were going to bring her to visit me.

Rites of naming

The continuation of family names is considered important for many people when they struggle with issues around being infertile: the family name symbolizes the relationship by blood to the lineage of the families involved. Naming ceremonies are themselves rites of passage which signify the identity of the person who is publicly named. There are cultural variations on this theme, such as with the Temiar people, with whom I did my anthropological fieldwork (Jennings, 1994). Temiar children were not named until they could walk independently and they then had an individual name unlike anyone else's; however, they were known in public by either nicknames or birth-order names, until such time as a woman became pregnant. Then, she and her partner were known by the word 'pregnant' until the child was born. Both parents were then known in relation to the gender of the eldest child, either parents of a boy or parents of a girl. In order to differentiate between several people having this same name, the name of the child was added on – so I was known as Litau Andy (parent of a boy, Andy), while Andy was known by his birth-order name, which was Along, for the firstborn. The Temiar example is an interesting one of the parents being known by the name of their children, rather than the reverse as in western culture when children carry the name of their parents. We can see here that naming is linked to fertility; that the name changes on conception. The Temiar have three major life stages: childhood; fertile years; years of wisdom.

Names change again after a person's childbearing years are past, when both men and women are thought to be wise people and are treated with growing respect. During the fertile years, men and women are a unit through having children, and are expected to adhere to certain taboos in food and behaviour in case of damage to any young child *in utero* or *in vivo*. However, whereas in western culture we exclude people because of their infertility (i.e. parents and infertile people), the Temiar include everyone who is of fertile years. So, as well as parents of a boy or girl, one can also be parents of no children, or parents of many stillborn births. The parental naming system is inclusive rather than exclusive. There are couples with no children who might 'borrow' children from other families, or adopt children who are orphaned. No child is left uncared-for and no individual is left childless. Many barren women themselves become midwives and have a special relationship which involves naming and gift-giving with all the children they deliver. This relationship continues into adulthood when people from time to time go and visit their midwife. I suppose the nearest approximation we would have is a godparent, where the relationship can continue into adulthood. Perhaps we can learn from the fertility rituals of other cultures to find ways of managing our own rather better, at least in terms of infertile people feeling that they are permanently excluded from mainstream society.

Ritual symbols of fertility, birth and death

When we observe the wedding rituals, we can note how many of them are in fact the ritualization of fertility: the throwing of rice and rose petals; bouquets of flowers; carrying the bride over the threshold, or the jumping-the-broom ceremony. Unions are expected to be fruitful and traditional medicine describes various treatments for newly-weds both to inculcate desire as well as to induce conception.

Entry into life, and exit from life, are the major transitions from womb to tomb, and share common symbols and rituals: flowers; clothes of the baby, or the corpse; a special resting place – crib and coffin; viewing of the baby or the body. Death can be seen as a rebirth or as a transition from being alive to being dead, which has greater importance for those left alive then for those who have died. Funeral and mortuary rites assist people to come to terms with death and enable them to move on after prescribed periods of mourning.

However, there are certain problems concerning the mourning of the child you have never had. How can you give form to this 'dream child' and ritualize an ending when there was no beginning? It has been suggested that it must be similar to losing a relative and their body not found so that a funeral would be an impossibility since there is no place for the corpse to be laid. However, it is more extreme for the loss of the 'dream' child as this child has never existed; there are no artifacts or photographs or memories that it once lived, even if a child lived for a few moments. The grieving of someone who is unable to have children is a very extreme form of grief over a type of death, made even more difficult because of new medical technologies. True, some people will have a child through technical means, but for the vast majority who have IVF or similar treatment (80% at least) there will be no take-home baby and hopes will have been dashed very cruelly since they were raised by the expectations of science. As one infertile person said, 'It's just me out there in an empty world, and there is nothing I can do about it.'

In the post-barren stage, or the reconciliation stage of counselling, it is important to have an understanding of death rituals. People need time to grieve, to express their feelings, and to lay 'the body' to rest in an appropriate way before moving into new spaces and new ideas.

People need time and space to make this transition, which is not only about the mourning for the child they never had, but is also about mourning the loss of the direct parenthood that they will never experience. Rituals of adjustment take time once the initial shock has been contained. We saw in case history 2 that this couple were able to help themselves through these feelings and, although not completely finished after their four sessions, they were certainly able to go home and manage their lives together. One function of ritual is to contain the event so that people can finish and move on, and we need to be careful not to impose yet more guilt if people feel repaired rather more quickly than we thought they would.

I usually find that once couples have made the decision to stop treatment or not to fantasize about winning money to pay for yet more treatment; once the actual admission is clear and articulated, it is a major step towards dealing with the issues. It is the people who get trapped into having 'just one more go', or when there is conflict between the couple as they disagree about decisions, where the grieving process is protracted. People need non-intrusive support while they are making the decision, where they feel they have made it for themselves, followed by reconciliation work, using ritualization where possible.

'Birthmasks'

I have developed a dramatherapy technique of using 'birthmasks' for people to come to terms with infertility. Masks are paradoxical because they both conceal and reveal, but most importantly they give form to feelings as well as acting as a container for things that cannot be expressed in other ways.

I usually use preformed blank masks that can be painted or stuck with other media, and allow people to spend some time with the blankness. One woman said, 'That's just how I feel; a nothing'. People then use the masks to create a 'mask of fertility' by painting and colouring. Most people very quickly get into using symbols on the mask, and all report how quickly the mask becomes an extension of themselves; the mask takes over and is able to 'say things' that they could not put into words. People then create a 'mask of infertility', not necessarily in the same session, unless it was a whole day workshop. People have thus expressed both their fertility as well as their infertility; the creating and wearing of the mask; speaking through the mask or dancing or dramatizing or creating a ritual – all are ways in which the fertile and infertile mask can be used. One must sense when people are ready to move on and create their 'mask of reconciliation': this is the third mask, which usually integrates images from the first two masks. Again, time is taken both in the creation as well as the wearing and experimentation of the third mask in dance and drama. I encourage people to keep a mask diary and record the stages of their feelings through faces rather than words, and if I am conducting an ongoing group, we may use it as a way of starting and finishing the sessions. Great care must be taken with people's masks: they are an extension of people's identity. One woman took her mask home and hung it behind the wardrobe door. She said, 'Now and again I look at it and realize that it was all very sad, but I can go on. This mask reminds me that I was never just a potential mother, even though I longed for a baby. I am other people as well.'

In this chapter I have looked at various aspects of fertility counselling through ideas drawn from anthropology, especially concerning rites of passage or the ritualization of life events. High-tech medicine has still to develop rituals that satisfy the participants, i.e. the patients, as well as satisfying the doctors and nurses, and shared cultural symbols need to be discovered.

I encourage the ideas of brief therapeutic intervention within a focused fertility context and suggest that a rite of passage that takes people through fertility, barrenness and reconciliation is a helpful model for constructing counselling.

Finally, I give examples of intervention where dramatherapy methods such as sculpting, sand-play, role charts, role-play, birthmasks can be used in unique and creative ways.

> You son of a clear-eyed mother, you far-sighted one, how you will see game one day, you who have strong arms and legs, you strong-limbed one, how surely you will shoot, plunder the Herreros, and bring your mother their fat cattle to eat, you child of a strong-thighed father, how you will subdue strong oxen between your thighs one day. You who have a mighty penis, how many and what mighty children you will beget!   A Hottentot song
> translated by Willard R. Trask

Chapter 9
Termination and Limitation: A Social Worker's Perspective

Hilary Everett

Introduction

Although the main focus of this book is on the counselling of people with infertility problems, in my opinion there are other areas connected with people's fertility that all counsellors and clinicians need to be aware of. The question of infertility and its treatment needs to be seen in relation both to the termination of pregnancy (and it is not unknown for women to request a termination after assisted conception), and also limitation of conception through the use of various forms of contraception. Writing as a social worker, I have to see counselling for infertility, termination and limitation etc. within the wider context of my social work role. This carries with it a comprehensive range of expectations, which include counselling as well as the assessment of clients and their situations.

In this chapter I therefore intend to highlight what seem to me to be two crucial areas: first, the counselling process in the context of termination of pregnancy; and second the importance of post-termination counselling. Along the way, I shall touch briefly on my own journey into counselling, followed by the definition of counselling within which I try to practise, and the aims of counselling in the context of termination. I shall look at the referral process and give an example of a day-care abortion service in action. I shall consider the impact of termination in various contexts such as different age groups, gender differences, fetal abnormality, trauma, effects on family members, cultural factors; and I shall also consider the potential for counselling around contraception. I would like to emphasize that my 'backcloth' includes respect for the work of colleagues in other disciplines and also the vital importance of self-knowledge on the part of the counsellor, more of which later.

Termination of pregnancy is still one of society's great taboo subjects. It is surrounded by an aura of secrecy and as such is vulnerable to assumptions – e.g. girls get pregnant and have terminations while they're still at school; it's a young woman's problem; some women use abortion as a form of contraception; some women are totally irresponsible – look at all those family planning clinics, there's no need for

151

anyone to have an unwanted pregnancy, and so on. I hope to indicate that the real situation is far more complex.

But it is no wonder that the women and their partners who actually make use of an abortion service are hypersensitive to any hint of disapproval, judgement or moral superiority on the part of the professionals they meet, and that of course includes the counsellor.

How many friends of yours have had terminations? Would you know anyway? Have you had a termination or been in a partnership where this has happened? Who did you tell? A friend of mine who is a part-time nursing sister in a day-care abortion clinic told me she is extremely wary about disclosing the nature of her job in a social context: you never quite know how even your best friend is going to react.

My journey into counselling

I trained in social work in the 1960s when there was considerable emphasis on specialization. My specialism was in probation and I look back on that specialist course with great affection, although at the time it was hard going. What I chiefly remember is that it helped me to lay the foundations for developing a skill in really listening, and for managing silences in sessions with clients. I have had subsequent opportunities to build on those foundations with further training courses (these may be an essential refreshment and stimulation for counsellors). I also began to experience working in a secondary setting, firstly as a probation officer in magistrates' and juvenile courts; and later, alongside teachers and psychologists in London comprehensive schools. I have worked in secondary settings ever since and greatly value multidisciplinary communication and contact.

A definition of counselling

Counselling is not telling people what to do or giving instructions. Rather, it is a process through which women and men are given the opportunity to discover and explore ways of living more creatively and satisfactorily. The counsellor is there to enable people to understand the circumstances that affect their lives and relationships, to help them identify choices and make decisions. The counsellor will be non-judgemental, open, warm and supportive. There may be a practical role to play, for example in this context it may be helpful if the counsellor has some knowledge (though not necessarily first-hand experience) of abortion procedures.

He or she will also need to be very clear about confidentiality and about boundaries. Mary Pipes, in her book *Understanding Abortion*, (1986), gives a very clear picture of the qualities consumers require in a counsellor. This gives us an admirable checklist.

There is general agreement that counselling should take place in private, be non-directive and non-judgemental in its approach, that counsellors should be empathetic, exhibit non-possessive warmth, be open-minded, attentive and able to listen, and that they should discuss the practical aspects of abortion as well as the emotional ones. In some cases counselling will also involve a discussion of contraception and the woman's attitude to future methods of birth control. At its best counselling should help us to make our own decision about the pregnancy, based on a realistic understanding of ourselves and our circumstances. (Pipes, p. 71)

Why counselling for termination?

I became interested in pregnancy counselling when I worked as a school-based social worker some years ago. Contrary to popular belief, every schoolgirl over the age of eleven is not getting pregnant. But on the occasions that this did happen, I tended to get involved on behalf of the pastoral staff. I quickly realized that nothing much had changed over the years. To find yourself pregnant (unless planned) can be scary and complicated. I hope the young women I saw during that time found it helpful to talk things through with someone who wanted to hear their point of view, consider with them pros and cons of termination, understand their ambivalence (not everyone opted for termination), and support them emotionally during and after the procedure. The context of my counselling work later changed and I see a much broader spectrum of women and partners. I am totally convinced of the value of offering non-judgemental, non-directive counselling around termination of pregnancy. This is especially important for people who may find the decision a difficult one for whatever reason. I am aware that a number of women make clear decisions for themselves and I hope that they will feel supported in this by clinics and legal systems.

The aims of counselling for termination

Counselling in this context is really no different from other areas of reproductive medicine. One needs to concentrate on the client; to listen carefully; to be sensitive; not to get drawn into giving advice – there can be a lot of pressure from a client to do this especially where the decision is difficult; and to go slowly – allow time and, if useful, further sessions before the client comes to a decision. This last point is particularly important if there are complex issues for the woman and her partner.

Case history
M. was a young woman in her mid-twenties who had three children and was on her own with them. She had become pregnant by a man whom she liked

very much but could not completely trust. He seemed to be pleased about the pregnancy but M. had been let down in the past and was fearful of being left alone with an additional child. She needed several sessions with the counsellor to talk about her past experiences and try to work out her feelings about this new man in her life. Eventually M. decided on a termination. This was an extremely difficult decision for her and she could not possibly have made it in one counselling session.

Cultural perspectives

There is still very little literature available on cross-cultural counselling. My own background is white British, middle-class, and mid-fifties. I am very aware of this. Sometimes I counsel women and men from different ethnic groups. I realize I know nothing about where they come from and what their experience of British society is like. I wonder if I even have the right to offer counselling in the wake of such ignorance.

This is a very complex area which is important for counsellors to think about. For example some women may come from a culture where termination of pregnancy is widely accepted. They may have had several terminations in the past and their perspective may be different from that of some members of a clinic team in this country. I have increasingly found it important to acknowledge my ethnic difference very openly with women and men I am counselling. Phrases such as 'there is a large part of your experience that is very different from mine . . . I may be a person you feel you can trust . . . if not, let's think about an alternative person . . . I am here to listen and help you come to a decision in whatever way is most useful to you.'

Respect for others' differences is a vital element of counselling. This is particularly relevant in the case of language and advocacy. There may be a key role for the counsellor, especially in a clinic setting, in working with team members to meet this need. My experience of counselling women via interpreters and family members led me to talk with colleagues about developing independent health advocacy for women. Women have the right to speak freely and receive counselling from a trained advocate who is familiar with their culture and who speaks their mother tongue. This is especially important when difficult decisions are about to be made, as in the context of termination.

Case history

An Asian woman who spoke no English came into hospital over a weekend for a very late termination of pregnancy and then went home alone afterwards. I was asked to follow her up as the ward staff felt very concerned about her. I was able to arrange a home visit in the company of a trained health advocate who came from the woman's ethnic background and spoke her language. We found that she was a young widow with children. She had been attacked in the street by a stranger and had been raped. She had told no-one in her social circle because she felt so ashamed. Eventually she went to her GP because she was pregnant as a result of the rape. It does not require much imagination to recognize the relief experienced by this woman to be able at last to receive the counselling in her own language that she so desperately needed.

Sensitivity to cultural and ethnic differences extends to written information, which should be readily available in this context for example in GP's surgeries, family planning clinics and well-women's clinics. It should be easily understood, without sounding patronizing, and should include information about counselling services (a useful exercise may be to pilot new information sheets among users before distributing). Written information should meet the needs of the local population in terms of language translation. It forms an essential part of an accessible service initiative in contacting their local hospital. Ideally, the professionals involved (including the counsellor) should reflect the population they serve in ethnic and cultural background. There is still some way to go, but these are issues for us all in developing equal opportunities and anti-discriminatory practices.

The context of counselling

There are a variety of settings in which pregnancy counselling may take place. For example a counsellor may be working quite independently in a private counselling practice; or she or he may be part of a team in a specialist setting such as a Brook or Pregnancy Advisory Service centre; or possibly working with a GP practice and receiving referrals from the doctors; and possibly part of a multidisciplinary hospital clinic team.

Whatever the setting, one thing seems certain – counselling is extremely emotive work and counsellors need to ensure they have access to professional support and consultation. In some settings, the counsellor may be very involved in supporting other colleagues – which is all the more reason, as a counsellor, for finding ways of taking care of yourself. Counsellors also need to be aware of the dangers of becoming desensitized. I feel that counselling for termination is difficult to do full-time and may combine with counselling part-time in a different area of women's health, but this is a personal view. In a model of pregnancy counselling I shall now describe, all members of the team spend part of their week in another area of work. Our experience suggests that this does help to maintain a continuing freshness of approach as well as conserving emotional energy and commitment in a demanding area of counselling.

A day-care abortion service in action

This particular clinic offers termination of pregnancy up to 12 weeks on a day basis, thereafter terminations are negotiated via the consultant gynaecologist. All the staff are women, though male doctors are sometimes involved – in fact, the service was initiated and run successfully by a male gynaecologist for a number of years.

The nursing sisters who run the thrice weekly clinics work on a job-share basis. They have all had some counselling training, and this is a key element in the service. They see every woman who comes to the clinic. Apart from taking a brief history, they spend some time talking with her (and sometimes her partner) about the pros and cons of possible termination as she perceives them. The woman will see the doctor for physical examination and further discussion.

It may be that the woman feels unclear, unready, distressed, or confused. As the back-up counsellor, I may be asked to see her either the same day or as soon as possible. Hopefully, by the time she reaches her decision, whichever way that goes, the woman will feel she has had sufficient time and support. If she opts for termination, it will happen within the next few days, under general anaesthetic – hospital in the morning, home the same day.

A multidisciplinary approach offers advantages to everyone, including:

(i) Policy issues may be discussed within the team, with an input from different perspectives, hopefully leading to consensus. Thus women considering termination should have access to a unified service.
(ii) Opportunities for the professionals to learn about one anothers' skills and to develop mutual respect and understanding.
(iii) The possibility of developing a support network for one another is enhanced.

I am very aware, as a counsellor, that I do not work 'hands-on'; i.e. I am not spending time in an operating theatre actually terminating pregnancies. Until two years ago, I had never seen the termination of a pregnancy. At that time I was in America and had the opportunity to spend half a day in a termination clinic where the doctor performed terminations well past 12 weeks (but strictly within the law) under local anaesthetic. I was thus able to talk with the women as they were literally undergoing their operation, and with the doctor at the same time. I gained a very useful insight into what a doctor has to do in this context. I also felt I had acquired some information about the physical aspects of termination that has been tremendously useful to me.

I am not advocating that every counsellor should have this experience – it is a very personal choice. I use this example to illustrate an earlier point – the need to respect the skills of other professionals and the stresses they may sometimes experience. Nurses on a ward where late terminations are carried out may have their own support system. They may also appreciate input from the counsellor, not just for the woman in their care but also for themselves. This need not be a formal counselling session, maybe a spoken acknowledgement by the counsellor of what that experience may mean for the nurses as they care for the woman through her termination.

Referral

Who refers to the counsellor?

It may be a self-referral. Sometimes women feel they need counselling and take the initiative in contacting their local hospital clinic. It may be a referral via friends, for example a woman who has felt she was helped by a counsellor may pass the name on to a friend who has become pregnant.

Referral may come via a general practitioner. In my experience, some GPs are extremely good at networking on behalf of their patients. The counsellor may be asked to see a woman prior to referral to a clinic, which I find particularly rewarding. I like to feel that a GP has confidence in the counselling process and I think that women appreciate the concern on the part of their doctor and the opportunity to share their feelings at an early stage.

Referral may also come via a hospital clinic within a gynaecology department. It may come from a family planning clinic or specialist young people's project. I offer back-up counselling to a hospital-based abortion clinic and the majority of my referrals comes from the doctors or nurses in that clinic. They in turn receive referrals from other departments within the hospital.

It is important to bear in mind the various aspects of the referral process in hand. For example, the counsellor may see a woman (and her partner) who have specifically requested counselling; she or he may see someone who may not feel they need or want counselling. The counselling approach needs to be geared to this. I used to feel rather daunted by women who couldn't or wouldn't speak when they arrived. I have developed a way to acknowledge this quite openly: I might say something like 'it feels as if it's difficult to talk at the moment . . .'; 'that's OK . . . maybe this isn't the right time or the right day . . .'; or I may not be the right person for you . . .'. I leave lots of spaces and always make sure clients go away with my name and work telephone number – no woman coming to counselling in this very difficult situation should ever feel rejected by the counsellor.

I never give out my home telephone number and I offer two reasons for this which may be helpful to consider: first, it is important for the counsellor to maintain professional boundaries in order to maximize energy and commitment to a wide variety of clients. We are not trying to be friends with them. And second, a major aspect of the counsellor's role with very anxious clients is to give them a sense of being 'contained' – that we can hear their distress and survive it to continue our work with them. It may be our own anxiety that we are trying to deal with in giving out personal telephone numbers, which would not be helpful to a client, so it is important to resist the temptation! It may, however, be useful to pass on information about helplines and other useful relevant organizations.

Confidentiality and termination

This is a very important ingredient in the referral process. The counsellor needs to be clear within himself or herself about this, and establish ground-rules with users of the counselling service and with other professionals. I feel quite strongly that women and men considering termination need a place to talk in absolute confidence, and that that is what a counsellor should be able to offer. However, it may be that information emerges in counselling which *should* be shared – for example an under-age young woman might have become pregnant as a result of incest or sexual attack. It is difficult to generalize – in the end each situation has to be talked through between the woman and the counsellor and, hopefully, a joint decision reached about any disclosure.

Other professionals need to be clear where the counsellor stands on confidentiality which is not always very comfortable. In my clinic setting, I am sometimes asked for social reports. These, of course, may enhance the understanding of professional colleagues and contribute towards more sensitive treatment. I like to work out with the woman I see what information she feels it would be helpful to her to share with team members who are caring for her.

Feelings

Sometimes there is so much going on in the woman's life that when she meets the counsellor for the first time she doesn't know where to start.

Case history

E was a woman in her late twenties, referred by her GP for counselling prior to her clinic appointment. Her feelings were very near the surface. She was furious with her boyfriend for leaving her to make the decision about possible termination; she was angry with herself because she felt she had trusted the relationship enough not to worry about using contraception one hundred per cent of the time; it looked as if her boyfriend might totally opt out and leave;

she was in an emotional turmoil. E eventually had a termination and spent the next twelve months in regular sessions with the counsellor while she sorted out other aspects of her life.

I think it is helpful for the counsellor to make clear at the start how long the session will last; I recommend one hour as a maximum. It is also helpful to indicate that this need not be a one-off session, which is the first step in the containment process referred to earlier. The counsellor then needs to be prepared to say very little for a while, to give the woman permission to let her feelings spill out all over the place. This can be quite difficult – I sometimes feel I am in danger of becoming over-whelmed myself. But it does give the counsellor the opportunity to hear the issues and to begin to get in touch with the woman's emotional pain.

There are a whole range of feelings around possible termination of pregnancy. As the woman comes to a decision, she may or may not be aware of them at a conscious level. The counsellor needs to know them, to identify them and to give the woman permission to experience and express them. This is especially important when considering with her how she may feel afterwards – a very relevant part of the counselling. My counselling check-list includes:

(a) relief
(b) loss
(c) permission to mourn
(d) truth
(e) knowledge – what actually happens with termination
(f) language
(g) information and the role of the counsellor.

To consider these in order:

Relief

It may be helpful to be explicit about this and to say 'one of the feelings you may experience is relief that it's about to be over, that the decision has been made.' Women sometimes need a lot of permission to feel that.

Loss

It is essential for the counsellor to be familiar with the processes of bereavement and to help women to understand that that may also be part of their current experience. This seems to me a key element in this context. Women sometimes acknowledge their grief and know that they will mourn the fetus. Again, they may not feel entitled to their feelings because they have chosen to abort it.

Permission to mourn

This links with the previous point. The counsellor may need to give a woman very clear permission to mourn in the context of what may have been an agonising decision for her.

Case history

K had found it extremely difficult to make a decision about her pregnancy. She was aware that part of her felt ready for a child, her long-term partner felt that he definitely did not want a child at this stage of his life, and K felt she could not have a child on her own. She eventually decided to have a termination. She devised her own ritual, the lighting and extinguishing of a candle. The counsellor encouraged K to feel that this was a very appropriate expression of her grief, which would help her in saying goodbye to what might have been her child, and which was an important stage in her grieving.

Being allowed to mourn the loss of the pregnancy is also a necessary part of the process which hopefully leads to self-forgiveness and moving on. I shall return to this when we consider post-termination counselling.

Truth

I have used the word fetus several times. In counselling it is helpful to listen to the way in which the woman describes her pregnancy. This gives clues to her sense of what is going on inside her body. She may describe it as a baby, as a bundle of cells, or 'just like a D & C really'. My experience leads me to feel that the counsellor should always be truthful, and always remember that in the end this is a life-and-death situation which you and the woman are talking and thinking about together. If you, the counsellor, cannot be open about that, the woman may also be inhibited, which in the long run may not be helpful to her.

Knowledge

The previous point raises the question of how much medical knowledge the counsellor requires. We can certainly be asked some very direct questions in counselling: For example – 'What happens at the operation?', 'Will I still be fertile?'; 'What happens to the fetus?'. If the counsellor has links with a particular clinic, it may be useful to have an idea what operative procedures they use, how they dispose of the fetus, whether it is used for research and so on.

Language

What words are being used by the woman in the counselling session?

Case history

P came to discuss the possibility of terminating her pregnancy. She already had two children and initially felt she could not cope with a third. She had just managed to get her work and child-care arrangements under control and another child at this stage seemed likely to disrupt all this. Her partner was apparently quite ambivalent and likely to leave the decision to her. Her use of the word 'murder' several times in relation to the fetus seemed to the counsellor to offer a clue to P's feelings. They talked together about the word and what it might mean. P realized that that was what termination meant to her and after much thought she telephoned the counsellor a few days later to say she had decided to continue with the pregnancy and felt relieved about her decision.

Information

It is essential that clinics and specialist centres make available relevant written information about procedures, risks, counselling services, etc., for the women and their partners using services. These should take into account their needs in terms of language translation; it may also be appropriate for the counsellor to share giving of information with the doctor or nurse, though some counsellors would not feel that was part of their counselling role. It may depend on the setting and professional relationships within it, but in the end women should be entitled to the information they feel they want and the support they may need in dealing with it. I still remember the gasp of horror from a woman who realized her fetus would be incinerated, and the help she required to talk through her feelings about it.

Fears and anxieties

It is important for the counsellor to understand what may lie behind the questions asked by women and their partners in terms of fear and anxieties. For example

- 'Will my fertility be affected by having a termination?'
- 'Will I have a miscarriage next time I get pregnant?'
- 'I wonder if my partner will still love me. I wonder what's going to happen to our relationship.'
- 'Am I going to be punished for this?' is a very important fear which is quite often expressed in the context of termination – a primitive sense of some sort of impending divine retribution.
- I have noticed that there may be special emotional difficulties for

women and men who already have a child. The woman has knowledge of the physical and psychological processes of fetal development from her experience of pregnancy and giving birth. Women
and men may find these memories disturbing when considering
termination. 'Could we have killed our son or daughter?'

There are no reassuring answers to these questions – the counsellor
needs to treat them seriously and understand their significance for the
women and men concerned.

Men and pregnancy termination

Much of what I have already written refers to women. The legislation
only mentions women and I think women themselves have a strong
political sense of the decision being theirs (the 'right to choose'),
hampered sometimes by the medical profession. So in this context men
may be marginalized; however, they should not be neglected in this
equation. Sometimes, of course they are not around or are unaware that
the woman is pregnant. I usually check out with the women I see
whether they are alone, whether there is a man around who might be
involved in the decision. Very often a woman will want her own time;
sometimes she will specifically ask for a joint session; occasionally men
will want some time on their own.

Case history

I saw S on her own for two sessions. She was very clear that she wanted a
termination. She had a good career under way and felt too unsure in the
relationship with P, her partner, to have a child together. She was aware that
P wanted to have the child. P made his own appointment to come to see me
and used the session to try to come to terms with what he realized was a very
firm decision on the part of S. The pregnancy was terminated.

A year later S contacted me again and we met. She was again pregnant by
the same partner. The relationship had survived the termination and to P's joy
this time S decided to have the baby. It seemed to be the right decision and
one which S felt was very much on her terms.

There is no doubt that some men grieve deeply over terminations and
feel that a part of themselves has been rejected in some way. Now and
again, men have revealed some of their feelings from the past, in the
context of another pregnancy. Women are sometimes very uncertain
how to deal with 'I'll support you either way, but it's your decision' from
their partners and can feel quite angry at what they perceive as opting
out.

This issue seems to me to involve a very delicate balance between a
woman's right to make decisions about her own body, and a man's

desire to have some say over a pregnancy which is partly his. As counsellors, we can only offer our skills, time and space as appropriate. My feeling is that we need to know much more about men's thoughts and fantasies in relation to pregnancy termination, and how they deal with their feelings.

Special contexts of termination

Termination and fetal abnormality

This is an extremely difficult area for everyone concerned: partly because a baby may have been very much wanted and planned; and partly because the results of some tests are not available until late on in a pregnancy, thus making possible termination a particularly traumatic procedure. One of the hardest tasks a doctor must have to face is to tell a woman and her partner there is something wrong with their baby – the impact of their anger, grief and perhaps above all, disbelief, may be extremely difficult to deal with.

Case history

I was asked to see M, a young woman on the ward who at first refused to go to the operating theatre for the termination of a hydrocephalic pregnancy. It emerged that she had had a routine scan the previous day. She had not seen the scan picture because the ultrasonographer had quickly realized something was badly wrong and turned the screen away. M, who desperately wanted this baby, her first, refused to believe what the doctor had to tell her. I spent some time with her, sitting beside her bed, and I listened carefully. It became apparent that M needed some confirmation that there truly was something wrong that could not be put right. It eventually became possible for M to be re-scanned, this time she was shown very carefully exactly what had happened. She had the pregnancy terminated, but she and her partner needed a great deal of follow-up counselling.

Impact on other children in a family

This is something counsellors need to be very aware of. We may be able to help parents find ways of responding to children's questions and sometimes changes in behaviour. Termination for abnormality can create enormous anxieties in other children about being 'alright' for their parents. Parents who go through the trauma of a termination may not be able to take account of their children's feelings. It is particularly helpful to offer post-termination counselling. There can be many repercussions on a family of a termination in this context.

Impact on medical and nursing staff

I would like to emphasize the need for support for medical and nursing staff who are involved in a very intimate way with the woman and her partner. There really needs to be a multidisciplinary team approach; a counsellor already involved in that setting may be able to facilitate this. Staff need to feel supported in order to offer that support to others. Termination for fetal abnormality touches deep feelings in all of us, not least the rights of such potential children to live or to die. As more and more tests are developed, so counselling skills and staff support systems will be increasingly important. In this context it is useful to remember the enormous contribution of self-help and other groups, a considerable resource for everyone concerned.

Regarding routine scans and termination of pregnancy, it is widely assumed that women considering termination would find it disturbing to be shown the fetus on a scan. That may generally be the case. However, interestingly, a woman recently told me she had seen her scan. She was pleased that she had recognized the pregnancy and felt that she now knew who she would say goodbye to – she felt this had in some way completed the process for her. She may be unusual, I do not know, but that incident highlights the need for flexibility and an awareness of what may be helpful to individual women.

Termination in the context of trauma

Women sometimes present for termination after a trauma such as physical violence or rape. The counsellor may find her or himself acting as a crisis counsellor in a very particular way. Especially in the case of rape, it is unfortunately likely that the woman will not have disclosed what happened to anyone official. She may not have spoken about it to anyone at all and may need a great deal of space and time to be able to talk about what has happened. The counsellor may be the first person in the setting to know the woman is pregnant because of having been raped. This has implications about confidentiality of information. It would undoubtedly be helpful if the doctor and nurse who examine her were aware of the rape – she could expect especially sensitive physical care, for example. In the end, it is for the woman to choose and the counsellor to respect her confidence.

It may sometimes be helpful to refer a woman on to a specialist agency such as Rape Crisis or a victim support network. But I feel it is important to be very careful about this. Women who have suffered in this way are hypersensitive to rejection. If a trusting relationship has begun to grow between the counsellor and the woman, she may not want to start all over again with someone else. It is a very delicate area. Rape is emotive for all of us. Counsellors may need to find *themselves* extra support, perhaps via a specialist agency. In this way, they may not feel too overwhelmed themselves to be able to focus on the needs of the women with whom they are working.

There may be situations where the confidentiality referred to earlier might have to be broken, such as in the rape of an under-age girl in an incestuous situation. The young woman and all the professionals involved would need a great deal of mutual support and good liaison with appropriate agencies.

Impact of termination of pregnancy in different age groups

Teenagers

My particular focus is on the possible needs of young women between 11 and 15 years of age. They may still be at home with a parent and the decision may sometimes seem to involve a number of people. How do they arrive? Sometimes they are referred by GPs, sometimes by clinic staff. Sometimes they appear with a boyfriend or with a girlfriend who may previously have been counselled. Sometimes they arrive with one or both parents.

Case history

H, a young Greek girl of 15, was brought to see me by her father at the suggestion of their family doctor. H had confided in her mother that she thought she was pregnant and her mother told H's father. He was determined that H would have a termination. She was still at school and he felt a child would bring disgrace on the family. I insisted on adhering to my rule, that whatever her age, a woman has a right to counselling time on her own; also that the decision in the end is hers, not that of her parents. It emerged that H was extremely frightened about the pregnancy and had no wish to have a child. Her father had forbidden her to have anything more to do with the young man concerned and H really wanted to have the whole episode out of the way. She had a termination and still keeps in touch with me from time to time.

I think it is extremely important to treat even the youngest pregnant woman as a person in her own right, separate from her parents – someone who may have her own ideas about her pregnancy and who deserves to be heard and listened to seriously. I stress the confidentiality of our session (although there may be times when that might have to be broken – see earlier in this chapter. Sometimes a young woman arrives with a parent who very much wants to be in the counselling session. I explain that I will see them later.

I have found that sometimes it is the mother who wants her daughter to continue with the pregnancy and her daughter who is resistant.

Case history

C came with her mother to discuss possible termination. C was just 16 years-old and it became clear that she did not want a child at this stage of her life with college and other possibilities ahead. I saw her mother separately. She had initially been shocked by C's pregnancy, but had begun to want her to keep the baby. 'I'll bring it up . . . it would be wonderful to have a baby in the house again . . .. She accompanied C to the hospital for the termination, very distressed. C, who continued to feel clearly that termination was right for her, had her operation and spent a lot of time comforting her mother.

Mothers sometimes use the occasion of their daughter's pregnancy to disclose to them details of terminations they have had themselves. They may be faced with unresolved feelings from the past and require counselling help for themselves. Disclosure may result in a sense of sharing between mothers and daughters; on the other hand it may engender quite confused feelings and fantasies on the part of the daughter, which the counsellor may need to help sort out. 'Did she really want me?'; 'Maybe I could have had a brother or sister'; 'I wonder what happened to the fetus/baby?'.

Older women with children

The situation with older women may be very different.

Case history

I recently counselled R, a married woman with two teenage children, who had become pregnant at the age of 43. She was extremely distressed that this had happened when she had hoped that one act of unprotected sexual inter-course would be 'safe' at her age. R was angry with herself and with her husband, but they had been able to talk it over and decide on a termination. She was very content with her children and could not contemplate starting all over again. R had cried a great deal (and wept again in our session) but felt she could move on in her life after termination. Her husband and she had decided he would have a vasectomy, which he had been considering anyway.

Sometimes woman have told children in the family that they are preg-nant and are having a termination. In this context, parents are some-times puzzled by their children's reaction. For example, a mother told me her teenage son had been very quiet and withdrawn about her termination though her other child, who was younger, had not seemed very bothered. It may be helpful for the counsellor to encourage parents to consider the possible impact of a termination on their children, as I mentioned earlier. Apart from anxieties about being wanted them-selves, there may be tensions and jealousies, sometimes subconscious, about their parents' sexual activities as evidenced by the pregnancy.

In a situation of fetal abnormality and termination, it may be very important to encourage parents to allow their children to share in grief and mourning, to see photographs and to share their fantasies about what has happened. Again, this can be quite difficult for grieving parents. The counsellor may be able to support them through this and in doing so, enable them to be supportive to their children.

Older women without children

The possibility of parenthood is by no means top of every woman's emotional agenda. There may be various reasons for this – we each have our own history and plans. An older woman who becomes pregnant may find the decision for or against termination an extremely difficult one. There may be implications for career-building and promotion; for a change in life-style; for possible adverse effects on a relationship; there maybe anxieties about possible fetal abnormality; above all, whether this is a one-off chance to have a child, which may never recur – 'If I don't take this chance, will I regret it for the rest of my life?'.

Counselling and contraception

This is a subject which evinces strong feelings. It is sometimes said that there is no reason for a woman to have an unwanted pregnancy. However, contraceptive failure is real. There seems to be no method of contraception which is entirely free from hazard. How many of the professionals involved in pregnancy termination have always acted safely within their own sexual relationships? How many children do we know whose conceptions were not exactly planned?

There is also the question of knowledge. Do women and men know where to go for contraceptive advice? Do they know how different methods work and possible risks? There is still considerable ignorance and a continuing need for accessible information. Myths persist; 'Unprotected sexual intercourse is safe if you do it standing up'; 'You only get pregnant if you have a climax'.

Women of every age have great anxiety about being perceived as 'being prepared for sex' – do they or do they not carry condoms as a matter of course? Is it sensible to be on the pill even if you're not in a sexual relationship? There may even be a need to test out one's fertility, sometimes at a subconscious level. It may be that a couple has set out to have a child, the relationship ends and the woman feels she cannot have this child alone.

It seems to me that if women and men are going to use whatever method of contraception effectively, they first need to be aware of themselves as sexual people; second need to feel good about themselves and their bodies; and third need to be actively concerned to take care of themselves and their fertility.

The counsellor's concern is not how effectively women and men may or may not have used contraception. Rather, it is to help them understand this aspect of their behaviour, perhaps at a deeper level. This is particularly relevant where a woman has had several terminations. She may be wary of possible disapproval. I try to encourage her to think about her experiences and her view of herself as a sexual person. Some women have very negative feelings about themselves as female and as potential mothers. This is likely to have originated in their earlier life. It may be some time before they feel self-confidence in the truest sense.

Counselling post-termination of pregnancy

If we are offering counselling pre- possible termination, we should certainly offer counselling post-termination or be able to suggest other agencies. Some clinics offer a medical check-up which might be a way of assessing with a woman how she is feeling; others do not. It would be a useful part of a clinic's written information to clarify what provision of post-termination counselling there is on offer. From my own experience, the majority of women experiencing termination do not return for counselling. I am not sure what this means – I think we can only offer a service and make it as available as possible.

Sometimes women book an appointment in advance. I have noticed this may link with a previous difficult experience following termination – possibly depression. Women may return on the anniversary of the termination or when the baby would have been born. The birth of a child may reactivate feelings lying dormant since a termination; or a woman may return in the context of something else.

Case history

A GP rang asking me to see D who had appeared in her surgery with a broken ankle. The doctor had picked up on her unhappiness relating to a termination some months previously. D came to see me. By the end of the session we were both aware that although the termination may have been the right decision, D was still experiencing much unresolved grief which was affecting her relationship with men and with members of her family. I saw her regularly for a year. She then referred a friend for counselling!

It may be that in the context of current infertility a woman remembers a past termination. This can be especially poignant.

Case history

In the course of counselling T and her partner for fertility difficulties, it emerged that what T really wanted to focus on was a termination of pregnancy she had had several years ago in a previous relationship. T's partner

was aware of her history. We decided that T and I would have some sessions
on our own. T brought along a photograph album from that part of her life.
We looked together at photographs of her taken then, around that time when
she was briefly pregnant and making her decision. She still felt it had been
right and the album with its photos helped her to get in touch with her feelings
and complete her grieving.

I wrote earlier on the need for the counsellor to have an understanding
of the process of bereavement. Many women who come for post-
termination counselling are experiencing grief that they did not really
anticipate. They may feel that they are not entitled to mourning since
they made the decision to end their pregnancy. They are terrified of
being overwhelmed by a complex tide of grief, guilt and sometimes
regret. It is extremely helpful if the counsellor can encourage a woman
to put these feelings into words. That shows her that she has been
understood and that the counsellor is not overwhelmed in the way she
fears for herself. Hopefully, the woman may begin to feel she can start
disclosing and exploring her feelings in a safe and accepting environment. She may use other means of expression: I still treasure the
photograph of a very moving painting, by means of which a woman I
counselled expressed her feelings about her termination.

Occasionally I have been aware that a woman needs to feel 'forgiven'
in a way that I cannot offer. In such circumstances if appropriate I have
been able to arrange for a *carefully chosen* priest to become involved.

Case history

O was a woman from a very strict Roman Catholic background who had a
termination. She was very distressed afterwards and I counselled her for
several sessions. I think this was helpful at one level, but O was very scared
about going to some sort of hell as the result of her action. The priest that I
found for her was able to help her in a very special way that I could not offer
her and she arrived at the inner peace she needed so badly.

Women may personalize the fetus, sometimes to the extent of giving it a
name. My feeling is that whatever helps a woman through the process
of grieving and self-acceptance should be accepted and supported by
the counsellor. The taboo nature of termination in British society means
that there are virtually no rituals associated with it. Hence in the aftermath women (and men) may experience loneliness and isolation.

Termination of a pregnancy sometimes acts as a catalyst. Women
begin to reexamine their lives, particularly their relationships, and find
ongoing counselling helpful. In this context the counsellor needs to be
very clear how much time she or he has available, because this process
may take months or longer. Personally, I find it an extremely interesting
and rewarding part of my counselling work. I am able to give it some
priority because it is a recognized part of the service I aim to offer.

Incidentally, I have noticed that hospitalization for gynaecological surgery may similarly be a point of crisis, leading a woman to reevaluation of her life.

In the context of post-termination counselling there have been a number of studies carried out to try and identify risk factors in terms of psychiatric or psychological disturbance. These seem so far to be inconclusive. Zolese & Blacker (1992) have surveyed the literature (see references) and it is a useful paper for anyone working in this area to read. For the counsellor, it is reassuring to have access to psychological or psychiatric services as appropriate. This may be for consultation, or referral on for more specialist care.

Know yourself

This concept is at the heart of the counselling process.

A medical colleague asked me recently how I found it personally possible to counsel women (and partners) who are considering termination of pregnancy, and women and men with fertility difficulties. The question took me by surprise. I suppose the superficial answer would be that this is all part of my job as the social worker-counsellor for a hospital gynaecology unit. But I thought about it and replied that I felt those two extremes were in fact part of a continuum – that women and men go through various experiences during their lives in relation to their bodies and their sexuality. I felt at ease with the offer of counselling in whatever situation arose along that continuum. At the times when I felt uncomfortable or out of my depth, I hope I would seek the consultation and support which I have referred to earlier.

If we take into account the aura of secrecy which surrounds termination of pregnancy, we will be aware that the counsellor's clientele is likely to be hypersensitive to any hint of disapproval, judgement or superiority on the part of any professional they meet. Hence, as a counsellor, 'Know yourself': get to grips with your feelings about termination of pregnancy – as a woman, as a man, as a political person, as a member of society. It is absolutely vital to be able to offer a non-judgemental, objective approach, without your personal emotional baggage getting in the way. That is not to say that there won't be times when we as counsellors don't feel a reverberation of something in our own souls. For example, I think I find termination of a twin pregnancy quite a difficult situation – but then so do our clients. It is a very delicate balance. My experience suggests that if as a counsellor you have a deep personal feeling that termination is wrong, that life at that stage is sacred, then counselling in this context may not be for you. It may be too personally traumatic and you do not have to be that hard on yourself.

Conclusion

The legislation which surrounds *in vitro* fertilization procedures makes the offer of counselling mandatory. In the context of termination of pregnancy there is no such requirement. However, this decision may be an extremely complex one, as I hope I have indicated. Women and their partners require the utmost care and sensitivity on the part of the professionals they meet. The work is highly emotive. Hence my emphasis on the need for counsellors to be very clear within themselves about their own feelings.

The model of clinical practice I described works on the basis of part-time hours and job-sharing – in this way everyone concerned is helped to maintain energy and commitment. Mutual support and consultation for the professionals are important at every level, to enable the professionals in turn to be supportive to women and their partners in a very vulnerable situation.

We know that a pregnancy may be an occasion for great joy. It may also engender feelings of ambivalence, uncertainty and sheer panic. The outcome touches on many aspects of a woman's life. The counsellor may be privileged to be part of that process.

Part II
The Wider Context

Part II deals with the wider perspective and context of infertility counselling; it documents its history as well as considering its future.

Chapter 10 (Blyth and Hunt) describes the history and development of infertility counselling in the UK and the various initiatives which provoked changes in the law. Chapter 11 (Doyal) takes us through some of the legal and ethical dilemmas and arguments regarding IVF treatment, using them as a focus against which many other treatment decisions need to be considered. Chapter 13 (Lenton) discusses who should actually be responsible for infertility counselling. Chapters 16 (Neuberg), 14 (Djahanbakhch, Saridogan and Kadva) and 15 (Taylor, Lower and Grudzinskas) are written by medical doctors and give varying views of counselling and its relevance to infertility treatment. Chapter 12 (Silman) challenges assumptions made by both doctors and counsellors, and provokes us to question what counselling actually is. Finally, Chapter 17 (McWhinnie) asks the question 'Why do we need counselling?' and looks at the experience and official reports not only from the UK but also from Australia and the USA.

Chapter 10
A History of Infertility Counselling in the United Kingdom

Eric Blyth & Jennifer Hunt

Introduction

Since the late 1970s there has been a rapid growth of government and public awareness in Britain concerning infertility treatments and choices. Increasingly the importance of the provision of adequate counselling has been recognized. This has been highlighted by the emergence of a professional organization, the British Infertility Counselling Association and by statutory recognition under the Human Fertilisation & Embryology Act. Nevertheless the development of infertility counselling has not been problem-free. This chapter considers infertility counselling past and present and concludes by identifying outstanding and future issues requiring consideration if 'proper' counselling is to be provided.

Recognition of the infertility counselling role

Despite recent developments in scientific and clinical aspects of reproductive biology, the contrast between the revolution in medical technology and the very slow pace of change in our understanding and handling of the psychological implications of infertility and involuntary childlessness is all too apparent. And despite a considerable literature on the emotional and social issues raised by infertility and involuntary childlessness, clinics in Britain providing infertility treatment in the early to mid-1980s remained largely unresponsive to such needs (Mathieson, 1986; Owens & Read, 1984). Pfeffer & Woollett quote one recipient of infertility 'counselling':

> I asked [the doctor] if there was any emotional counselling. She said, had I been told about the legal aspects. I said no, and repeated my question. She said, well the legal side is very important. I said, I'm sure it is, but I can't change the law. I don't call that counselling, I call that giving information. (Pfeffer & Woollett, 1983 p. 71)

Elsewhere, counselling provision was not immune from the critical feminist gaze that was increasingly being applied to assisted conception; Spallone & Steinberg (1987) in particular accuse some counselling as being little more than a euphemism for genetic screening.

The emergence of infertility counselling as a specialism

Unsurprisingly, there have been increasing demands for a new approach to the treatment of infertility, the focus on infertility as a social and not exclusively (or even predominantly) a medical problem, because it arises from an attempt to create a social relationship – not only that of parent and child, but a child in the context of the extended family network (Pfeffer & Quick, 1988). The 'problem' in its social context is more appropriately perceived as childlessness, rather than infertility which describes only the biological relationship and not the social status of the people concerned (Matthews & Matthews, 1986). Even more important is the need to integrate the biomedical revolution with an equivalent revolution in our psychosocial services, and be warned that 'any single approach to human behaviour can only be reductionist' (Bydlowski & Dayon-Lintzer, 1988).

The beginnings of official recognition of the need for and possible role of counselling in infertility may be discerned in the report of the Warnock Committee (see also Introduction and Chapter 17) which recommended that counselling should be available to ensure that 'couples and donors fully understand the implications of what they are embarking on, what rights and duties they may have, and where they may expect to experience difficulty' (DHSS, 1984, 3.3.).

The Warnock Report was also clear about the sort of counselling that should be provided and by whom it should be provided. 'The counselling that we envisage is essentially non-directional. It is aimed at helping individuals to understand their situation, and to make their own decisions about what steps should be taken next' (DHSS, 1984, 3.4).

Despite this fairly unequivocal mandate, the Warnock Report hinted at issues that would come to cloud the provision of counselling in infertility treatment, in particular the relationship between the counsellor and other members of the multidisciplinary team, and the tension between the provision of 'non-directional' counselling and the role of the counsellor in determining who should receive treatment.

In between publication of the Warnock Report and the implementation of legislation, several developments of relevance to infertility counselling in the United Kingdom took place. For convenience of presentation, these are presented separately, but in reality they interconnect chronologically. The aspects considered here are first the consultation process initiated by the Government to translate the Warnock Committee recommendations into legislation; second the establishment of a voluntary regulatory system for certain infertility treatments; and third the development of a professional body representing infertility counsellors.

The Government consultation process

In 1986 the Government published a Consultation Document (DHSS, 1986) crystallizing the issues that had been raised in response to the Warnock Report and identifying the areas in which the government considered legislation to be feasible. That the Consultation Document endorsed proposals that couples should receive counselling is clearly of little surprise. Perhaps more surprising (and contentious), though, is the explicit link made between the provision of counselling and the need for centres providing infertility services to have regard for the welfare of the child who might be born following DI or other treatments.

The ensuing White Paper proposed two strands for the counselling of couples (DHSS, 1987):

(1) Counselling should enable them to understand the options available and the kind of stresses they might face if they opt for treatment, so that they can make an informed decision, and
(2) (Where donated genetic material is used) [it should] explore the implications for the future family of having a child which is not genetically theirs.

Counselling for donors would aim to explain the implications of donation, particularly the legal framework.

The White Paper made clear the Government's intention to require centres providing licensed treatments to make counselling available to all couples considering infertility treatment and that the statutory licensing authority (HFEA) would take account of the quality of counselling services when considering whether to issue a licence. The counselling envisaged in the White Paper 'should be distinct from discussions with a doctor of any medical treatment he proposes and should be carried out by somebody different, preferably a qualified counsellor'. The White Paper also indicated the Government's intention to require the HFEA to ensure the availability of counselling to those born following the use of donated gametes who subsequently seek information about their genetic origins.

As with the Consultation Document, the White Paper linked counselling with the assessment of a couple's eligibility for treatment, though concluding that 'a formal statutory procedure to assess suitability would (not) be appropriate'. (Somewhat ambiguously, the HFEA would be required to take account of centres' procedures for deciding whether to offer treatment to particular couples in determining licence applications).

IVF and voluntary regulation

Given that the Warnock Committee had recommended a formal regulatory system for centres providing certain types of infertility treatment, but also recognizing that it would be some time before such a system was in place, the Medical Research Council and the Royal College of Obstetricians and Gynaecologists jointly established the Voluntary Licensing Authority for human *in vitro* fertilization and embryology (VLA) in 1985. In 1989, exasperated at government delay in implementing a statutory framework, the Authority redesignated itself as the Interim Licensing Authority, explicitly emphasizing its intended temporary status.

Although the VLA was not an exclusively medical or scientific body its concerns were primarily clinical and scientific. Its composition ensured that clinical and scientific interests were well represented, and at no time in its existence did it include a practising infertility counsellor. The VLA's first annual report discussed counselling as follows:

> In all centres the medical staff are involved in the initial counselling of patients, but subsequently follow-up discussions are frequently arranged with the qualified nursing staff involved in the programme. Some centres employ specially-trained counsellors. Most centres also go to some considerable trouble to ensure that patients who fail to achieve a pregnancy have the opportunity to discuss their problems and decide on future treatment with either the medical or nursing staff. In general, the care which staff take over their patients is most impressive. (VLA, 1986, p. 16).

This brief summary highlights some of the tensions that have subsequently become apparent as the precise nature of infertility counselling has been teased out. What is counselling if it can be provided by untrained medical and nursing staff (who are also providing the clinical treatment) and if it is focused primarily on treatment failure? Situations requiring special counselling care singled out by the VLA included sister/sister egg and pre-embryo donation, seen as procedures that should be carried out 'only under exceptional circumstances and only after very careful counselling of both donor and recipient' (VLA, 1986, p. 15). (The alert reader may have great difficulty in believing that the last sentence of the VLA's observations could possibly be referring to the same sorts of services described at the beginning of this chapter!)

It is, perhaps, indicative of the perceived standing of counselling at this time that the initial set of guidelines for both clinical and research applications of IVF devised by the VLA contained no mention of counselling services. This was rectified a year later, and centres were required to have 'appropriate counselling facilities with access to properly trained independent counselling staff' (VLA, 1987, p. 35). However, a summary of counselling provision in licensed centres two years later indicated that this ideal had yet to be achieved:

> The current provision made for counselling in IVF clinics varies considerably despite there being a general appreciation that counselling is essential for the well-being of all those associated with treatment programmes. In more than 50% of the IVF centres presently licensed by the ILA, the clinicians play a major role in counselling. This may include talking to the patients before treatment commences, as well as sessions during the IVF programme. Nursing staff may also put aside time for counselling; a number of centres have nurse counsellors who are responsible for counselling. There may be facilities for patients to ring the day-ward if they have worries or queries. (Frew, 1989 p. 4).

The situation was not set to improve significantly in the short term either. In 1990 Harriet Harman published the results of a survey conducted on behalf of the Labour Party. The general state of infertility counselling services can be summed up in the reply from one Health Authority: 'The colposcopy nurse at Margate is very good at talking to patients but she is not a fully trained counsellor' (Harman, 1990 p. 6).

Given such an indictment, it is hard to square this with the complacency evident in the 1986 report. It also raises questions about the substance of the VLA's claim that each centre is 'specifically questioned to ensure that the Guidelines are being followed' (VLA, 1987 p. 10) and that centres unable to confirm their adherence to the new Guidelines will have their approval withdrawn (VLA, 1987 p. 18). To our knowledge no centre lost its VLA approval on the grounds of inadequate counselling provision during the entire period that the Authority's counselling guideline was in operation (i.e. between 1987 and 1991). We can only speculate what impact a tougher stand by the Authority might have exerted on the subsequent quality of counselling provision, given later comments from the Authority about the provision of counselling, which included:

> There is confusion about the definition of counselling ... Proper counselling is possible only if space and time are available to the couple in a neutral atmosphere with a *fully-trained* counsellor.
> (VLA, 1988, p. 15) [our emphasis];

> We have been disturbed at the increase in the number of small IVF centres seeking to establish themselves without the necessary facilities, adequately trained staff or the requisite specialist supervision.
> (ILA, 1990 p. 2);

There is a shortage ... of trained counsellors

(Donaldson, 1991 p. 5).

Infertility counselling – an emerging professional base

The organization that was to become the British Infertility Counselling Association (BICA) had its origins in an *ad hoc* meeting of interested individuals in London in May 1988. It was convened by one of the authors who had previously worked as an infertility counsellor in an Australian hospital. Valuing the supportive peer-group network, the absence of such a network was particularly noticeable upon her return to the UK to commence work as an infertility counsellor in a London IVF unit. The lack of a single authoritative professional body that could speak for infertility counselling was all the more significant given the contemporary context and the proposals for introducing legislation for infertility treatments in the UK.

Participants at the May meeting were a group of virtual strangers drawn from a wide variety of professional fields, including psychiatry, social work, psychology, psychotherapy, nursing, education, theology and medicine. They decided to establish a professional association, provisionally entitled the National Association for Infertility Counselling (NAIC), and set up a steering committee, and the Association was formally launched five months later.

The initial agenda for the Association was daunting to say the least. Coming into existence over four years after the Warnock Report had been published, many of its terms were already set. Nevertheless the Association quickly made contact with the DHSS and was given the opportunity to contribute to consultations concerning the implementation of legislation. The support of senior civil servants and financial assistance from the Department were also crucial to the viability of the fledgling Association. At the same time the Association offered the DHSS (and hence the Government) an opportunity, so far lacking, of hearing the views of the only body that could claim to represent infertility counselling in all its guises.

Given the range of backgrounds and orientations of its membership, the Association was quick to articulate the confusion over what infertility counselling actually was. Less speedy, inevitably, was the task of defining counselling in a way that could be accepted by at least the majority of its members. It was 1991 before the Association published its definitive Infertility Counselling Guidelines (BICA, 1991 – see Appendix 3).

However, within its first year of operation, the Association undertook work outlining a model infertility training programme, provided a response to the White Paper and to a DHSS Checklist for the Training of Infertility Counsellors (DHSS, 1988), produced a bibliography of literature and research concerning psychological and social issues in infertility, and established a newsletter for members (BICA, 1989). More recently, the Association has ascertained members' views on various issues (such as whether information about genetic origins should be made available to those born following the use of donated gametes, and also the role of counsellors in assessing potential clients for suitability for treatment). It has also undertaken an audit of infertility counselling training (Dustin & Waugh, 1991), as well as seeking opportunities to contribute to the legislative and regulatory process concerning infertility treatment.

Despite the difficulty in clarifying the role and task of infertility counselling, the Association nailed its colours to the mast early on with respect to the relationship between counselling and assessment for treatment. It accepted that discussion of a client's affairs, including their financial situation, employment and career prospects, marital and sexual adjustment, psychological and personal adjustment, family and social relationships and physical health, formed part of the agenda for counselling. But it also made it clear that: 'it is *not* suggested that consideration of these issues should take place in the context of assessment of a couple's/individual's suitability for treatment' (NAIC, 1988).

Nevertheless the role of the counsellor in the assessment for treatment process was to remain controversial. A survey of BICA members undertaken in 1990 (in relation to treatment involving donated gametes) indicated that 33% considered there should be some form of assessment, 46% believed there should not, whilst the remaining 21% were unsure. 40% also considered that social workers, counsellors or psychologists were professionally best equipped to undertake assessment, 25% advocated a multidisciplinary approach (which included medical and nursing staff) as the most appropriate model for assessment, whilst 26% were either uncertain or considered that no professional group could take responsibility for such assessment (BICA, 1990).

An early attempt to gauge the state of infertility counselling in the UK concluded that counselling is 'thin on the ground' and there was very little training or supervision (BICA, 1989). Another study undertaken to ascertain levels of counselling provision in the 25 clinics then licensed by the ILA revealed considerable variation in the provision and availability of counselling (Inglis, 1989). Most clinics did not offer a professional counselling service: in only a quarter was counselling provided by a designated counsellor, whilst in 65% of the clinics counselling was provided by a nurse and in 60% by a doctor. Not surprisingly, the survey also revealed considerable confusion concerning perceptions of what constitutes counselling.

Meanwhile the Association's Newsletter provided a forum for the discussion of controversial issues or those at risk of neglect. Appleton's paper on the potential role for counsellors in surrogacy arrangements (Appleton, 1990) and Crawshaw's warning of the neglect of counselling provision in outpatient gynaecology clinics or GP's surgeries – where the bulk of people having fertility difficulties actually go (Crawshaw, 1990) are typical examples of these.

When in November 1989 the Government introduced the Human Fertilisation & Embryology Bill in the House of Lords the Association lobbied to ensure that the final legislation would adequately address the need for the provision of counselling, primarily in conjunction with the British Association of Social Workers and British Agencies for Adoption and Fostering.

'Proper' counselling – a statutory base

The Human Fertilisation and Embryology Act 1990 requires that a suitable opportunity to receive 'proper' counselling should be offered to the following (though there is no obligation on anyone to take up the offer of counselling):

(1) prospective recipients of treatment services
(2) prospective donors of gametes and embryos
(3) those who seek information from the HFEA concerning their genetic origins.

Membership of the HFEA is by appointment by the Secretary of State for Health. Although the Act ensures that membership reflects the interests of the medical and scientific community this does not extend to infertility counselling; it is probably indicative of the still-marginal status of counselling that no-one with direct current involvement in infertility counselling has been appointed as a member of the Authority. Similarly Latarche (1992) notes that although BICA was approached by the Authority to nominate members to complete the inspectorate teams, none of the BICA nominees were appointed.

As part of its responsibilities under the Act, the HFEA was required to produce a code of practice and to consider the quality of centres' counselling facilities in determining whether licensing conditions were being met. To facilitate this work the Department of Health requested the assistance of the King's Fund Centre (see also Chapter 15), which established a ten-member interdisciplinary committee of specialists whose terms of reference were:

> To provide advice for the consideration of the Human Fertilisation and Embryology Authority on the counselling needs relating to the provision of infertility services for couples considering any of the regulated infertility treatments; for children born following gamete or

embryo donation who seek information about their origins, and for all
donors, (King's Fund Centre, 1991)

Though the committee included nursing, medical and patient interests
(amongst others), the fact that three of its members were professionally
qualified, experienced social workers presented the best opportunity so
far offered for that particular professional group to make its concerted
voice heard, and may well account for the tone and direction of the
committee's report, especially its emphasis on the rights and needs of
children born as a result of assisted conception.

The committee noted there were ' "significant differences" of interpretation and emphasis as to what the term "proper counselling" means
. . . between counsellors, those providing treatment, infertile people, the
general public and among professional people possessing qualifications
in and knowledge from other disciplines. It also noted that these
discrepancies were almost taken for granted'. The committee therefore
identified four elements integral to the provision of counselling:

(1) The welfare of the resultant child and other children who may be
    affected.
(2) The needs of infertile people.
(3) The needs of the prospective donor.
(4) The desire for assurance at a societal level that the infertility services
    are 'conducted responsibly'.

The committee made several unambiguous statements about the relationship between counselling and the protection of the child's interests,
for example: 'In our view it will be impossible to separate the process of
counselling from consideration of the welfare of the child' (King's Fund
Centre, 1991, p. 13).

Such a focus had obvious implications for the counsellor's role in
assessing potential treatment recipients and donors, and the King's
Fund Committee had no doubts that the counsellor should play a central
part in this.

Implicitly at least the committee were beginning to identify the
distinction between the provision of counselling and the role of the
counsellor. Whilst the counsellor necessarily provided counselling,
counselling did not encompass all the counsellor's activities or responsibilities. In the committee's eyes 'proper counselling' was seen to
include: first giving relevant information, second, providing an opportunity to discuss and explore the personal implications associated with
this information; and, third, providing an opportunity to come to an
informed and considered decision concerning the choice to be made
amongst the alternative options.

Noting that giving of information and counselling about the implications of treatment are differentiated in the Act, the committee therefore identified four specific components of 'proper counselling':

(1) *Information counselling.* (The combination of information, advice and discussion which may be provided by 'any suitable member of the infertility team, not necessarily requiring formal training and qualification in counselling').

(2) *Implications counselling.* (The exploration of personal and family implications of infertility and infertility treatments and gamete donation, requiring the high skill levels of a trained infertility counsellor).

(3) *Support counselling.* (The provision of emotional support throughout the process of diagnosis, investigation and treatment and gamete donation, which may be provided by the range of professionals working in the infertility team).

(4) *Therapeutic counselling.* (A treatment process in its own right, 'focusing on healing, on the gradual adjustment of expectations and on the eventual acceptance of life circumstances'. Although the committee does not make it clear who it considers should be providing such counselling within centres, it acknowledges the need for counsellors to be sufficiently skilled to know when clients require the particular skills of counsellors in other specialized settings).

In the long term, the King's Fund Committee proposed that all centres should employ at least one trained infertility counsellor, and further counsellors in line with any HFEA-recommended patient/counsellor ratio (though so far, no such recommendation exists).

Recognizing the practical problems of providing adequate 'proper' counselling in terms of its own definition, the committee proposed a training programme designed to ensure that from 1997 all infertility counsellors should hold a general professional counselling qualification and demonstrate evidence of successful completion of a short specialist training course, for which it produced an outline curriculum.

The committee produced an agenda for the monitoring and evaluation of infertility counselling that could be taken into consideration by the HFEA as part of its inspection and licence-awarding responsibilities. The information considered important by the committee included:

- the number of staff and staffing structure
- the number of counsellors
- the qualifications of counsellors
- the presence and quality of a training programme for counsellors
- the size of the budget for the training of counsellors
- arrangements for the employment/availability of counsellors
- the provision of written information for patients/donors

- the number of patients referred to the treatment centre
- the number of patients seen by the counsellor
- the number of patients referred to specialist agencies following a problem identified during counselling
- the number of patients withdrawing from treatment after counselling.

Further, the HFEA's inspection visits were expected to provide opportunities to inspect counselling facilities, see samples of counselling records and engage in detailed discussion of work with individual counsellors and elicit the perceptions of counselling provision held by recipients and other team members. The King's Fund Committee also suggested that some centres might acquire the facilities to enable unobtrusive observation of counselling (with the patient's permission).

The Human Fertilisation & Embryology Authority

The HFEA has exercised an impact on infertility counselling in three specific ways; through its Code of Practice; through licensing and inspection; and through the establishment of a working group on training for infertility counsellors.

The HFEA produced its first Code of Practice in 1992 and a second revised code in 1993. Drawing on the King's Fund Committee, the Code of Practice considers counselling services in some detail to give centres a clear idea of its expectations. The Code outlines the essential ingredients of implications, support and therapeutic counselling, specifies the required qualifications and experience of counsellors and their role in assessment of potential treatment recipients and gamete donors, and emphasizes the need for centres to establish systems for monitoring, improving and updating standards for services, including counselling provision. The Authority took the opportunity in presenting the Code to assert that: 'Health professionals are not normally trained to have the necessary skills (in counselling)' (HFEA, 1991, p. 3).

Although the Authority recognized the contribution of the King's Fund Committee to its own thoughts on infertility counselling, it departed from the Committee in several crucial respects. Chief amongst these was the emphasis on the welfare of the child. Whilst the HFEA noted the main concern to avoid treatment being provided where there is reason to suppose there is a risk of harm to the child, it specifically recorded its own view that neither the wishes and needs of those seeking treatment nor the needs of any children who may be involved is paramount over the other.

The Code is also less stringent than the King's Fund Committee on the availability of a suitably qualified counsellor in centres, by failing to ensure that counselling for prospective and actual treatment recipients and donors will necessarily be offered by an appropriately qualified and experienced counsellor.

Other tensions inherent in earlier debates are evident in the Code. On the one hand it re-affirmed the emphasis on 'the specialist and non-directional' nature of infertility counselling (HFEA, 1991 p. 8) and the distinction between counselling and the process of assessing prospective treatment recipients or donors (HFEA, 1993, 6.2) whilst on the other noted that: 'the views of all those at the centre who have been involved with the prospective parents should be taken into account when deciding whether or not to offer treatment', (HFEA, 1993a, 3.26).

For the counsellor in licensed centres, therefore, there is an evident tension between the requirements to provide 'proper counselling' and the implications of membership of the multidisciplinary team – especially in relation to multidisciplinary assessment and consideration of the welfare of the child. Similarly the counsellor was expected to be a member of the multidisciplinary team at the same time as being independent of it.

The Code of Practice adopts the King's Fund Committee's notions of implications, support and therapeutic counselling; though it does not separately identify information counselling. (It is important to note that this distinction is potentially confusing, since all three aspects of counselling could, in practice, be provided concurrently, possibly even during a single interview.)

In its first annual report the HFEA conceded that the counselling requirements of the Code of Practice 'are greater than some centres are at present able to meet, not least because of the shortage of appropriately trained or qualified infertility counsellors' and acknowledged its responsibility to 'see what needs to be done' (HFEA, 1992 p. 30).

Although, as noted earlier, BICA had expressed its disappointment about the composition of the Authority's original inspection teams, by 1993 a small number of practising infertility counsellors had been appointed as inspectors. However, since there is no specific 'counsellor' category for HFEA inspectors, such individuals have ostensibly been appointed as 'lay' members. They do not adequately represent the interests of either infertility counsellors or 'lay' people. And, as a consequence of the relatively large pool of 'lay' inspectors appointed by the HFEA, the experience of inspection is thinly distributed amongst inspectors who are counsellors. Equally, the focus on counselling services by inspection teams is likely to be variable, depending on the composition of the team. Without sufficient practice opportunities or clear guidance on the qualitative criteria to be used in assessing standards, it will be some time before inspection teams become universally skilled in this work.

The HFEA's inspection and licensing process represents the most critical means of ensuring the maintenance of standards and, although the specific guidance issued to inspection teams by the Authority is not publicly available, a summary of the process is outlined in the Authority's second annual report (HFEA, 1993).

All centres permitted to operate under the Act's transitional arrangements were inspected between November 1991 and July 1992. As the Act requires, the inspection includes consideration of the counselling provision. The 1993 Report indicates that five licence applications (including two research applications) were refused following inspection. The report does not indicate whether the adequacy of counselling services played a part in any of these decisions. However the report indicates that in an unspecified number of instances licences were issued with conditions attached: 'It is not surprising that many of the conditions relate to counselling, confidentiality and security, the welfare of the child and information for patients' (HFEA, 1993 p. 7).

Evidence, about the inspection of counselling services by the Authority is therefore limited. Certainly the inspection team will not always contain anyone who is conversant with counselling. Regarding the first round of inspections the Authority notes that: 'In most cases the inspection team consisted of a clinician, a scientist and an inspector with skills in nursing, counselling or a background relevant to the Authority's work' (HFEA, 1993 p. 5).

Our view that the extent to which counselling is adequately addressed is likely to depend upon the interests of the 'lay' person inspecting, and will therefore vary according to the composition of each inspection team, appears to be borne out by counsellors themselves. At the end of 1992, BICA distributed a questionnaire to all members working in a counselling capacity in a licensed clinic (Crawshaw, 1993). The 23 questionnaires returned revealed that less than 40% of respondents were present for half or more of the inspection, and only 22% were present throughout the inspection. In four instances, the counsellor was not present for any part of the inspection. Three respondents were unable to give details concerning the composition of the inspection team. Of the remainder, 55% of the inspection teams included a counsellor, whilst 45% did not.

Respondents' views concerning the rigour of the inspection were varied. 22% considered that the inspection had been 'thorough'; 30% thought it had not been thorough; 26% felt it had been 'fairly thorough' and a rather large 19% were unable to comment.

It is perhaps not surprising that most respondents did not know what to expect of the inspections, since only those centres providing IVF treatment would have previously experienced an inspection under the VLA arrangements and there are no publicly available records of these inspections. Nevertheless particular comments about the quality of inspection focused on points such as: 'concerns about the paucity of questioning about professional counselling skills; about the apparent uncertainty among inspectors about what they were looking for and the lack of expertise among inspectors; about inadequate attention to detail; and about inadequate attention being paid to egg donation counselling' (Crawshaw, 1993 pp. 2–3).

Sixty-five per cent of counsellors had not seen the inspection report and just over a quarter did not know whether the report had made any conditions about counselling in granting the licence. Of those who had seen the report three said that licences were granted with recommendations about counselling – two were to improve the accommodation and one was to appoint a counsellor! For example, 'There were a number who commented that they felt that only lip service was being paid to counselling in their clinics with raised attention prior to the inspection and slipping away again soon afterwards' (Crawshaw, 1993, p. 4).

Whilst the views expressed in this survey may not be representative of all centres and all inspections, our earlier reservations about the focus on counselling during inspections appear to be substantiated; there is clearly much to be done if the inspection and licensing process is to exert a substantial impact on standards.

In February 1993, following consultation with interested groups, the HFEA organized a conference on training in infertility counselling to examine the current availability of suitable training in this area. By that time the lack of consensus on standards in training by which the Authority's inspectors could judge any particular individual's level of competence had become apparent. At the conference it was decided that a working group be established to examine the provision of training in infertility counselling. At the time of writing this group, representing a broad range of counselling interests and expertise, had produced a report which was under consideration by the Authority. It is anticipated that the work of the group will clearly be influential in establishing the future directions of infertility counselling in the UK.

Conclusions

In conclusion we aim to draw together some of the threads of the earlier discussion to outline what the future for infertility counselling might look like, in the light of its past. Essentially, the remaining issues centre on the general concerns of the nature of the counselling task and the counsellor's role and, secondly, areas of particular practice that have so far received little attention.

As may have been inferred from this chapter issues concerning equal opportunities and the rights and needs of minority ethnic groups have not so far received much explicit attention, although it is equally evident that the provision of 'proper' counselling needs to be informed by, and take account of, contemporary debates concerning measures to combat discrimination.

Infertility counsellors will need to find ways of accommodating the inherent tension between the requirement to be both integral members of a multidisciplinary team and yet independent of it. As the HFEA notes, an essential ingredient of integration is the presentation of counselling as a routine activity and not simply for those who have problems. Yet the experience of many counsellors themselves is that counselling is not taken seriously by other colleagues, that there are too few practising counsellors for counselling to be genuinely offered as a routine service to all, and that, in many instances, clinical staff in reality do regard the counsellor as the person to whom the 'problem cases' should be sent. Counsellors themselves can play an important educational role in promoting the integration of medical, nursing and counselling approaches to infertility and assisted conception. A further theme in relation to the multidisciplinary approach is the proposal contained in the Government's review of adoption laws, that licensed centres and local authorities should cooperate to establish infertility counselling services (DoH, 1992).

Inevitably, counsellors must be involved in assessing client and donor suitability. Whilst counselling is specifically distinguished from centres' assessment arrangements, the counsellor is clearly expected, as a member of the multidisciplinary team, to contribute to the final decision on whom to accept as a client or donor. Given that counsellors do not encounter all those seeking treatment or offering to become donors, their involvement in such a process can only be partial. Inevitably, though, their advice will be sought, particularly in difficult cases where clinicians themselves have doubts and reservations.

Finally, we address some areas of particular practice that have so far received little or no consideration, but will (or should) become items on the counselling agenda in the not-too-distant future.

We have already referred to the counselling role in surrogacy, which is seen by many as a somewhat dubious means of achieving a family, (for a fuller discussion see Blyth, 1993). Nevertheless it is a 'treatment' that is provided in some centres, and consequently it needs to be addressed by centres' counsellors. Arguably, if surrogacy is an especially problematic enterprise – as most seem to assume – then 'proper' counselling concerning its potential implications is even more necessary for all those contemplating such a step. A self-help organization for those considering surrogacy, Childlessness Overcome Through Surrogacy, has already begun to seek out counsellors who may be prepared to provide an independent and private counselling service (COTS, 1993).

It is necessary to consider the particular needs of those people who are contemplating the storage of gametes because of particular medical conditions or in advance of certain treatments. Expertise in some of these areas – e.g. oncology and genetics counselling – may already be accessible elsewhere, but are unlikely to be readily available within infertility treatment centres.

There is also the need to provide 'proper' counselling for those people who may have been born following the use of donated gametes and who seek information concerning their genetic origins. In many respects, the requirements for such counselling may not be much different from that already provided for adoptees and there is probably much to learn from the experience of post-adoption counselling. In one key respect, however, there is a crucial difference. As the King's Fund Committee noted, the restrictions on access to available birth information afforded by statute to those born following the use of donated gametes 'may prove to be very difficult' in counselling, the focus of which may well prove to be 'the distress and frustration flowing from a refusal to provide this available information' (King's Fund Committee, 1991 p. 19). Whilst those eligible to seek this information will be able to do so from the year 2006, the necessary preparation needs to be undertaken now, including gathering information about donors. Elsewhere it has been argued that the HFEA's attention to this has been less than adequate, though individual centres are able to address these shortcomings within current legislation (Blyth, forthcoming).

Also, as we have previously indicated, the attention given to counselling in licensed centres is not currently matched by that given to counselling provision outside the formally-regulated sector. As it is unlikely that services in this area will be subject to externally-established standards, counsellors, as individual practitioners and responsible professionals, will need to demand and ensure the maintenance of quality control.

This brief historical account has indicated that infertility counselling has travelled a long way since the early, if somewhat naïve, recognition of it as beneficial. As a consequence of the detailed scrutiny and refinement of the task of counselling it is now seen to be an especially complex and contentious activity.

For a summary of major events in the history of infertility counselling please see Appendix 7.

Chapter 11
Infertility Counselling and IVF: The Moral and Legal Background

Len Doyal

Introduction

The scientific and moral dimensions of clinical care go hand in hand. Nowhere is this more obvious than with reproductive technologies, especially IVF. Health professionals within reproductive medicine may often have enormous technical expertise but may well lack understanding of or even interest in the moral issues to which this technology can give rise. For example, a clinician may know perfectly well how to implant a human embryo into a woman but still abuse her right to a reasonable standard of information about her condition and to an informed choice about whether or not she wishes to proceed with the implantation. To ignore such issues poses risks for all concerned, including the resulting child – if there is one.

Counsellors working with infertile couples or individuals face particular responsibility for facilitating informed choice about reproductive alternatives, but what do we really mean by 'informed choice' in this context? Given the large amount of information which might be communicated about such a choice, how much is appropriate for good professional practice? In view of the fact that clients vary widely in their ability and willingness to listen – especially in the face of what is sometimes an overwhelming desire for therapeutic success – how should counsellors assure themselves that the information which they have attempted to communicate has actually been understood to an acceptable standard?

Equally, even if it is assumed that the communication of clinical information has been entirely successful, counsellors still have the task of helping clients to explore their emotional responses to such information. Here, good practice entails not only a clear understanding of clinical issues; but it also requires a sensitivity to the moral dilemmas which prospective parents can face when public opinion is divided. In other words, the role of the counsellor is not just emotional, demanding sensitivity and empathy. It is also educational, calling for an ability to present balanced accounts of whatever moral arguments are creating concern and distress. Suppose, for example, if someone tearfully asks a

191

counsellor: 'If I have a baby in this way, aren't I murdering my embryos which haven't been implanted?'. The counsellor should be able to frame an informed response.

This chapter will address these issues through a discussion of the moral and legal duties and debates associated with good counselling practice for clients who have made a provisional decision to proceed with IVF. Focusing on this in the context of infertility counselling is justified because of the unique dilemmas to which the use of IVF gives rise. However, the analysis does not just apply to IVF: many of the debates and much of the information we will outline also apply to other types of reproductive technologies and to the effective counselling of those who receive them.

The primary duties of care for health-care professionals

Although there is now a vast literature concerning the moral and legal responsibilities of health professionals, much of its content can be summarized within two moral principles. First, the life and health of patients should be protected to the highest standard – 'high' being defined by what is regarded as best practice endorsed by experienced professional opinion. Second, the autonomy of patients – their right to as much self-determination as they are capable of – should be respected. This means that clinicians have a duty to obtain the patient's informed consent to treatment and to maintain confidentiality about information communicated for purposes of treatment (Doyal, 1990).

The general implications of this are clear. Clinical staff should do nothing which they know might cause serious harm to their patients, including allowing others who are inexperienced or inept to 'practise' on them. Further, patients must not be deceived or manipulated into doing what clinicians believe to be best rather than being allowed to choose for themselves.

Similar implications follow for good practice in reproductive counselling. Counsellors should be sensitive to the educational and emotional needs of their clients. Accepted therapeutic and communication skills should be used to maximize informed choice and to minimize the psychological trauma associated with infertility and infertility treatment. Counsellors should act as facilitators, respecting autonomy through helping clients to articulate their own aims and beliefs and to express and explore their associated emotions (Shaw, 1991). The beliefs of counsellors should not be focused on clients. Otherwise, they may embark upon actions which could bring potential harm to them and to any resulting children.

So, as with other forms of medical treatment, the goal of good IVF counselling should be consent which really is 'informed'. This entails communicating clear information about the reasons for infertility, the ways in which technology might solve such problems and the associated physical and emotional risks of using such technology. The feelings of clients about unsuccessful treatment or about ceasing treatment should also be explored. Of course, what counsellors should do in principle and what they can accomplish in practice are not necessarily equivalent. The educational and emotional needs of clients will vary enormously, with some being more receptive to information and discussion than others. In order to maintain some sort of consistency, counsellors should employ what might be called the 'prudent client' model, always critically comparing their existing practice with what they believe an average, knowledgable person would wish to know in the same circumstances (Kennedy, 1988).

The goals of protecting health and respecting autonomy can indeed sometimes conflict. For example, a patient may disagree with their clinician about what is in their best interests; the same applies to IVF counselling. In our culture, it is increasingly accepted that when such conflict occurs, the right to informed consent has priority over the judgement of the 'carer' or medical expert in this case. Individual rights are what are sometimes called 'strict' entitlements – they 'trump' the desires, expectations and preferences of others, no matter how well intentioned those others may be. Because this understanding of human rights has now become widespread, the 'paternalism' which characterized the practice of medicine for so long in Britain is declining (Doyal, 1993). The high value placed by professional counsellors on respecting the wants and needs of clients has also contributed to this decline (Oldfield, 1983).

Yet despite this increasing emphasis on individual rights, they should not be regarded as absolute. It is widely held that individual rights should be curtailed at the point at which respect for them places others at serious risk of harm. For example, though there are many things which I am entitled to do with my private property, I am not entitled to injure you with it. This is just another way of saying that whatever my moral rights, my moral duties include doing nothing which is knowingly injurious to others. This is true whether I am acting as a patient/client or reproductive counsellor (Lesser & Pickup, 1990).

The duty to abstain from harm to others goes to the heart of so many of the dilemmas which confront IVF counsellors. For, in trying to provide help, they can succeed in causing unhappiness. On the one hand, the conflict between an infertile couple is often imbedded deep in the psyches of each partner. Help for one half of the couple can sometimes lead to distress for the other, especially if one or both decide not to proceed with implantation (Greil *et al.*, 1988). In talking this through, for example, couples often come to understand that their wish to conceive a child is really an attempt to resolve other problems in their relationship. On the other hand, and perhaps even more importantly, there can be genuine confusion on the part of clients and counsellor about the potential harm which infertility treatment itself can cause. Unsuccessful intervention can add dramatically to whatever trauma is already present as a result of infertility. Even successful treatment raises the question again of the harm done regarding fertilized embryos which are deliberately not implanted, as well as concern about the future welfare of any resulting children from those that are (Adler *et al.*, 1990).

The potential harm of unsuccessful treatment to the client can be minimized by ensuring that the decision to proceed is as informed as is practically possible (King's Fund Centre, 1991). Of particular importance will be clear communication about the high risks of failure and typical emotional responses to it, as well as strategic advice about what can be done in the face of such reactions. During such discussions, potential recipients and partners can reveal anxieties about the ethics of their intended actions. To help, counsellors must understand the general structure and content of opposing moral arguments. Constructively addressing potential conflicts between the interests of the parent(s) and the potential child(ren) will require similar understanding.

Why IVF?

Infertility can be as disabling as many diseases. It affects more than one in ten couples attempting to conceive children and can lead to chronic unhappiness, depression and the destruction of relationships. While it is true that the success rates of IVF remain low, it does offer some people a significant hope of successful pregnancy. On the face of it, therefore, the procedure can be morally defended because of its potential beneficial consequences and the right of those in need to access to these possible benefits. It also assumes the availability of donated ova (Overall, 1991).

Standard IVF procedures (see Appendix 2) involve the removal of several ova either from the recipient or another female donor. Each of these eggs is then fertilized with the sperm of the partner or another male donor – assuming for the moment that it is the woman and not the man who is infertile. In Britain, usually two and at most three embryos with the best embryological characteristics are then implanted (HFEA, 1991). These are the embryos which have no obvious genetic abnormalities and which appear to stand the best chance of successful implantation. Since many more than three eggs are fertilized for the purposes of such selection, the remainder are either frozen for future treatment cycles or simply discarded.

Some fertilized eggs may also be used for research and great benefit has already been derived from such work. For example, aside from improved success rates for IVF itself, embryonic tissue may be useful in the study of genetic diseases and the development of more and better screening programmes. Other therapeutic uses to which it can now or potentially be put include cancer research and tissue transplantation (Trounson, 1990). Despite all of these benefits, some people argue that discarding or experimenting upon human embryos may count as the deliberate taking of human life.

On the face of it, it could be argued that these spare embryos have only a questionable claim to have their lives protected. Ordinarily, we associate the possession of rights with preconditions for personhood – with the capacity to claim rights in appropriate circumstances. For example, we generally distinguish between persons and animals through arguing that it is only the former which possess human attributes. These include the ability to use language to conceptualize and communicate, to formulate aims and beliefs, to make choices about future courses of action and to be held morally responsible for one's actions on the basis of such choice (Harris, 1990). Equally, when these attributes are radically diminished due to age or severe illness then the allocation of rights may be reduced accordingly. For example, very young children, the severely mentally handicapped, the severely mentally ill and those suffering permanent unconsciousness from severe brain injury, all may be seen to lack the right to informed consent, and in some situations even to life-saving treatment itself (Doyal & Wilsher, 1994).

Moral arguments against IVF

Most arguments against IVF reject the preceding views concerning the moral status of the human embryo. Those who believe that it is morally wrong to kill embryos *in vitro* argue that even though the embryos do not possess the attributes of personhood at present, they still possess the *potential* for them in the future. This is what guarantees their human right to be protected from premeditated killing, in the same way that it can be argued that the fetus should also be protected from abortion. If we believe it to be our duty to protect and nourish children because of their potential to flourish as adults, should this argument not be taken back to the beginning of life (Marshall, 1990)?

There is a further possible theological argument which reinforces the above. A Christian version maintains that a person is formed at conception through a process of 'ensoulment'. The soul is presumably not reducible to a collection of a few cells: it embodies the personal identity which the embryo has the potential to become. Therefore, the destruction of these cells is tantamount to killing that person even though physically and mentally they do not yet fully exist. To the degree that this or a similar argument is accepted, the immorality of killing spare embryos directly follows. Not only would one be taking the life of a potential human but, morally speaking, that of a human in the here-and-now (Reidy, 1982).

The final argument often presented against IVF has both a religious and a secular variant. In the first, it is claimed that the creation of human embryos *in vitro* is 'unnatural' and 'against God's will'. Surely, it is said, it is the height of human arrogance to meddle in God's design – by attempting the creation of life itself. In such circumstances health professionals who ordinarily have a professional duty to preserve human life can find themselves under an obligation to 'take' it. Equally, it is claimed that the relationship of partners and potential children will inevitably be damaged by artificial breaches of the natural reproductive process (DeMarco, 1987). Even in the second viewpoint, IVF is still often represented as creating a slippery slope towards consequences which will be socially damaging and dangerous for everyone. For example, it is argued that the more desensitized we become to the taking of human life *in vitro*, the more likely it is that we will feel the same about human life in general.

The same arguments are applied to research on human embryos, which some also believe to be morally wrong. The deliberate taking of human life for instrumental purposes in the interests of others cannot be justified. Even if somehow it could, the potential benefits would not outweigh the risks. For the knowledge that we might gain must be balanced against the greater danger of a 'brave new world' of reproductive technology and genetic engineering spinning out of moral control. Among other things, the fear is that the quest for reproductive perfection will lead to the general devaluation of human individuality and dignity.

Moral arguments in favour of IVF

We have seen that opponents of IVF argue that there is no moral difference between the spare embryo, the human fetus and the young infant. Since it is widely accepted that the latter has the right not be killed arbitrarily, why should we not say the same for the former. To see how such reasoning might be countered, consider the biological development of the embryo.

Initially, the embryo is a small group of cells with no identifiably human characteristics. For example, it is impossible at this stage to tell which cells from the group will become fetal and which placental. It is equally uncertain whether or not the embryo will successfully implant, develop into one or more fetuses, or even take the form of an abnormal growth – for example, a cancerous mole. None of this becomes clear until around 14 days when the nervous system or 'primitive streak' begins to develop. Even then, the potential of the successfully implanted embryo remains indeterminate. For example, it may still spontaneously abort, suffer a fatal injury during pregnancy or even be deliberately terminated.

Thus it is just not possible to say with certainty whether or not any particular embryo will become a successfully evolving fetus, much less a born infant and adult person (Singer & Dawson, 1990). Yet this moral indeterminacy does not apply to the groups of cells identified as a spare embryo *in vitro* which will not be implanted. With these it is certain that, with no nervous system, embryos at this stage can experience nothing. They have only one potential – at present to live well under 14 days and then to die either as a result of being discarded or experimented upon. Consequently, one of the most powerful arguments of the opponents of IVF appears to evaporate. Or does it?

Opponents who support the benefits of IVF but continue to support the moral rights of the embryo still argue that there is no necessity to create spares. Only eggs which are going to be implanted or frozen for implantation should be fertilized, they maintain. This policy would respect whatever human potential the embryos do possess while not arbitrarily depriving redundant embryos of the opportunity to achieve their potential (Lee, 1986). This chance should certainly be afforded if one believes that all embryos possess souls and in this sense contain an individual human identity from the point of fertilization. To create a situation where some embryos will inevitably be denied the opportunity for self-development cannot be morally or theologically justified.

However, there are two problems with this argument. First, just because something has the potential for being human does not necessarily mean that we have to respect that potential. All healthy sperm and eggs have this potential when combined, but we do not feel obligated to make sure that every sperm or ovum produced can combine. Equally, we now accept that in some circumstances abortion can be morally justified and the potential for human life can be outweighed by other considerations like the life and health of the mother. Spare embryos are created with similar aims in mind – to optimize the success of implantation and thereby the health of the mother (Harris, 1990).

Second, the God cited in these arguments would presumably only want things otherwise if there were some necessity in believing that the soul is present from the point of fertilization. However, we have seen that the embryo only becomes an identifiable human fetus around 14 days. Would it not be more logical to accept that 'ensoulment' occurs here? Some Christian theologians have endorsed such arguments (Dyson, 1990). In any case, given the uncertainty of the moral status of the embryo at conception – compared with adult persons who can potentially benefit from IVF – the actual interests of the adult should not necessarily be outweighed by the possible interests of the embryo (Brazier, 1990).

Finally, is the use of IVF unnatural and the beginning of a slippery slope toward the cheapening of human life and dignity? Few would accept such an argument simply on the grounds that this technology makes certain things happen in nature which would otherwise not. To do so would entail the rejection of all other forms of medical treatment and other technologies which most of us would wish to retain – everything from antibiotics to airplanes. Of course, technological innovation inevitably creates risks of abuse, going right back to the discovery of how to make fire. The trick is socially to control technology which is potentially dangerous, rather than turning our backs on it (Doyal, 1992). There is no evidence to suggest such control is impossible. Indeed, the successful regulation of modern medicine confirms this possibility. Why should the same potential not apply to the new reproductive technology?

The professional and legal regulation of IVF

In countries where IVF is practised it is now subject to varying degrees of legal regulation. While details vary, there is a wide consensus about central issues. In the UK, the history of public scrutiny begins with the Warnock Committee which met in the early 1980s with the aim of exploring the ethical dilemmas posed by this new technology and to formulate proposals for acceptable clinical and experimental practice. Members of the Committee were selected both for their expertise and to represent different sectors of professional and public opinion. Compromise was inevitable over some moral issues, but this did ensure that its final conclusions stood a reasonable chance of political implementation. Generally speaking, the practice of IVF and experimentation on spare embryos was endorsed, subject to strict controls (Morgan & Lee, 1991).

The conclusions of the Warnock Commission were published as the Warnock Report in 1984 and formed the moral basis for constructing the current legislation in Britain: the 1990 Human Fertilisation and Embryology Act (Warnock, 1985). This created a number of specific statutes, along with an authority (the HFEA) responsible for licensing and regulating clinics where IVF and embryo experimentation are undertaken. The HFEA publishes guidelines for acceptable practice and has an inspectorate whose job it is to ensure that clinics adhere to the provisions of the law.

As regards IVF, the most important of these guidelines are as follows:

(1) All IVF, including the storage of gametes or embryos must be done in licensed clinics.
(2) Gametes cannot be stored for more than ten years, embryos for more than five.
(3) All recipients must have the opportunity for counselling and must give their *informed* consent to treatment, along with the storage or donation of gametes and embryos.

(4) Irrespective of their genetic relationship, the woman carrying the child will at birth be its legal mother.
(5) The partner of the recipient (if any) will be regarded as the legal father of the child provided that he has given his informed consent to the procedure beforehand. (This applies equally to artificial insemination.)

The violation of any of these regulations could lead to the suspension of a clinic's license and to the criminal prosecution of those responsible for the offence (Human Fertilisation & Embryology Act, 1990, 3.1; 14.3.4; Schedule 3; 27.1.; 28.1,2).

Equally stringent provisions were enacted for experiments on human embryos. These must only be done to improve treatment and/or understanding of infertility, congenital disease, miscarriage and contraception, along with the detection of genetic abnormalities before implantation. Among actions forbidden are:

(1) Experiments on human embryos of over 14 days.
(2) Research on embryos without the informed consent of donors.
(3) Attempts to clone the cells of human embryos – i.e. replacing their nuclei with those from other humans.
(4) Attempts to create human and animal hybrids (aside from the hamster test for establishing fertility and the destruction of resulting embryos).

Internationally, there is more variation among regulations concerning embryo experimentation than those relating to IVF. For example, some countries (e.g. Germany) do not permit it at all; while others allow more discretion about what research can be performed and when (e.g. Britain – see the HF & E Act 1990, 3.4; Schedule 3.2,c; Schedule 3.3,d; Schedule 4.1,c).

The role of the HFEA is not just to enforce the law but also to interpret it. To do this the Authority publishes a code of practice which articulates and updates good practice regarded as consistent with the relevant legislation. This covers a wide range of issues, including evaluating staff facilities, assessing clients and donors with the welfare of the child in mind, providing information, obtaining informed consent, controlling the various uses of gametes and embryos, storing and handling gametes, embryos, research, records and complaints. For example, comprehensive information must be provided for the purposes of obtaining consent and it is made clear that 'the woman should be given the opportunity to decide whether she wishes to consent to all stages of her IVF ... before it begins'. In the case of research, 'Centres within the NHS should refer research projects to the Local Research Ethics

Committee of the relevant District Health Authority' (HFEA, 1993, 9.7).

The role of the HFEA as an interpreter of the law cannot be over-estimated. It must be flexible enough to apply the spirit of the law to new technological developments and to other problems not necessarily envisaged by the original legislation. It must also carry out its regulatory tasks in ways which are both understanding of the practical difficulties often facing clinics, as well as being fair to the public with whose 'safety' it is entrusted. For example, after concern about the numbers of multiple births from IVF treatment, the Authority has restricted the numbers of eggs which can be implanted to three (HFEA, 1993, 7.9). The positive role of the Authority is also illustrated by its constructive involvement in recent British debates about the maximum age of IVF recipients and the use of ovarian tissue from aborted fetuses to provide ova for implantation. There can be little doubt that the scope and drama of its regulatory problems will continue to expand with further technological innovation.

The interests of the potential child

One of the most perplexing dilemmas facing the reproductive counsellor is the degree to which they should address the interests of resulting children when their primary concern is the interest of their client or clients. We have seen that our rights stop at the point at which their exercise risks harm to others. Children created by the exercise of the right to appropriate reproductive health-care are no exception. But what should this moral principle mean in practice? At one extreme are those who argue for a strict system of vetting future parents, one analogous to that traditionally associated with adoption. Those at the other extreme deny the force of the analogy and claim that IVF is simply an extension of the ordinary reproductive process which should be left to the private choice of the individuals concerned.

The Warnock Commission wrestled with this question and concluded that consideration of the child's interest should lead to some prospective parents being refused treatment. This view was incorporated into the 1990 Act in the form of the following statement: 'A woman shall not be provided with treatment services unless account has been taken of the welfare of any child who may be born as a result of the treatment (including the need of that child for a father), and of any other child who may be affected by the birth' (Human Fertilisation & Embryology Act 1990, 13.5.). Note that this ruling has two different components: one which focuses on the interests of the child and the other on the child's suggested need for a father. As regards the former, there can be little debate about practical implications. For example, a clinic should not give IVF to someone who is discovered to have been convicted of child abuse or who for other reasons (e.g. a large already-existing and/or troubled family) appears incapable of properly looking after any child that results. Indeed, in one famous case a former prostitute sought unsuccessfully a judicial review of the clinic's decision to refuse her treatment on similar grounds (Brazier, 1992).

This said, most dispute about the interest of resulting children has focused on the latter component of the provision concerning the child's best interests – the supposed need for a father. On the face of it, the rule appears to forbid IVF to single women, even if it is accepted that they might subsequently develop a partnership with a man. Lesbian women would certainly seem to be excluded. Such an interpretation is endorsed by those who think that only a childhood within a nuclear family can be a healthy one (Scritchfield, 1989). The popularity of this argument is understandable in a culture so influenced by ideas about the importance of the father generally and by Freudian ideas about the importance of the father in the formation of sexual identity and also infected by varying degrees of homophobia. But are there arguments strong enough to merit denying IVF to a single heterosexual or homosexual woman who wants a child desperately enough to embark on such an often harrowing procedure?

We have already argued that infertile women can be seriously harmed by their condition. There is, as yet, no convincing evidence to suggest that children who grow up in single-parent families face comparative risks. There is some indication that they may suffer disadvantages but these appear at present to be more related to the poverty often associated with such families than to the lack of a father. Further, the converse does seem to hold. That is to say, much of the physical and emotional damage which many children encounter is firmly rooted in the traditional nuclear family. Therefore, if we are going to regulate reproduction with reference to family structure, it makes more sense to concentrate our attention on the suitability of heterosexual couples than on single parents of whatever sexual orientation. The question to ask is, which is worse: for a potential child to run the risks of growing up with a single parent or never having the opportunity to exist at all? The answer seems clear (Doyal, 1992).

The remaining arguments for excluding single women from receiving IVF are religious. Irrespective of the issue of the child's best interest, it is claimed by some that to have children out of wedlock is morally wrong. This might be another version of the belief that assisted reproduction in these circumstances is 'unnatural'. If so, we must return to our previous arguments about the consequences of such arguments for the morality of the whole of modern technology. If the immorality is justified by nothing other than reference to scripture then it simply becomes an article of faith about which rational debate becomes impossible (Dyson, 1990). Suffice it to say that many single women are excellent parents, highly religious and raise their children to be the same. Should they be less respected than other believers just because they are single?

On the basis of arguments like the preceding, the licensing authority has now decided not to ban IVF for single women. Rather it now states: 'Centres are required to have regard to the child's need for a father and should pay particular attention to the prospective mother's ability to meet the child's needs throughout his or her childhood, and where appropriate whether there is anyone else within the prospective mother's family and social circle who is willing and able to share the responsibility for meeting those needs and for bringing up, maintaining and caring for the child.' (HFEA 1993, 3.18). In short, the issue is not the physical presence of a father but the degree to which the traditional role of a father can be met by others. Here, there may indeed be questions to be explored about the absence of any extended family or friends.

Tensions within IVF counselling and other reproductive counselling

The dilemmas which we have examined raise difficult and complex questions which were widely debated before the HFE Act was passed. It is hardly surprising, therefore, that not only candidates for IVF but also their counsellors will at times find the same problems both perplexing and distressing. Counsellors will have their own beliefs. Yet their role is not to impose these upon their clients. Rather, they are charged with helping potential recipients to explore their own beliefs and emotions, as well as trying to ensure that treatment which proceeds will do so on the basis of optimal emotional and intellectual understanding. To achieve both therapeutic and educational aims again will require fluency in articulating the opposing arguments which we have examined above.

Assuming that this requirement is met, what role, if any, does the counsellor play in evaluating the interests of the future child. It might be argued that counsellors should be involved since they will know more about personal details of potential recipients of treatment than their clinicians. Yet this would create enormous contradictions in their professional relationships with clients. Thus the HFEA Code of Practice makes it clear that 'Counselling should be clearly distinguished from . . . the process of assessing people in order to decide whether to accept them as a client or donor . . .' (HFEA, 1993, 6.2). The reasons for this are clear. The honesty between counsellors and clients which is crucial for a successful professional relationship would be impossible if the latter thought that they were being morally judged. Failure would also result from any doubts about the confidentiality of the counselling process. Indeed, in the context of IVF, confidentiality is legally backed up by the Act.

This still leaves open the question of how parental assessment should be done. That it should occur in some way seems clear. Parental rights do not trump the moral obligation to offer protection to potential children whom we believe really will be at risk of serious harm if they are born. Yet the focus of such assessment should not be on individual details revealed in the counselling process but primarily on more general information about the personal background of the parent. This should be made available to the clinic for consideration *before* treatment or counselling are offered. As part of a multidisciplinary team, counsellors are and should be involved in assessment at this pre-counselling stage of potential treatment. They also play a particularly important role in helping to explain why treatment has been refused.

Another dilemma may face the counsellor who is given information which might seriously jeopardize the future interests of an infant. This is a rare situation. However, if it does occur, a breach of confidence might be justified. It is probable that such a client will not have revealed information about themselves and their personal circumstances when first approaching the clinic. If so, they may reasonably be rejected for treatment on these grounds alone without further assessment being an issue. Where this is not the case, a counsellor might reason in a similar way to GPs who have the discretion to report epileptics to the DVLC when they know the patients have not done so themselves. In both cases, if a breach of confidence is contemplated, the patient should be informed.

The difference between the two circumstances is that in the case of the counsellor, the only people who would be informed are clinical staff also involved in the client's care. Thus, according to our codes of ethics and practice, counsellors should do their best to respect the privacy of their clients. Yet they should not feel strictly obligated to keep secrets from clinical colleagues which could severely damage the health and safety of future children. In all other respects, however, confidentiality remains sacrosanct in fertility treatment, only to be broken with the consent of the patient or in order to protect her life and health when she is unable to consent.

Finally, many of the issues raised here about IVF could be applicable to other types of reproductive counselling. Thus questions about the interests of potential children are also raised in relation to regulating the availability of medically managed DI (Doyal & Lesley, 1994). The preceding discussion and conclusions apply equally here, especially those concerning the marital status and sexual preference of a minority of potential single mothers. Also, in discussions about the morality of abortion, arguments about fetal rights pose similar problems to those concerning the rights of embryos.

We have far from exhausted moral debates about IVF, let alone other forms of assisted conception. Issues which have not been discussed concern the appropriateness of artificially conceiving children in an 'over-populated world'; the acceptability of expending scarce medical resources on IVF in the face of other types of more acute medical need; and the problems of assuming that women can give their informed consent to the procedure in light of their psychosocial conditioning in a social environment which links their so-called normality to their reproductive potential and potential as good parents (Warren, 1990).

One of the answers to the over-population argument is that the numbers of children born through IVF are very small due to its low success rate. In the case of resource allocation, much will depend upon how disabling infertility actually is. To the degree that the parental benefits can be shown empirically to be comparable to other forms of accepted medical care then there seems no reason to discriminate against it. With respect to informed consent, the fact that women seem to be socialized into having children does not mean that they are incapable of choosing whether or not to do so. As Overall says: 'We attack the manipulation of women's desires by current medical/ scientific reproductive practices. But we can also resist the too-simple depiction of infertile women as nothing but dupes or victims.' (Overall, 1991). Counsellors should be especially sensitive to the possible coercion some fertile women may be subjected to by poorly fertile husbands to have their biological children (Lorber, 1989).

Conclusion

In this chapter, the focus throughout has been on infertile women and men who have chosen to try to have children through IVF. 'Good counselling' for them will depend upon the seriousness with which counsellors take their client's attempts to control their own reproductive destinies.

We have explored arguments concerning the morality and legality of IVF and, to a lesser extent, experimentation on spare embryos. These arguments have been outlined to shed light on the kinds of questions and dilemmas which often emerge in counselling potential parents, and in debates among counsellors and others. The aim has not been to derive a correct solution to the moral problems posed but to allow the arguments to speak for themselves. To this extent, some conclusions will no doubt seem more reasonable than others.

We have summarized key components of the law concerning IVF and embryo experimentation, highlighting differences between moral and legal issues and showing how the HFEA works at the interface of both. Aspects of good practice in IVF counselling have been discussed, especially the importance of distinguishing between the role of the counsellor and assessor in deciding who should not receive IVF treatment. Throughout, the aim has been to emphasize the intellectual and educational role of reproductive counselling in order to balance the more traditional emphasis on therapy and support.

Chapter 12
What is Fertility Counselling?

Robert Silman

Introduction

To understand fertility counselling is to understand counselling. Understanding counselling is not as simple as it seems.

Doctors have a distorted view of what it entails. On the whole, doctors believe counselling is an elaborate way of referring to good communication, and that counsellors are needed instead of doctors because doctors do not have enough time to spend with their patients. The counsellor is entrusted with the lesser task of hand-holding and sympathy, which the doctor would love to do, if only there were more time in the day. In other words, counselling is a good bedside manner. It is a belittling view, because it supposes that counsellors have no autonomous skills, and that counselling is not a discipline.

It is easy enough to understand why doctors have a hard time understanding counselling. What is surprising is that counsellors also have a belittling view of their own profession. The insistence on something called 'therapeutic counselling' is an indication of this problem. Counsellors are driven to satisfy the positivist ethic of 'healing' and 'cure'. They are intimidated by the accusation that if there is no sickness why bother? But the virtue of counselling, what makes it different from medical advice and therapy, is that it needs no sickness. Counselling is a discipline in its own right which owes nothing to doctors and therapists.

Fertility counselling, and the role of the counsellor in the fertility clinic, present an opportunity to investigate these issues in depth, and to arrive at a definition of counselling which proclaims its specificity and originality.

A statutory definition

The recent legislation governing fertility services in the Human Fertilisation and Embryology Act (1990) makes it mandatory that patients be provided with the opportunity for counselling. The HFEA, the statutory body empowered to enforce the act, has provided guidelines for ensuring that this is done and these guidelines lay down a definition of counselling, of which there are three distinct types (see Introduction and Chapter 17): implications counselling; support counselling; therapeutic counselling.

In addition to defining what counselling is, the HFEA also deems it necessary to spell out what fertility counselling is not: 'Counselling should be clearly distinguished from: ... information which is given to everyone ...; the normal relationship between the clinician and the person offering donation or seeking storage or treatment, which includes giving professional advice; and the process of assessing people in order to decide whether to accept them as a client or donor...'.

It is remarkable that a statutory body should need to define the contents of a discipline. It leads one to suspect that the discipline is one which contains areas of ambiguity and confusion.

I believe there are two reasons for this. On the one hand, there is a group of professionals, doctors, who think they are counsellors by right. On the other, there is a group of professionals, counsellors, who think they are therapists by right. It is my contention that both groups are wrong in their assumptions and this has led to the corresponding ambiguity and confusion which bedevils counselling. Of course nobody would argue that doctors cannot be counsellors, or that counsellors cannot be therapists; but the pity is that counselling, as an autonomous discipline, should be deprived of its specificity by being reduced to either a medical or a therapeutic model.

The medical model of counselling

The HFEA is addressing itself primarily to doctors when it lays down guidelines for what does not constitute counselling. It spells out that counselling is not 'information which is to be given to everyone', nor is it 'the normal relationship' between physician and patient, nor is it 'professional advice'. The reason why the HFEA has to spell this out, is that most doctors have no idea about counselling. Why should they? Medical education does not include counselling in the curriculum. Left to their own devices, most doctors believe that counselling is just a fancy word for a sympathetic ear and sound medical advice. In other words, the HFEA is correct in assuming that doctors confuse counselling with good medical practice, and is well advised to point out the distinction.

All the same, we need to examine the distinction. Why is medical advice different from counselling? What is there about the doctor–patient relationship, at its best, which is different from the counsellor client relationship, at its best? When a patient brings a problem to the doctor, the patient is entitled to expect that the doctor will provide a diagnosis and offer a treatment. It is part of the technical expertise of a doctor to arrive at a diagnosis and identify the best form of treatment. But good medical practice does not stop at technical expertise, it also includes communication. It is the doctor's duty to inform their patients, and to present them with all sensible options concerning the reliability of diagnosis and the efficacy of treatment. The process of giving information is part and parcel of the doctor's duty. The purpose of such communication is to ensure that patients are in a position to make informed choices as to what, if anything, they wish the doctor to do on their behalf. The empowering of patients, in the doctor–patient relationship, is good medical practice: but it is not counselling.

What the doctor gives is not counselling, but expert advice: and advice is only advice if it is understood. Moreover, the fact that it is understood, (and the patient has the means to make an informed choice), does not preclude the doctor from recommending a course of action. On the contrary, the patient is likely to feel cheated if the doctor stands back from the information, and refuses to offer a firm opinion. 'What would you do, doctor?' is a sensible question for a patient to ask; and 'I would do X, Y or Z' is an appropriate answer for a doctor to give. Thus the doctor–patient relationship is not about counselling, it is about giving and receiving advice, and it is none the worse for being just that.

The counsellor, of course, offers no expert advice to the client. It is the other way round: the client is the expert, an expert on their own desire. There is no question of empowering the client in the counsellor–client relationship: the client is already empowered. If there is no empowerment there can be no counselling.

It is probably a good thing that doctors are not counsellors. The roles of doctor and counsellor are different and if practised by the same individual there can be a conflict of interests. The doctor's role is to give expert medical advice and ensure that the advice is properly understood. For the most part, there is no need for counselling in the doctor–patient relationship. But sometimes medical advice is just one part of a complex equation: this is particularly true with fertility treatment. The counsellor's role, unlike the doctor's, is to help the client explore the complexity. Medical problems and solutions can obfuscate other considerations. Where doctors are professionally bound to place the patient's medical problems and treatments in the medical context, counsellors are professionally bound to place the medical problems and treatments in the client context. For a single individual to act as both doctor and counsellor is therefore a hazardous enterprise. The HFEA wisely recommends: 'Centres should offer people the opportunity to be counselled by someone other than the clinician responsible for their treatment'.

Unfortunately, there exists an area of medicine where doctors are half expected to be counsellors: this is the realm of 'informed consent'. When a patient gives informed consent, it should mean that the patient has (i) understood the medical problem, (ii) weighed the treatment option against other treatment options, and (iii) weighed the treatment option against other (non-medical) considerations. As we have discussed, the doctor is only truly competent to deal with the first two issues. Indeed, given the nature of the doctor–patient relationship, it may even be improper for the doctor to go into the third. Doctors are not counsellors, and doctors who proffer advice on non-medical matters are patronizing their patients. But there are all sorts of personal and social pressures which patients have to take into account before consent is agreed, and on the whole, patients are left to deal with these on their own. There is nothing wrong in that, and patients are free to exercise their autonomy as they see fit.

But sometimes they need help. The legislation governing fertility treatment gives a lead for a code of practice in this respect. In the best of all possible worlds, informed consent should mean that a patient has understood the medical problem (communicated by the doctor), has weighed the treatment option against all other treatment options (discussed with doctor), has weighed the treatment options against other non medical considerations. e.g. the implications of the proposed course of action for himself or herself, for his or her family (with the possible assistance of a counsellor), and has consented to the suggested treatment option. In other words, what the HFEA says about fertility services can be extended to medicine in general. 'Centres must make implications counselling available to everyone', with the necessary proviso that no-one is obliged to accept counselling.

The therapeutic model

The purpose of therapy is the cure or alleviation of an ailment; psychotherapy is a form of therapy, its object is the mind (or consciousness). Though there are a wide variety of theoretical therapeutic models, and an even wider variety of practices, the overall purpose of such theory and practice is the remedy of a disorder of the psyche.

Let us consider the Freudian model when applied in a therapeutic context. Here the disorder can be a neurosis and the theoretical model understands the neurosis as being the consequence of an unresolved conflict in childhood – for example the Oedipus complex – leading to the repression of desire. Repressed desire may then manifest itself in later life in a censored form.

However the repressed desire cannot achieve its goals and seeks surrogate expression in neurotic activity, e.g. anxiety, fetishism, etc. The tool of 'cure' is verbal – the patient talks. By talking, the unconscious is made conscious, the perpetual quest to satisfy an impossible desire is purged, and the patient is 'cured'.

Psychotherapy assumes that manifest desire is in some way suspect. It is essentially a reductionist process. It is reductionist on the part of both therapist and patient. 'Your/my apparent desire for X is in fact your/my real desire for Y'. The goal in psychotherapy is to find the Y behind the X and, by reducing X to Y, to purge X from the psyche. Psychotherapy is not counselling because it assumes that: (i) there is a psychological disorder which needs to be resolved, (ii) the psychological disorder is not what it seems, and (iii) the psychological disorder is resolved when it is exposed for what it is.

Is there a place for therapeutic counselling?

This is the fundamental question, and I believe the answer is an unambiguous 'no'. The conjuncture of 'therapeutic' and 'counselling' creates confusion. If we accept our starting premise that the purpose of therapy is to cure (or alleviate) a disorder; and that psychotherapy, of whatever school, is concerned with curing or alleviating a disorder of the mind, then we are entitled to ask of therapeutic counselling 'where is the disorder?'. If patients have blocked tubes or low sperm counts, there is clearly a physical disorder. That is why they come to a fertility clinic. But the fact of a physical disorder does not necessarily entail a psychological counterpart. The patient is entitled to confront the therapeutic counsellor with the question, 'what gives you the right to assume that I have a disorder?'

Consider the definition of 'therapeutic counselling' proposed by the HFEA: its aim is defined as (i) 'to help people to cope with the consequences of infertility and treatment', (ii) 'to help them resolve the problems which these may cause', and (iii) to help people 'to adjust their expectations and to accept their situation'. In what way are such aims 'therapeutic'? The first (helping people to cope with the consequences of treatment) is surely another form of 'support counselling', i.e. helping someone to support an indignity. Since there is no endogenous disorder, there is no need for therapy, unless therapy is a word without meaning. The second definition (helping them to resolve the problems of treatment) is an extension of the first, i.e. a more complex expression of 'support counselling'. Again, if there is no disorder, just problems, why do we bother with the word 'therapy'? Why is there a need to confuse problems, which we all suffer to a greater (abandoned by a lover) or lesser (kettle not working) extent every day of our lives, with disorders (inappropriate depression or anxiety)? This is not a semantic point, or, if it is semantic, it conceals a truth – that counsellors feel a need to be therapists. If that is true, it is a shame as counselling is a noble profession, which is diminished by being reduced to something other than itself.

It is with the HFEA's third example (helping people to adjust their expectations, and to accept their situation) that therapy takes on a real meaning. What is implied by this definition is that people may have unrealistic and inappropriate expectations of their treatment. If that is true (and it may be true for some patients), it suggests that there is an underlying disorder, and if there is disorder, therapy may be in order.

But why call it counselling? There is a perfectly good word to describe such treatment: it is 'psychotherapy'.

The specificity of counselling

By removing 'therapeutic counselling' from the list, it seems we limit counselling to two activities, implications counselling and support counselling. But there is a third type of counselling which takes place, although the HFEA does not give a name to it: it makes the others trivial in comparison. I will call this counselling, 'desire analysis'.

Determining a desire

The first task of a counsellor is to help the client determine what it is they seek. This does not mean that people do not know what they want, it means that sometimes people need a guide to help them explore their desire and reflect on its object.

If we consider the childless couple at a fertility clinic, it may appear self-evident that they desire a child. However the child is not a desire, the child is the object of desire: this distinction is crucial. The desire might be being a parent; satisfying the expectations of others; proving the male partner's masculinity or the female partner's femininity; attaining companionship in later life; or any combination of any number of such desires, all of which can seek expression in the object 'baby'. It is commonplace in human behaviour that our actions are over-determined, and that there cannot be a one-to-one equation between desire and its object. Determining a desire is therefore performing a desire analysis, working through a panorama (or hierarchy) of parallel (or competing) desires.

Why should this be part of counselling? The role of the counsellor is to be a sort of 'alter-ego', another self, with whom the client can enter into an intimate debate. The first area of such debate is going to be around the question 'what do I really want?', and the consequence of such debate should ensure that the object of desire truly satisfies the desire. Unlike my understanding of psychotherapy, the desire of the client is never suspect. However the object of desire is always a compromise and, as with all compromises, its suitability can be questioned.

Exploring the implications of a desire

When the suitability of the object of desire has been affirmed, the task of the counsellor is to explore the implications, both physical and spiritual, of its achievement, particularly over matters which might be neglected in the 'excitement of the chase'. In the case of a child, this can cover mundane considerations of financial hardship, and social isolation, to more complex issues such as the impact of a newcomer (the child) on existing social, familial and affective relationships.

Of course, these are matters which are dealt with in day-to-day life without reference to counselling. However, the particular area where fertility counsellors can be of assistance is exploring those substantive issues which are unfamiliar to the client, such as the demands of treatment, or, the more than likely, failure of treatment.

Supporting the implementation of a desire

Determining a desire and exploring the implications of achieving that desire are processes which are designed to test the object of desire. In other words they are designed to raise the question, 'Do I really want a baby?' The answer is very often 'Yes', and therefore the major role of the counsellor is to offer support in its implementation. At its simplest, this is offering a shoulder to cry on – the reassurance that the patient, in moments of stress of despair, can have a friend who has no other interest at that moment than the patient. But the friend is a professional and will be knowledgeable in seeking support strategies which are not dependent on false hopes or false misgivings.

The fertility clinic

The fertility counsellor is a counsellor whose clients have a specific object of desire, a baby. But fertility counsellors also have a specific social context in which their clients seek a baby, namely the fertility clinic. The specific task of the fertility counsellor is to ensure that the object of desire remains that of the client rather than that of the clinic.

Medical enthusiasm and new technology

For a clinic, objects of desire can be 'high conception rates', or 'pioneering new technology' and so on. So long as the desires of the clinic are compatible with those of the patient, there need be no problem: in other words, the satisfaction of the clinic in providing assisted conception is matched by the satisfaction of the patient in having a baby.

But these aims and desires can be mismatched. For example: there can be satisfaction in the clinic for a successful conception, even though it did not proceed to term, whereas for the patient this might be a more terrible outcome than not having conceived at all. Or, the clinic might propose donor sperm or donor eggs as a means of achieving the object of desire 'baby', whereas for the patient this might negate the object of desire 'my baby'.

Therefore an important role for the fertility counsellor, in supporting the patient through the trials of assisted conception, is to protect the patient from being overwhelmed by the 'desire of others'. The enthusiasm of doctors is infectious, also patients do not like to 'disappoint' their doctors. By encouraging patients to reassert and reaffirm their desires, the fertility counsellor can help to counterbalance such pressures. This does not mean that the fertility counsellor is a patient advocate, i.e. someone who represents or argues a case on behalf of a patient. On the contrary, the job of the fertility counsellor is to support autonomy in an environment where it can be eroded.

Unsuccessful outcomes

It is self-evident that doctors will be happier in the company of patients whom they have treated successfully. Unfortunately, the success rate for assisted conception is low, and most patients will leave without a baby. Hence a successful outcome is doubly satisfying: the patient leaves with the cherished baby; and the patient leaves in the glow of the clinic's contentment at a difficult job satisfactorily concluded.

The corollary is that an unsuccessful outcome is doubly distressing: the patient leaves without the cherished baby; and the patient may be seen as a clinic 'failure'. Because the success rate for assisted conception is low, most patients will end up in this position. It is therefore important that the fertility counsellor help the client find other objects of desire, when it becomes apparent that the quest for a baby is doomed. Also, and just as important, the fertility counsellor must help the client resist the implication that the clinic failure is their failure.

Conclusion: the legitimacy of desire

Unlike the doctor, the counsellor does not attempt to identify an illness nor suggest a means to cure it. Unlike the psychotherapist, the counsellor does not seek a disorder of the mind. If there is not disorder, there is no need for therapy. We dispose of the concept of 'therapeutic counselling' to free counselling to express its true specificity; it is the reverse of 'therapy'. Therapy questions the legitimacy of desire, counselling accepts it. We find that therapy seeks to purge the patient of inappropriate and unrealistic desire, whereas counselling seeks to make desire free by rendering it appropriate and realistic. The purpose of 'therapy' is to purge the patient of unfortunate desires, the purpose of 'desire analysis' is to assist all desire to fortune.

Chapter 13

Who Should Give Fertility Counselling?

Elizabeth A. Lenton

Introduction

As the Director of an IVF unit, I am well aware of the directions given in the HFEA's Code of Practice on the need for counselling provision for patients undergoing IVF treatment. It is evident that patients about to embark on complex infertility treatment do require some form of counselling: but exactly what, by whom, and when, is not yet clear. But it is probably also true that all infertility patients should have access to some form of counselling from the time of their first visit to an infertility clinic.

The HFEA has divided the area of fertility counselling into four main types: information-giving, implications counselling, support and therapeutic counselling. Each of these needs to be considered separately, in the context of who should actually deliver the counselling.

Information-giving

Of the four counselling sub-types, information-giving is the one most universally required and should, I believe, be provided in a structured and systematic way to all patients at all levels of fertility investigation and treatment. The specialist infertility nurse is the best person to provide information in a way and at a level that the patients can understand. She or he is used to talking to the patients, is familiar with all the procedures, and is less likely to become bored by the repetitive nature of the exchange. The infertility nurse has more time available than the medical staff and that time is less costly. He or she is quite capable of operating a structured and systematic interview and of noting specific points of concern expressed by the patient. Indeed, the patient is more likely to express their concerns in an informal interview with the nurse than in a doctor–patient situation. Later on, it is likely that the same nurse (or the same team of nurses) will be heavily involved in the patient's management enabling an element of continuity to operate.

Implications counselling

The infertility 'nurse-counsellor' is also well placed to offer implications counselling. He or she should be familiar with the success rates of the various assisted conception treatments, and as part of the infertility care team, will be able to reflect any recent changes in the management schedules. The nurse should be able to reinforce previous written and verbal information on the hazards and/or side effects of treatment – for example to explain why triplets might not be a good idea, when many patients are initially delighted at the possibility. If she is a woman (and has children herself) she can identify more directly with the patients and has the time and may have the insight to help couples consider the implications of 'success' as meaning more than just a pregnancy (i.e. proof of their fertility) but as the creation of another human life. The implications of failure also need to be explored. Furthermore, it is not unheard of for IVF patients to become acutely anxious if they do find themselves pregnant, even to the point of considering a termination because they had become so dedicated to the pursuit of treatment for infertility that they had never stopped to contemplate how they would cope with fertility. This situation could be construed as just as much a failure of the implications counselling, as the case of a couple who are quite convinced that IVF will work first time for them, and that consequently the ensuing normal menstrual period must be a miscarriage.

Support counselling

The need for support during and after treatment is required to different degrees by different couples. Most couples remain confident during the initial treatment, and the egg collection procedure itself. However, difficulties are often experienced whilst waiting to hear whether fertilization has occurred and many patients find the interval between embryo replacement and pregnancy-testing the most difficult to endure. It is also possible that the marked hormone changes which occur as a result of ovarian stimulation exacerbate feelings of depression, in a manner not dissimilar to transient post-natal depression.

Support counselling should in someway be provided by all members of the infertility care team, from the receptionist through the infertility nurses to the clinicians. It is possible that more could be done in terms of patient managed self-help or support groups and certainly patients should not be deterred from contacting clinic staff for advice. This can be greatly facilitated if the clinic has sufficient manned telephone lines and nurse-counsellors available to ensure that patients are not discouraged from requesting support. A few patients will experience a major domestic or emotional crisis at this time, often precipitated by the demands of assisted conception treatment, and these couples should always be offered rapid (i.e. within 24 hours) contact with the independent infertility counsellor attached to the unit, at no extra charge.

Therapeutic counselling

A small proportion of couples will actually need specialist therapeutic counselling either before, during or after treatment. These couples will generally have been identified by the clinical personnel or the trained counsellor and will probably require referral to the social work agency. Lists of local appropriately qualified agencies should be available in all clinics, as recommended by the HFEA.

The counselling environment

A number of counselling locations are required as appropriate to the various components and types of counselling. Most doctor–patient consultations are traditionally rather formal affairs, with the doctor 'protected' behind a desk, and the couple sitting in front of him. Though eye-to-eye contact can readily be established, the physical barrier helps to keep the patients remote and the doctor detached. This may prevent patients from speaking freely and asking trivial questions; they will often make comments like 'the doctor seemed a busy man and I didn't like to bother him'.

Information-giving and implications counselling can be provided in a less formal setting, for example using easy chairs in a small comfortably furnished sitting room by a nurse-counsellor. Cups of tea or coffee could be available and the only table permitted would be a small coffee table. Couples could be left alone in the room to discuss issues raised between themselves and there should be no pressure on them to hurry even though there may be a waiting room full of people outside.

This same environment could be equally suitable for specific support counselling, though much of this would take place during normal clinic interactions, for example during blood sampling, ultrasound scanning and so on.

The counselling staff identification

The concept of the nurse-counsellor has already been alluded to. Since such a person is clearly part of the health-care team, she needs to be seen to represent the clinic and so should wear the appropriate clinic uniform, with name badge. The clinicians too will generally be in a white coat or something similar, again with name badges. The infertility counsellor, however needs to present an independent demeanour and therefore should not wear uniform.

All infertility clinic personnel must appreciate that they too are in a way part of the counselling team, from the receptionists through to the biologists, and training for all of them in the management of distressed clients would be advantageous.

Written information

It is freely acknowledged that most patients are only able to retain a fraction of the information presented verbally during a consultation and so each clinic should have detailed, user-friendly written information which can be provided either in advance or at counselling itself. These information sheets can also be used to explain the system and to provide details of telephone contacts and helplines. Production of such material is however difficult and not many clinics have yet addressed the problem satisfactorily.

Chapter 14
The Doctor's View of the Counsellor

O. Djahanbakhch, E. Saridogan & A. Kadva

Introduction

The early days of my involvement in the field of subfertility are still vivid in my mind. I recall the busy subfertility clinic on Monday afternoons. The long narrow corridor was lined with several chairs occupied by couples waiting to see the doctors. They sat silently with anxious and concerned faces. The clinic was organized very efficiently and it was very precise and mechanical in its approach to patients. My duty as a junior doctor was to complete the history and clinical examination in the short span of twenty minutes. This would be followed by microscopic examination of a vaginal swab. In the absence of obvious infection, a very crude technique of tubal insufflation was performed that same day. If the fallopian tube was blocked, a hysterosalpingogram was performed and the couple was seen by a senior doctor at the next visit, and considered for tubal surgery. If an ovulatory disorder was suspected, induction of ovulation therapy was started.

These were the only two modes of treatment available. If they failed, there was nothing further to consider, and the patient was then discharged from the clinic with precious little to look forward to. In those days we were trained to perform tubal surgery, and monitor induction of ovulation with proficiency, but the training sadly lacked in providing any form of instruction in the psychological aspects of subfertility or infertility. I cannot recall a single lecture on this subject. If, however, the female partner suffered from any obvious psychiatric disorder, she was promptly referred to the hospital psychiatrist.

Over the past two decades investigative and therapeutic procedures in the field of subfertility have progressed in leaps and bounds. Laparoscopy has become a routine procedure, and endocrinological testing is now freely available. The culmination of this progress was in the birth of the first test-tube baby in 1978. This exciting new development opened an avenue for those women with tubal disorders who until then had practically no hope of conceiving.

Although the technique brought great hope it also raised doubts among sceptics, some of whom even suggested that the such an embryo could be the result of a parthenogenetic process rather than an *in vitro* fertilized egg. These doubts were prevalent despite the work of those such as Chang (1959), who was the first to provide convincing evidence that fertilization could occur *in vitro*.

There were moral, ethical and scientific concerns that the technique might produce an abnormal embryo. If the experts were confounded, one can imagine how perplexed the public was. Nobody was prepared to provide any funds or grants for research into these issues. In 1979, I was appointed, with a group of scientists at the Reproductive Biology Unit of the Medical Research Council in Edinburgh, to study the incidence of chromosomal abnormalities following *in vitro* fertilization. During that time our work was also involved in improving the techniques of monitoring follicular development, measuring the luteinising hormone surge, and predicting the exact timing of ovulation. Very little was known of the size of the pre-ovulatory oocyte (potential egg), or the desired internal diameter of the oocyte aspiration needle. All this vital information came to light and offered great potential for the many IVF units which were growing rapidly. While the work was in progress, we found that babies born after IVF were indeed normal which allayed fears about chromosomal abnormalities.

However, the success rate of IVF were still very poor. Scientists and clinicians were continually striving to develop newer techniques to achieve better success. One of the alternatives to *in vitro* fertilization was the introduction of sperm and oocyte directly into the cavity of the uterus without prior fertilization. Although pregnancies did occur as a result of this technique, success rates were still rather poor. As a clinician, I was fascinated by these phenomenal discoveries, and while all these revolutionary discoveries captured the imagination of the medical profession, the public remained confused and unsettled. But those infertile women who realized and accepted that this was the only hope for them travelled far and wide to seek such treatment.

The lay press not only served to bring these developments to everyone's attention but also succeeded in sensationalizing the treatment. Newspaper headlines such as 'first IVF twin pregnancy', '... first IVF triplets,' accompanied by photographs of babies, doctors and scientists, were often seen. Some clinicians and scientists were unhappy about this because it created an unnecessary element of competition among various units. Sometimes, in order to achieve higher success, more embryos were replaced into the uterus. This resulted in multiple pregnancies, an increase in spontaneous miscarriages, premature births, and some severely handicapped children as a direct consequence of the premature births.

For the subfertile parents and couples this was a time of great excitement and confusion. It was inevitable that all attention was then focused on improving clinical and scientific standards, and very little heed was given to the attitudes and feelings of the patients themselves. Those who were seen in general gynaecology clinics would have their clinical examination, often in the presence of medical students and untrained nursing staff. Very little attention was paid towards the emotional needs of these patients. Couples often waited up to three years to see the specialist for the first visit, followed by another two to three-year period on a waiting list, for a procedure which offered only 15–20% chance of success. All of this uncertainty would have had a significant psychological impact on these individuals.

All clinicians now appear to acknowledge the enormous emotional and psychological impact of subfertility. The question is, who should be the one to attend to this psychological impact with professionalism and sympathy? Should it be the doctor, the patient coordinator, a qualified nurse, a professionally trained psychologist or counsellor, or should it be a family member or friend?

Although various members (doctors and nurses) of the infertility medical team may contribute towards counselling, their involvement mainly extends to giving information about and explaining the technical complexities of various investigations and procedures. Furthermore the doctors, who play a major part in the decision-making process of the couple's management, are not detached enough to allow the couple the freedom of unreserved expression of their true feelings and fears. The couple may still have some difficulty in comprehending all the technical terms, and the implications of the treatment that lies ahead. They may also feel diffident or embarrassed about questioning 'the doctor' or indeed, about the treatment itself. It is important to give them every opportunity to discuss their misgivings and misconceptions, and to convey to them that they are not merely egg- and sperm-producing robots. They should be made to feel part of the decision-making process itself; and also prepared for the real possibility of failure.

It is of great importance to emphasize that the psychology of infertility is very individual to each couple. It is intricately related to their own cultural attitudes, country of origin, and ethnic and religious beliefs, and some writers are now addressing these intercultural issues. The cultural attitude of the community that the couple live in is also very important: for example, in some cultures having a family with a large number of children is the norm, and failure to procreate brings shame on the infertile couple and undermines their role within the community. Cultural differences may also affect the acceptability of some investigations and treatment options: there are some men who do not want to be investigated at all, because in some cultures, it is usually assumed that infertility is always due to a female problem, and investigation of the male partner would imply that his sexual prowess and ability is questioned. For this reason, women from such backgrounds are usually sent alone or with their mother or mother-in-law for the first consultation. Similarly, this attitude would render many treatment options unacceptable, and donor insemination especially would be entirely out of question. Therefore, azoospermia has profound psychological and social implications in those countries and religious sects where donor insemination is not only taboo but illegal. Sadly, the inability to conceive, in such societies, gives the husband grounds for divorce or the right to have another wife.

Careful consideration of all these factors not only facilitates the investigation and management of such couples, but gives them the ability to cope with their situation. There are instances where counselling is difficult or impossible even for a professionally trained and experienced counsellor. It is not rare to see patients from countries where assisted reproduction technology is either not readily available or where the use of donor gametes is illegal. These are the couples who need the greatest support and counselling because either the decision has already been made for them or, the decision they are about to make goes against their traditional beliefs and culture. The task of the counsellor, in this situation, is made almost impossible when compounded with a language barrier and lack of background knowledge – very few counsellors have any training in anthropology. Such patients, therefore, may end up undergoing treatment without proper communication between themselves and the medical staff.

In the West, infertile patients are referred for psychological support to a counsellor. The role of the counsellor is that of cushioning the 'blow' at each step of this uncertain time of their lives. The counsellor is also a subtle 'bridge' between the infertile couple and the medical team. The aim of establishing this rapport is to inspire confidence in the couple to make them feel that we, the doctors, are on their side and, that the team as a whole understands their individual problem.

In the East, the majority of patients get support from their family members and friends, which can in some cases be as effective as professional counselling. Furthermore, it is important to recognize that many patients consider their thoughts and emotions to be very private and personal and do not wish to express them to strangers. We cite the example of a recent case of donor insemination, where all the emotional care and support in each treatment cycle was provided by the patient's mother. Her contribution was highly appreciated by both the couple and the medical staff. Nonetheless, such a situation is rare. The question of who should provide counselling for a particular patient cannot be answered simply, and should be considered on an individual basis.

It is important to perceive the role of the counsellor as not one who is there to screen the couple for inclusion or exclusion into a treatment programme. At the same time, the interest of the unborn child have to be protected. Undoubtedly the confidentiality between patient and counsellor should not be breached, but if the counsellor's impression is that the couple is not ready for parenthood, then all team members have to assess whether delaying treatment would be appropriate. The counsellor is not the assessor; rather that is the role of the multi-professional team.

Conclusion

In this chapter we have highlighted some developments which have contributed to the recognition of the psychological needs of people suffering subfertility or infertility. Whereas medical and nursing staff are well placed to provide information, advice and treatment, counsellors are needed to give psychological support. The importance of increased cultural awareness should be recognized, and in particular, the differences between East and West in relation to family support systems. In this regard, it is important to understand that the counsellor's role can also be fulfilled by a supportive, sympathetic and understanding person who may or may not be professionally trained.

Chapter 15
The Doctor as Counsellor

J. Q. Norman-Taylor, A. M. Lower & J. G. Grudzinskas

Introduction

The doctor occupies a powerful position in society and is sometimes even thought of as a giver or taker of life. With this degree of power, the relationship with the patient is such that advice is given on the assumption that the doctor knows what is in the patient's best interest and that the patient is likely to do his or her best to take the advice or carry out the treatment.

For the subfertile couple the role of the doctor is subtly changed. The couple are not ill as such and will have more control of the situation. If they do not seek treatment it is unlikely that any physical harm will result. Equally if they choose not to follow the treatment or guidelines suggested by the doctor, the consequences for the couple will not be a deterioration of their health. The role of the doctor is changed from the provider of health care to that of provider of advice for the couple, in other words the doctor becomes their 'counsellor'.

High levels of stress are associated with reduced conception rates in subfertile couples, not least because of reduced sexual activity. Any visit to a doctor is associated with anxiety, and it is particularly important that the doctor treating couples for fertility-related disorders seeks to reduce this stress as far as possible. The doctor must build up a relationship of trust with the couple as medical therapies with potentially serious side-effects may be administered, or potentially dangerous procedures may be undertaken. Equally, the couple must have complete faith in the confidentiality practised by the doctor and the information kept in the records, if a complete and accurate history is going to be obtained.

However, no matter how approachable the doctor might be, there may be some things that a couple feel unable to discuss with the doctor, but may raise with a coordinating nurse, embryologist or counsellor. Liaison with the rest of the team is therefore a vital aspect of the doctor's role. Good feedback and discussion among team members (without breaking confidentiality) ensures that the most appropriate input is provided to the couple at all stages of their treatment. The doctor, whilst using counselling skills, is not a trained counsellor. In other words, if after assessment the doctor feels that the couple would benefit from counselling or further exploratory work of a psychological nature, then an appropriate and efficient referral can be made to the most suitable person on the team to deal with this.

Communication

Most communication between the doctor and a couple seeking treatment will take place in an outpatient situation. In these consultations, both the doctor and the couple will have their own agenda. The doctor's agenda is to take a history, perform an examination, carry out tests, make a diagnosis and, analysing the couple's needs, formulate a management plan. The couple's agenda is based upon the expectation of a conception and what they need to do is conceive, with the associated complications of financial, emotional and social costs. Whilst there is usually a broad overlap in these aims, this is not always the case. The doctor and the couple will try to come to terms with this through verbal negotiation and develop a relationship through which they can communicate: this is known as the doctor–patient 'relationship'.

The doctor–patient relationship

The question of whether we get better more quickly because of good relationship with a doctor is a difficult one to answer. Whether pregnancy is more likely to occur when a couple are attended to by a doctor they like or have respect for poses even more difficult questions.

There is some evidence which suggests that speed of recovery from operation and illness is related to the level of confidence that a patient has with a doctor, possibly because of the interpretation of symptoms or the likelihood of taking medication. Faith does seem to play some role in most medical interactions. In the past, the recovery was based almost entirely on faith when subjects were bled, purged, sweated, fumigated, had leeches attached, were administered concoctions, potions or elixirs. However patients seemed to recover regardless of what was done to them.

In any human interaction there will be some reaction on the social level; a doctor with a good bedside manner will generate much more confidence than one with a poor one, and may hope to get a speedier recovery. Certainly, episodes of humiliation or degrading aspects of treatment, if not minimized, will have the opposite effect. The patients' perception of a medical interaction will depend upon the manner of the doctor concerned and this may be related to status. A more authoritarian attitude will be expected from the consultant specialist, but may not be tolerated from the junior house doctor: nevertheless, it must be emphasized that an authoritarian attitude that reduces the patient to a state of fear would be detrimental to any patient.

The doctor–patient relationship can be broadly categorised into four areas:

(1) The active doctor and the passive patient scenario is obviously desirable when the patient is comatose, under anaesthetic or dangerously ill. In other settings, an authoritarian structure would be uncomfortable for most patients, as most individuals wish to have some degree of control in their medical management.

(2) A doctor–patient relationship of guidance and cooperation is a paternalistic relationship, where the expert medic gives advice to the willing patient which he or she is expected to follow. This is suitable in many cases of medical interaction, for example an acute infection for which the patient is expected to take the antibiotics.

(3) Mutual participation is an interaction where there is mutual cooperation in which power is more evenly distributed. Though this is rare in most medical interactions, in the fertility setting this is often the most appropriate.

(4) A fourth unusual type of relationship may develop, in particular, in people who have had a lot of exposure to physicians. This is one of 'doctor as technician', where the patient or client knows what he or she wants and the doctor is merely the facilitator of this. In the subfertile couple, the woman, after the latest of several IVF attempts, may just want her prescription and her operation, feeling that there is not much else to be discussed.

The structure of a medical interview

Medical decision-making is directed at making a diagnosis through the use of a complicated and highly specialized set of rules. These will include taking a history, which in order that all the relevant questions are asked with no important points missing always follows a specific pattern. Although different doctors will vary the approach somewhat, the pattern will remain much the same. Following the taking of a history, it is usual for the patient to be physically examined. This is in order to confirm the suspicions that the doctor already has about the condition of the patient and in order to exclude any other unexpected findings. Lastly, the patient may be subject to investigations. Within this format the infertility specialist will be making a social and psychological as well as a biological assessment of the patient and couple.

In order for the doctor to obtain a history properly, a couple must feel able to part with all the information, and all physical and psychological barriers to this communication must be removed. The interview will usually start with a set of closed questions i.e., questions that have simple, factual and to-the-point answers. The doctor must avoid the use of jargon in order not to confuse the couple, and should try to keep the interview on a narrow track at first. Once an understanding of the background to a couple's problems has been established, the questioning will broaden out towards open questions with the use of silence and space to allow the couple to be able to communicate their fears and feelings freely. Gradually, the questions will come from the couple and information will begin to flow in the other direction.

Giving information

A consultation is the two-way exchange of information and an important a part of any interview will include an explanation, diagnosis or treatment plan. It is important to note that in a general medical consultation, most patients will forget the majority of what has been said, including how to take therapy or the plan of action.

The degree of explanation needed for sometimes complex pieces of information will vary between patients, and may depend upon their own level of education and their willingness to understand the workings of their own body. Certainly some women and men would rather not know too much detail about their bodies. The doctor needs to balance the amount of information giving, avoiding patronizing the couple, or giving too much information and causing confusion.

The language used by doctors is very different from that used by lay people. Even what doctors might regard as the simplest of medical phrases may be meaningless to many, even educated people. It is important to use non-medical terminology as much as possible and to find a suitable level of common and medical language for both doctor and patients.

The adage that a picture can be worth a thousand words is very true in this situation, and stylized diagrams can be very helpful. Couples must be allowed to feel free to make notes during a consultation and many practitioners will make up a short summary for a couple to take away with them which would include the important points covered. Books and informative leaflets in plain language can also be helpful.

The clinical setting

The traditional setting of the doctor facing the patient across a large oak desk is not optimal for the establishment of a relationship based on trust and frankness with a subfertile couple. A desk is generally required because of the need to make formal notes, therefore most subfertility clinics are set up so that the couple can be interviewed across the angle of a desk. The room styles are often clinical in nature which will not contribute to the relaxation of the couple. Clinical settings may have the detrimental effect of sterilizing the process of procreation, when a fertile effect is being looked for. Attempts should be made to 'desanitize' the surroundings and to convert the clinic into a 'fertile ground', (see Chapter 6).

Because of the nature of the fertility problem, several clinic visits will often be required. If possible the couple should always see the same physician and if this physician is not the senior doctor, then they must understand that their case will be discussed with and managed according to the protocol of the senior doctor. This will allow for the development of a relationship between the couple and the doctor, and avoid the need for a frustrating repetition of their clinical history.

A common situation that couples will face is that there will often be other people e.g. medical students or doctors in training in the room. Most doctors feel that the teaching of students and junior doctors is an essential part of their role. They must be aware that this will provide an added stress for some patients and must be sensitive to the wishes of some of the couples not to have a student present.

Time waiting for appointment

Even though a couple may have waited many months before making a decision to seek medical help, once the decision is made, most would prefer to move ahead with medical treatment as quickly as possible. Many will feel that their life is 'on hold' whilst this problem is sorted out, and will feel unable to make other life decisions whilst no progress is made in terms of conception. Long waiting-times before treatment should generally be avoided.

However, in some circumstances, the delay may prove to be beneficial, as some couples will be seeking treatment at too soon a time interval and conception may well occur spontaneously without intervention. The appropriate length of this time interval is generally held to be 12 months, though this is open to discussion. For example, a 37 year-old woman in a new relationship who knows that she has bilateral tubal damage should be seen sooner than a 25 year-old who has failed to conceive after six months of marriage. Whilst the psychological problems faced by both may be equally pressing, the time factor is clearly on the younger woman's side and her chances of spontaneous conception much greater.

Time allowed for the visit

As long waiting lists to be seen in a fertility clinic are common, it is inevitable that, within the NHS, there is pressure on the time available and the length of time available for each consultation is therefore rationed. The physician may feel at times that the consultation has not been complete but must also be aware that there is a waiting room of other couples outside who equally have been waiting for their consultation. In order to balance these priorities the doctor must be able to seek the help of other individuals within the clinic set-up, such as the nurses or the counselling staff.

Conclusion of the interview

A couple may feel that there are aspects of their care that have not been fully explored during a consultation. If they have had to wait many months before they are seen and then feel that their consultation is incomplete it may be difficult to terminate the interview. Again the liaison with other members of the team may help to resolve this issue.

Expectations of patients

The first visit to see the hospital doctor will be a time of great expectation. A couple will often hope that the doctor will be able to suggest a simple remedy which will result in immediate conception. This is of course most unlikely and whilst most couples will not expect this in reality, it will remain a hope. When the true situation becomes apparent, anger and resentment may be expressed unless a careful explanation is given together with the outline of treatment options.

This situation is magnified when the couple are at tertiary referral stage – in other words, they have already been reviewed and undergone treatment in their local hospital and have been referred to one of the major centres. The couple may be expecting to see an eminent physician and, on meeting him or her, may find the experience daunting. Conversely, seeing one of the junior staff may result in resentment, and a feeling that they have some how been cheated.

It is important therefore that, right from the beginning of a period of consultation, a couple do not have unrealistic expectations of the doctor and that they understand what is the likely course of events and possible outcome of their treatment.

Hiding information from the doctor

This can be a common problem encountered in the initial consultation with the couple. There can be a host of reasons why couples conceal important information regarding their past history both from the doctor and from their partners, an obvious example being the failure to disclose a previous termination of pregnancy, or any sexually transmitted disease suffered. The area of conception and fertility is obviously a sensitive and emotive area and couples may be embarrassed and worried about revealing aspects of their personal history in this manner.

They may be anxious that revealing certain facts pertinent to the situation may cause problems in their relationship, which is already under some potential strain since undergoing fertility treatment; or they may feel that in some way true revelation may jeopardize their place on the programme. This problem certainly needs sensitive handling and emphasizes the importance of thorough history-taking.

Permission to give up or defer treatment

Once a couple have attended the infertility clinic they may perceive themselves to be on a treadmill of time-consuming, emotionally draining and expensive treatment, which is difficult to get off. It will often seem easier for the couple to continue with medical therapy as that does not require a finite decision as such, whereas a conscious decision to discontinue or defer treatment may be more painful. Also, a couple may feel that they will offend the members of the team who have been treating them, and that so much work has already been carried out on their behalf that it would be rude to stop now. It is important, therefore, that each couple is fully aware of their options which must always include one of no active medical treatment. Couples must also not feel as if they should continue treatment to please the doctor.

Dealing with anger

Although every effort will have been made to discuss the options with the couple, it is inevitable that the breaking of bad news regarding unsuccessful conception will be a major role of the doctor in such a consultation. This is not a straightforward task for the clinician. The couple are likely to be experiencing a culmination of bewildering feelings and emotions. They may feel an extreme feeling of failure, despondency and guilt. At the same time, they may wish to direct a lot of these feelings towards the doctor, whom they may perceive to be the main counsellor of their potential conception. It is therefore important for the doctor to be perceptive to these feelings and whilst the doctor may not be the most appropriate provider of more thorough counselling for the couple, discussion with the doctor at this stage is necessary for a discussion and referral to the team member who can provide this service.

Treatment protocols

All clinics require protocols which outline diagnostic and treatment strategies for the management of their patients. An important aspect of this protocol is to ensure the existence of adequate lines of communication. Regular meetings involving all members of the team are essential. The doctor will commonly take the convenor's role at these meetings, but this does not always have to be the case. The setting-up of these rules ensures a fair distribution of the available resources. These protocols should be established in advance with all members of the fertility team. Another important aspect of team liaison is to ensure that all the correct procedures involved in the treatment of the couple are maintained and implemented.

Accepting responsibility

Most fertility clinics have been established by one of the medical staff within the team. It is the medical staff who have to take clinical responsibility for the treatment that the couple undergo, and who are most likely to take legal responsibility for their care. For these reasons, most teams working in the fertility arena will look to a member of the medical team as their leader and with this role, other responsibilities will often have to be accepted. The couple often will look to the doctor as the one responsible if things go wrong, or for explanation should treatment be refused or if there is bad news to be explained. The doctor must remember that he or she is not necessarily the best person to deal with those matters when they arise, and have a ready channel of communication to other members of the team who may be better equipped.

Conclusions

For a doctor working in the area of fertility there are a great many rewards on offer. He or she can practise his or her skills as a clinician, surgeon and counsellor. Great ethical debates can be entered into in which his or her words will be carefully listened to. With success comes the greatest reward of all, the creation of a new life. However, the doctor must remember that he or she is just one member of a team of people that go to make up a successful clinic, where success may not necessarily be measured in terms of pregnancies per couple.

Chapter 16
Infertility Counselling: A Consultant's Personal View

Roger Neuberg

Introduction

Ask most consultant physicians and surgeons if they counsel their patients, and the reply will be: 'Of course, it's part of the job, we do it all the time.' They are right, it is, but do they really?

Traditionally the consultant's role has been to give an informed opinion based on physical findings and investigations, to advise on the most appropriate action to be taken, and then to carry out the proposed treatment. The patient will usually be given information on the nature of the treatment and, if fortunate, be told something of the implications and consequences of being so treated. As far as the patient is concerned, our role as consultants is to diagnose, explain and treat. We certainly advise and give guidance, which is the dictionary definition of counselling. We *tell* the patient what should be done for their particular medical problem; this enables patients to give informed consent, possibly, but does not constitute true counselling.

This distinction was brought home to me recently. I asked the counsellor on the Assisted Conception Unit to help a distraught patient of mine whose very pre-term baby had just died on the intensive care neonatal unit. My patient most willingly agreed to see the counsellor, who went up to the neonatal unit to give some initial support with a view to offering bereavement counselling. Upon her arrival on the unit, the counsellor was challenged by the senior registrar with the enquiry 'Who are you?' She introduced herself saying that she was the counsellor who had come to help my patient. The reply was mind-boggling: 'But I've already counselled her. I've explained what has happened and we will be seeing her again in six-weeks time in the outpatients clinic.'

Virtually all gynaecologists will see infertile couples in their outpatient clinics and would accept that the investigation and basic correction of infertility was part of the service they had to offer. Indeed, they have no choice, as infertility is now the commonest reason for referral to a gynaecologist. All gynaecologists would agree that infertility is upsetting to the couple, but I am confident that most will not truly appreciate how the anguish, despair and bitterness experienced by many infertile couples can devastate their lives and even destroy otherwise loving relationships.

Although I had run my own infertility clinic for 15 years, it was not until I became involved in *in vitro* fertilization (IVF) some four years ago that I really recognized the grief-state associated with infertility. At first I found it difficult to accept that a failed IVF treatment cycle was a cause for grieving. I had always recognized that miscarriage was a dreadful experience and could understand the grief associated with that event: and surely a stillbirth was worse, and what about a cot death or the death of an older child? How could a failed IVF cycle compare with the loss of an actual pregnancy, or of a child? I argued that IVF was basically a treatment which was, admittedly, complex, that failure was distressing, but it was something which could always be attempted again, hopefully with success next time. How wrong I was.

Unlike any other member of the animal kingdom, the human has the ability to hope. In an IVF treatment cycle, in particular, there are so many hurdles for the patient to pass: will the follicles grow?; will the sperm preparation be alright?; will the eggs be retrieved?; will they fertilize?; will good embryos result?; (couples see their embryos down the microscope – their potential babies); will the embryo transfer go well?; will it all work? The 'dream' baby implants in their minds even though they know they should not hope, and that the chances of failure are far higher than success. The coming of the woman's first period after an attempted treatment is like a kick in the teeth, and the dream baby that never was is lost. Even though I take them through this sequence of events, I also warn them that it will not prepare them for the shock of failure. Many couples will, after the initial upset, recover their perspective and normal outlook on life. But for others a true grief-state follows.

Practising doctors are generally very poor counsellors. After all, we are not trained to carry out this work. We are trained to assess and come to a decision and tell the patient of that decision. For a doctor to be a good counsellor, that medical role must be unlearned. As an infertility specialist I discuss treatment options, and carry out information, implication and consequence counselling every day. But I am not a bereavement counsellor although I have experienced bereavement. I know that I have become a better doctor since my mother died. It is much easier now for me to put an arm around a distressed person and offer comfort. But I have not been trained to counsel patients in how to cope with their grief.

In accordance with the HFEA Code of Practice, counselling is always offered before any licensed treatment is carried out. It is interesting that most couples are more than happy with the information they receive from the infertility medical specialist and infertility nurse specialist during the preparation before treatments such as donor insemination and IVF and may therefore decline the offer of counselling. I have found that the take-up of the offer of free counselling (even in the private sector) before treatment is less than 10%. Although assisted conception units are advised not to push patients into counselling, there are always situations when the specialist will inform a patient that counselling will be a requirement before a particular treatment can be offered. This would apply for example to single women without a partner, homosexual couples, in cases of possible surrogacy and particularly where there may be concerns for the welfare of the child resulting from treatment. The need to counsel the donors of eggs, sperm and embryos is clear-cut.

I do know that a number of specialists are irritated by the emphasis that the HFEA put upon the need for trained infertility counselling. They argue that most patients don't want it and don't need it, and they complain that sometimes the HFEA gives the impression that counselling is of such paramount importance that it is even more important than the treatment itself. To the resentful specialist, counselling has become an 'in-thing' getting in the way of treatment.

Conclusion

I am convinced that the problems people face in infertility require the skills of the trained counsellor, as much as any other more obvious branch of medicine. Unlike any other speciality, the condition of infertility does not generally have any lethal consequences nor affect life-expectancy. But unfocused grief, the sense of loss and feelings of inadequacy can affect the quality of the rest of a couple's life together. Sadly, for many infertile couples, coming to terms with their infertility is the only goal they can hope to reach. Counselling is an essential requirement in helping to restore such a couple's perspective on life and help them to channel the love they have to offer into other fulfilling directions. In this sense the counsellor has an awesome responsibility indeed.

Chapter 17
Reproductive Medicine: Why Do We Need Counselling?

Alexina McWhinnie

This chapter deals with how counselling has come to be seen as an important part of infertility services in general, and assisted conception programmes in particular. Using the experience and official reports commissioned and written in UK, Australia and USA, developments in the thinking about the task of counselling in this area are explored. The change in emphasis and the widening of concern from the purely medical and scientific into the social and ethical consequences are demonstrated. Legislation has incorporated counselling into its provisions in the UK and in some states in Australia, but no such legislative counselling provision has been made in the USA. The counselling issues for participants in all these countries are examined.

Although the main emphasis to date has been on the infertile adults, there should be equal concern for the needs and potential difficulties for donors of making donations and for the children created by medical reproductive technology. Society's fears and concern to have a say in what is acceptable are also addressed. The controversies about the provision and status of counselling expertise and its potential contribution to different aspects of service provision are addressed, as too is the question of training for infertility counsellors.

Introduction

Why do we need counselling in reproductive medicine? The answer to this depends on the perspective of those asking the question. For the person experiencing the pain of infertility, with its loss of hope of parenthood, the answer may be apparently straightforward – to help them deal with the pain, to suggest options, to support people as they embark on medical intervention strategies, either high-technological or low-technological.

Other chapters in this book deal primarily with the 'therapeutic' aspect of infertility counselling, how it has developed in the UK, the counselling done by doctor, nurse and counsellor and the skills they may need to do this. There are also case examples of counsellors' work. In short, the book has presented the views and increasing experience of the professional experts. There is a burgeoning literature about this type of multidisciplinary work, though basic texts about the psychological aspects of infertility are still few. So there is much still to be explored, learnt and understood.

There is, however, another perspective to counselling in this particular area which should not and cannot be ignored. This is counselling as a kind of intermediary between the rapid advances in medical technology and what contemporary communities find is acceptable. Some would also see it as having a protective role for vulnerable, infertile people against possible exploitation by unscrupulous medical scientists. So within the question, 'Why do we need counselling?', there are in fact at least four perspectives to consider. This chapter will address these in turn and will use the UK experience of public debate, legislation and clinical and participant experience to do this. The UK is unique in the stance it has taken on legislation in this area, offering regulation and control regarding research, practice, clinical and scientific and counselling. Legislation elsewhere, on the whole has concentrated on the scientific and research aspects.

Public debate

The pressure to consider legislation came from a series of committees of inquiry and from extensive debate and discussions, both in the UK and elsewhere, from the 1970s onwards. To highlight how a view has developed about the value and role of counselling in reproductive medicine, it is useful to consider how it has been referred to in these reports.

The concerns in the 1970s were about the ethics of *in vitro* fertilization (IVF), the ethics of experimenting with human embryos, the moral status of the embryo and whether the children born in this way would be abnormal. There was also a fear of a Huxley's *Brave New World* and of a eugenically planned population. This was conceptualized by Mary Warnock in an introduction to the Warnock Report (Warnock, 1984) p. xiii, (see also Chapter 9). She argued that the public expect research method and outcome to be monitored and be subject to public scrutiny: 'Society, insofar as it is a single identifiable body, has here, perhaps uniquely, a corporate reaction. It is one of fear. People generally believe that science may be up to no good . . .'

Alongside the concern about the ethics of the research being done to develop the effectiveness of the technique of IVF, was a concern about how participants' consent was obtained. Was it ethical to ask for this under the format reported as being used by Steptoe and Edwards. 'Your only hope is to help us ...' (Ramsey, 1971).

In 1977 in the USA an Ethics Advisory Board was set up to consider the ethical acceptance of IVF and to clarify the legal status of the child. The birth of the first IVF child in 1978 resulted at once in a widening of this remit to consider the social issues surrounding IVF. In the UK, a Medical Research Council Advisory Council in 1979 similarly added to its scientific concerns by including the question of 'informed consent'. By 1982 this Council had been reconvened and was reviewing work on genetic manipulation. It suggested that there was a need to develop a way of monitoring worldwide the children born as a result of IVF. One of the other issues discussed was, 'Does a couple have an absolute right to have a child?'

In Australia in 1979 a Committee of Inquiry in Victoria, the state within which much of the pioneering medical and scientific work had been developed, considered legislation for IVF. Their report, the Waller Report (1984), resulted in immediate legislation and introduced compulsory counselling.

The Warnock Report

In the UK there was pressure to address this area and to consider legislation. But it was 1982 before the Government ultimately responded with a Committee of Inquiry into Human Embryology chaired by Mary Warnock. The remit of this committee was to:

> ... consider recent and potential developments in medicine and science related to human fertilisation and embryology; to consider what policies and safeguards should be applied, including consideration of the social, ethical and legal implications of these developments; and to make recommendations.
>
> (The Warnock Report, 1984, 1.2).

This remit is relevant. It shows how gradually social aspects had come higher up the agenda. In the USA the Ethics Board remit had added 'social issues' right at the end of its list of non-medical matters. By 1982, the Warnock Committee's emphasis was – 'the social, ethical and legal implications'. This showed an awareness that the human consequences of these new developments were as significant as the immediate concerns about the morality of the procedures themselves. The composition of the Warnock Committee also reflected a change of emphasis: more than half its members were non-medical. Warnock argued that it was not intended as a committee of experts. Its task was rather '... to attempt to discover the public good, in the widest sense, and to make recommendations ...' (The Warnock Report, Foreword).

The Committee extended its consideration beyond IVF to all aspects of assisted reproduction which were causing public concern: donor insemination, egg and embryo donation and surrogacy were thus also included.

The Committee's conclusions (Warnock, 1984 p. 95) greatly influenced subsequent developments and ultimately led to legislation in the UK. It also had a major impact on counselling practice in infertility services. Its main recommendation was that there should be a statutory authority to regulate research and services and to license approved clinics. The recommendation about counselling was that: '... counselling should be available to all infertile couples and third parties at any stage of the treatment, both as an integral part of National Health Service care and in the private sector.' (Warnock, 1984, 3.3).

Under the heading of counselling was included 'Advice, information and discussion'. Recognizing that the issues were complex, it recommended that those seeking treatment and those donating needed to be given careful consideration over a period of time: 'In particular, the task of the doctor and the counsellor must be to ensure that couples and donors fully understand the implications of what they are embarking on, what rights and duties they may have and where they may expect to experience difficulties.' (Warnock, 1984, 3.3). This envisaged counselling going far beyond the immediacy of the stress of treatment.

The recommendations also stated that counselling '... should be carried out in a neutral atmosphere and involve a skilled, fully trained counsellor.' (Warnock, 1984, 3.4).

Counselling was seen as being 'essentially non-directional'. Its aim was to help individuals 'to understand their situation and to make their own decisions about what steps should be taken next' (Warnock, 1984, 3.4).

The Report in practice

How to put these ideas into practice has been the substance of much of the continuing debate in UK about counselling provisions in infertility services. The Report and its recommendations were viewed as controversial and aroused heated debate and hostility. Pending a decision about possible legislation to ban or accept the new fertility treatment techniques, the medical profession decided to regulate its practices itself and thus offer reassurances to the public about where research and practice might be leading.

A system of voluntary control was set up with the Voluntary Licensing Authority (VLA) which lasted for six years. It produced guidelines and created a forum for debate about controversial issues, social as well as medical and scientific. In the guidelines it recommended that infertile couples should have access to 'good independent counselling to help them decide whether to continue with treatment or to come to terms with treatment failure.' (Gunning and English, 1993 p. 54). Skilled and independent counselling for donors was also recommended: 'Clinicians were expected to explain the implications of treatment and nursing staff to deal with day-to-day anxieties but counselling was considered best undertaken by properly trained third parties.' (Gunning and English, 1993, p. 54).

However, there was confusion about the definition of counselling and many clinicians interpreted it as meaning giving information regarding procedures, 'rather than helping couples come to a better under-standing of themselves as well as the treatment' (Gunning and English, 1993 p. 54). The provision of counselling over this six-year period was variable. The VLA was powerless to do much about the situation because of the shortage of qualified counsellors and of available training. Its powers were by persuasion and peer pressure.

A further aspect of the social implications of the new reproductive techniques appears in a 1983 BMA report, (British Medical Journal, 1983, **286** 1594–5), i.e. a year before the publication of the Warnock Report. It stated that before being offered treatment 'a couple seeking IVF should be assessed as to the stability of the family relationship and the sincerity of their intentions to accept the responsibilities of parent-hood' (Gunning and English, 1993 p. 30).

The issue of assessment was not addressed directly in the Warnock Report, although it would have been presented to the committee for discussion. Whether assessment is an issue for the counsellor, the whole team or the 'person responsible' for the administration of the clinic or unit is a contemporary issue which will be discussed later. It certainly became an issue during parliamentary discussion of the White Paper proposing legislation which was introduced early in 1988. The princi-ples behind the White Paper were set out as follows:

> ... that due respect must be given in law to the presence of human life, the desire not to cut off hope unnecessarily from infertile couples and others who may be helped by the new development and that the welfare of children born as a result of such treatments must be of paramount importance. (Hansard, 1988, col. 1204)

Legislation

It was the first time in the UK that there was a public assertion about the paramount importance of the welfare of the child in this context, although such a principle now permeates most child-welfare legislation in the UK. The legislation that was eventually agreed and enacted in the Human Fertilisation & Embryology Act 1990 retreated from the paramountcy principle and declared that:

> A woman shall not be provided with treatment services unless account has been taken of the welfare of any child who may be born as a result of the treatment (including the need of that child for a father), and of any other child who may be affected by the birth.
>
> (Human Fertilisation & Embryology Act 1990, 13.5 – see also Chapter 9).

The wording of this paragraph and the comment about the need for a father for a child were written in as amendments to the original bill as a result of public controversy at the time about whether single women and lesbian couples, should be included in infertility service provisions ('Virgin Birth' headlines in national newspapers, March 1991).

How this provision of 'taking account of the welfare of the child and of any other child' will be interpreted and covered in clinic practice, and whether or not counsellors have a role in this, is an area of contemporary controversy. It certainly indicates a retreat from saying that the welfare of the child is paramount. It opens the door, however, to taking the debate beyond the morality of the scientific techniques and the treatment processes themselves into the arena of the social consequences when the treatment is successful.

On counselling provision, the Human Fertilisation & Embryology Act states:

> People seeking licensed treatment (i.e. *in vitro* fertilization or treatment using donated gametes) or consenting to the use or storage of embryos, or to the donation or storage of gametes, *must* be given 'a suitable opportunity to receive proper counselling about the implications of taking the proposed steps', before they consent. (HFEA Code of Practice, **6.1**. HF&E Act 1990, s 13(6) & Sch 3 **3(1)a.**)

The counselling requirement is thus very specific in one sense and open-ended in another. It must be made available, but it is not compulsory for those attending assisted reproduction centres to participate in it. In this it is in marked contrast to the provision under the Australian Victoria state legislation where counselling is compulsory for participants before starting IVF treatment, (The Infertility (Medical Procedures) Act 1984 based on the Waller Committee Report in the State of Victoria, Australia). It is open-ended about what counselling should or might cover and about how it should be done and by whom.

The King's Fund Centre Counselling Committee

In order to offer guidance on how to define counselling services, the King's Fund Centre, at the request of the Department of Health, set up a small multidisciplinary working party. Their terms of reference were:

> To provide advice for the consideration of the Human Fertilisation and Embryology Authority on the counselling needs relating to the provision of infertility services for couples considering any of the regulated infertility treatments; for children born following gametes or embryo donation who seek information about their origins, and for all donors.'
>
> (King's Fund Centre Counselling Committee Report, 1991 – see also Chapters 9 and 10)

The fact that this Committee was to address all three perspectives regarding counselling needs was a clear indication that the welfare of the child had now to be more formally addressed. The Report recognized the three perspectives and included a fourth perspective: '. . . the desire for assurance at societal level that the infertility services are conducted responsibly and in accordance with the provisions contained in current legislation'. (King's Fund Committee Report, 1991 Section 1, 1.3).

This implies that ethical and social safeguards are fully integrated with the services and it corresponds to the societal fear that 'science may be up to no good' mentioned earlier in this chapter.

The HFEA Code of Practice

Most of the King's Fund Committee's recommendations were used by the HFEA in its Code of Practice in relation to counselling, published in July 1991 and revised in June 1993. This code spells out the areas for counselling and relates them to what is prescribed in law. It states that counselling should be clearly distinguished from the information which has to be given to everyone, from the clinician/patient relationship of giving advice, and from the process of assessment to decide whether to accept them as client or donor. It also states that: 'no-one is obliged to accept counselling. However, it is generally recognised as beneficial.' (HFEA, Code of Practice of the HF&EA, 1991, revised June 1993, **6.3**).

Three distinct types of counselling are described and should be made available – implications counselling; support counselling; and therapeutic counselling.

It is not envisaged that these should be provided by three separate counsellors. The division was originally made by the King's Fund Committee to indicate the different strands or levels of the task of meeting the counselling needs of participants on these programmes.

Implications counselling

> This should be available to everyone. It includes not only the medical but the social implications too:

>> the implications of the proposed course of action for himself or herself, for his or her family, and for any children born as a result.
>>   (HFEA Code of Practice 1991, **6.4a**).

Support counselling

>> . . . this aims to give emotional support at times of particular stress, for example, when there is a failure to achieve a pregnancy.
>>   (HFEA Code of Practice, **6.4b**).

Therapeutic counselling

>> . . . aims to help people to cope with the consequences of infertility and treatment, and to help them to resolve the problems these may cause. It includes helping people to adjust their expectations and to accept their situation.   (HFEA Code of Practice **6.4c**).

What the HFEA Code of Practice does not cover is the need for counselling before and after treatment at a licensed clinic, or for those experiencing infertility who never get as far as a clinic. It does, however, set out a clearly defined counselling package in reproductive medicine, albeit one tied to regulated centres as defined by the provision of this in the Human Fertilisation & Embryology Act. It can be asked how far does this meet the expressed needs of those experiencing infertility, and how does it compare with the counselling agendas in reproductive medicine being developed elsewhere?

The assumption behind the package of counselling is that it is beneficial. But why is its provision prescribed by law, when counselling is not so prescribed where other high technology medical procedures are involved or where the consequences of medical intervention are equally dramatic – as in abortion. The Asche Report (1985) gave it as their view that the crucial difference lay in the fact that life was being created:

> Reproductive technology differs fundamentally from other developments in science, technology and bio-technology in that it enables the creation of new life, the creation of a child who would not otherwise be born.   (Asche Report, 1985)

The international perspective

Australia

An Australian report on reproductive technology counselling sets counselling in a wider context than the UK sources quoted so far. It argues that counselling is both beneficial and cost-effective, that it should be provided routinely on programmes and be more available, along with education, in the community for those experiencing infertility but not embarked on any reproductive technology programme. It also states that: 'Community education about the causes, nature, incidence and treatment of infertility is necessary. (National Bio-ethics Consultative Committee Report, 1991 **3**, 3.3).

This report, based on nationwide consultation, indicates that although most of the legislation introduced in the different states in Australia has acknowledged the value of counselling, the provision of this throughout is patchy. It is also clear that an issue in Australia is confusion about counselling; how to define it; what should be included in its role concerning informed consent, decision-making, assessment and screening; where should the counsellor be located – as part of the clinic team or independent of the treatment programme?

This confusion and debate also mirrors UK experience. The legislation enacted in the state of Victoria is described as having 'international importance'. It is the most specific in its provisions about counselling. Under the Australian Infertility (Medical Procedures) Act 1984, all reproductive technology programmes are required to provide 'counselling by accredited counsellors'. The Act also prescribes certain matters about which counselling must be provided to all prospective clients of such programmes, and to prospective gamete donors before they can enter the programme. The compulsory nature of this provision is criticized by some as inimical to the counselling relationship, and by others as possibly resulting in a restrictive approach. But some argue that it has the advantage for clients that an early contact is established with a trained counsellor.

Different states in Australia have come up with different decisions and divisions about what should be included in the counselling role. The report from the National Bio-ethics Consultative Committee (1991) is quite clear in its recommendations. It sees counselling as separate from assessment and screening, and separate from the process of consent to treatment. It further agrees that within counselling on reproductive programmes, four activities can be identified (Section 7, Paras 4.4.1– 4):

(1) the provision of information
(2) the facilitation of decision-making

(3) the provision of personal and emotional support
(4) the provision of therapeutic counselling.

These divisions are very similar to those formulated by the King's Fund Counselling Committee.

The USA

In the USA there has not been a similar clarification of roles and tasks within infertility counselling. In fact, counselling has not been on the agenda in discussions about legislation and regulation. Three of the 50 USA states have passed laws to regulate aspects of reproductive medicine, but there seems little possibility of anything similar developing on a federal basis. There have been discussions about setting up something similar to the Voluntary Licensing Authority that was in operation in the UK before the Human Fertilisation & Embryology Act; however, no specific proposals have emerged (personal communication with Dr Howard W Jones, 1993).

As far as counselling is concerned, the American Fertility Society has produced recommended guidelines, which were originally published in 1986, updated in 1990 and were due for further updating again in 1994. (Fertility & Sterility, 1986 and 1990). The driving force in this is the Psychological Special Interest Group of the American Fertility Society. This group has been considering both the level of expertise needed for counselling and the content of specialist training. It appears that, on the whole, the medical practitioners do not yet see the need for or the value of counselling, nor of having a mental health professional on the staff or available for consultation (personal communication with Dr Linda Hammer Burns, 1993). This is clearly in marked contrast to the acceptance of counselling in both the UK and Australia, although marked differences of opinion about this remain in both countries.

So far this chapter has looked at how the concept of counselling in reproductive medicine has evolved historically, particularly in the UK, Australia and the USA. The perspectives in this review have included the concept of the 'public good', and public morality and ethics; the need for society to be involved in monitoring such dramatic scientific developments; the need to offer protection to potentially vulnerable people, hoping that their dream about having children will be fulfilled; and a concern about the health and welfare of children thus created. Gradually there has been a shift in emphasis; an increased acknowledgement of the needs and psychological problems of infertile people; a growing concern for the donors making their donation of sperm or eggs; and an awareness about issues affecting the welfare into adulthood of the children conceived through these programmes, with a particular need for counselling and consideration for those who learn or suspect that 50% of their genetic inheritance was from an unknown donor.

Do counselling services meet public need?

The next section of this chapter will look at whether the counselling services recommended or prescribed will meet the needs of these three groups of participants.

Counselling and the family

Most people throughout the world grow up within a family, whether nuclear or extended, or within a wider kinship group; and the family, though frequently imperfect, is seen as playing an important role 'in conveying a sense of security and protection and a notion of belonging which contribute to one's sense of identity' (National Bio-ethics Consultative Committee Report, 1991 **3**, 3.1).

And while there have been marked changes in family composition in recent years: 'founding a family through conceiving, bearing, nurturing and rearing one or more children is still regarded as an important stage in human development and a "rite of passage" to adulthood ...' (National Bio-ethics Consultative Committee Report, 1991, S 3, para 3.1.).

In the social climate of most western-style cultures, many young men and women expect and are expected to reproduce and the majority take their fertility for granted; parenthood produces a certain status and community of interest. In many non-western style cultures having a child can be even more important. In some cultures it is seen as essential in a marriage, and the inability to conceive constitutes grounds for divorce. In this context, children are valued: when they are wanted and the adults involved find they are unable to conceive, their concepts of their own sexuality, self-image and self-esteem are challenged.

Although there has long been an interest and literature on population studies and policies, there has been surprisingly little written about infertility. Studies about those who are unable to have children have so far mainly concentrated on the medical factors in infertility. However, over the past decade, studies relating to the psycho-social aspects have emerged.

Menning (1980) was the first to write specifically about the 'infertility life crisis'. She described it as a block to the developmental task of procreation and generativity. Others have commented on the mourning process of infertility and that the difficulties for the mourners and for others in their world are twofold: the loss is not evident to others and it cannot be easily communicated. Another barrier is community attitudes. A man is quoted in one study as saying: 'Talking about infertility is like Victorian sex. Nice people don't do it.' (Covington, 1988).

Mahlstedt (1980) identified eight areas of loss in infertility, as follows: loss of real and of fantasy relationships; loss of health; loss of status (as perceived by the community); loss of self-esteem and confidence; loss of security (others are in 'control' of the treatment process); and loss of hope, both for the immediate time and for the future years. She comments: 'Any one of these losses could precipitate a depressive reaction in an adult. The experience of infertility involves them all.' (Mahlstedt, 1980.)

Infertility, as well as being a taboo subject for general conversation, has many myths. A common one is that by and large this is a woman's problem. However, figures now available show that it is as likely to be caused by factors in the male. A survey of infertility referrals to a specialist centre (Randall & Templeton, 1991) showed male infertility, including referral for DI, was the largest clinical diagnostic group with primary infertility, affecting 39.2% of all couples referred. It should be noted, however, that this figure concerns only referrals and does not necessarily represent the causes of infertility as experienced by the general adult population, many of whom will not seek referral to a specialist clinic. However, figures for infertility causation quoted in North American studies are similar: female factors are approximately 40%, male factors also 40%, combined male/female factors or unknown factors are 20% (Valentine, 1988).

Options and choices available

It is argued that counselling can help people to grieve for the losses identified by Mahlstedt and begin to consider what is the appropriate option for them. Some will opt for continuing with infertility treatments over many years, moving from one specialist to another. Some will apply to be adopters or to become foster parents, some will opt for a child-free lifestyle, seeking fulfilment and satisfaction in their lives in other ways. Some infertile marriages or partnerships do not survive the discovery of infertility. In the anguish that follows, the suggestion that the fertile partner should seek another mate is nearly always raised – either openly expressed or wondered about (McWhinnie, 1993). Some will decide to pursue their desire for children through one of the new assisted conception programmes. Which of the various options within such a programme they choose will depend on the cause of the infertility, whether it is within the female or male partner, or shared between them, or alternatively, whether the reason for the infertility may have no known or establishable cause.

A final deciding factor will be their personal financial resources. How far this dominates their personal decisions will vary between individuals but will also depend on how such programmes are provided and financed in their respective countries. Frequently private medical insurance cover does not include these programmes. In the UK, infertility services as such are provided generally within the NHS, although the level of such provision is uneven throughout the country. The more specific assisted conception programmes are, however, not generally available under the NHS and increasingly are provided in the private sector. The cost incurred on IVF and GIFT (Gamete Intra-Fallopian Transfer) treatment programmes are considerable (GIFT treatment is not covered by the Human Fertilisation & Embryology Act, but is a medical option available on assisted conception programmes). Those centres providing DI treatment are less expensive because it is not high technology medicine and, although sperm donors are paid, the sums involved are limited. Donors of eggs, on the other hand, may receive medical treatment for themselves in return for donations.

Surrogacy is also an option in the UK. Commercial surrogacy is banned by law, but non-commercial surrogacy is increasingly being practised. Amendments to regulations under Section 30 of the Human Fertilisation & Embryology Act 1990, are being considered to accommodate this.

Factors affecting choice

Which option it is appropriate for infertile people to consider will thus depend on a range of factors:

- the medical diagnosis
- their financial resources
- their commitment to becoming parents and their perseverance in this respect
- and finally, whether their commitment within the partnership is to parent a child, either from within the relationship or, if that is not possible, someone else's child, or whether becoming a parent must also include experiencing a pregnancy.

They will need to consider both how they can respond to the implications of each of the pathways and also what are the chances of success on each – success being defined as 'the take-home baby rate'.

The kind of questions that they will need to ask themselves were spelt out in the Asche Report (1985, p. 57):

- Whose problem is infertility? Mine? My partner's? Society's?

- Is infertility a problem at all? For me? For us?
- Is our infertility resolved by having a child? Do I/we want to have a child by means of reproductive technology? Is the use of donor gametes acceptable to both of us?
- What might it mean to me, for my partner, for us, to raise a child who is not biologically ours?
- What will we tell the child as she or he gets older?
- Should our artificially-conceived child have the right to know his or her origins?

To these can be added:

- If my/our religion does not approve of artificial intervention and the process involved, should I seek advice from my religious adviser or decide these issues for myself? Can I live with the consequences? How will I resolve this in the religious upbringing of any child I/we may parent?
- If there are spare embryos, what decision will each of us make about how/if they should be used in the future? To whom do they belong if our relationship ends in separation or divorce?
- Will our kinship group and friends agree with my/our decision and support me/us in the future, whichever pathway we go down?
- How open and frank, secretive or reticent will I/we be about the infertility and the decisions we make, both now and in all the years ahead when I/we will live with the consequences?
- Will there be health hazards for me/us as a result of the draconian drug dosages and the invasiveness of some of the medical procedures?
- How much of our financial resources will I/we commit to this quest to becoming parents? Will I/we set a limit or will I/we go on hoping for success? (McWhinnie, 1993)

These are the kind of questions that are hard both to address and to resolve, both individually and in a partnership. The acknowledged poor success rate of IVF and GIFT adds another dimension: the temptation is not to look at these figures too realistically in case all hope that the treatment might succeed becomes extinguished. Figures vary from centre to centre, but an average success rate of 15%–25% is frequently quoted, giving the resulting failure rate of 75%–85%. In the case of DI, the pregnancy rate is reported to be much higher and in fact more nearly that of the average fertility rate (McWhinnie, 1992).

One option is not to seek admission to a specialist programme, either from choice or necessity, for example because there are no programmes available in the area, or their cost is unaffordable. In such cases, infertile couples may apply to adopt or to foster children. In the

UK there are few babies needing adoptive parents – under 1000 per year. Older children or sibling groups or children with special needs do need adoptive parents, but not all those seeking parenthood feel that they can respond to that kind of challenge. Fostering children is also a possibility but it too has its own particular challenges. It frequently involves a continuing personal involvement with the birth parents as part of the day-to-day care of the children, and regular contact with supervising social workers.

The role of counselling

It is not surprising that, faced with such diversity of choice, together with uncertainties of outcome and potential risks for the future, many people report their need for counselling and support in the early stages of learning that there is a fertility problem (McWhinnie, 1993).

Those who go on to participate in assisted conception programmes will have faced some of the questions already posed. Once on a programme, they will experience the stress of the programme regime itself. Attendance on such programmes, with the need for timed injections which correspond to ovulation times, attendance at centres at particular times, both for the woman and the man, disrupts the routine of daily living and can adversely affect personal and sexual relationships. If this continues over a considerable period, and also involves travelling considerable distances, then the medical treatment can be reported (McWhinnie, 1993) as 'taking over our lives'. Where treatment fails, the level of disappointment is often acute; and then with each renewed attempt, hope is revived, to be followed by increasing despair and desperation if failure recurs. Many find it difficult to ask for the emotional support they need and would value. When there is repeated failure, many find it hard to make the decision to stop treatment. The arguments they put forward are that they have already spent many years of their lives trying to have children, invested their time and their money, given up career prospects, social life, and so on and next time it might work.

Attendances at DI clinics are much less invasive of patients' lives. However, keeping the attendance 'secret' and anonymous – which many practise – has its own hazards. It is more manageable at a clinic in a city than one in a small town or a rural area.

The donor's perspective

Much of the emphasis so far in this chapter, and in the literature, has been on those experiencing the infertility and treatment programmes. Much less has been written about the perspective of those who donate gametes. What, for example, are the factors that motivate donors to do this and what are the long-term psychological implications for them? Do they wonder about the children born from their donations? Do they keep their involvement a secret? Do they tell any future partner, or any children they may have themselves that they may have half-siblings somewhere? Are they concerned about any ethical aspects? Does the involvement and the process offend against their religious faith?

Counselling donors

Counselling sessions should be available to explore such issues with donors. Many of these issues are included in details given in the HFEA Code of Practice of the HF&E Authority (see para 6.16, revised June 1993). Not all donors on UK programmes, however, opt to accept counselling. In practice, to date, the emphasis, particularly with sperm donors, has been on assessing their suitability as donors and whether they are aware of and understand the procedures that will be used; the need for a personal and family medical history; the possible implications if a child born from their donation is disabled; the number of children their donations are allowed to create; anonymity; and their legal position (HFEA Code of Practice, para 4.5). A question that has been addressed by research is their attitudes to the possibility of contact being made with them in later life by children from their donations. These studies show a much larger proportion of donors willing to accept such contact and ready to understand the needs of such children than is generally assumed or recognized by those providing this service (Daniels & Taylor, 1993, pp. 155–170).

Counselling DI adults

In the UK, the Human Fertilisation & Embryology Act specifies that a person aged 18 can apply to the Authority for information about their possible gamete donation origins. If the applicant has been, or may have been born in consequence of this, they must be given a suitable opportunity to receive proper counselling about the implications of compliance with this request. (Human Fertilisation & Embryology Act, 1990, para 31.3b). An enquiry can also be made as to whether anyone they propose to marry might or might not be related because of gamete donation. However, it is important to note that the person applying can be told whether they may be from donated gametes, but given no further information: 'Regulations cannot require the Authority to give any information as to the identity of a person whose gametes have been used or from whom an embryo has been taken . . .' (Human Fertilisation & Embryology Act, 1990, para 31.5).

There has been, as yet, no discussion of how this clause will be interpreted in practice. Donors are being assured that if there are changes to these regulations in the future, that they will not be retro-spective in effect. This, of course, appears to protect the interests of donors; it does nothing to address the needs of those donor-offspring who find that they personally want and need more certain information about their origins. The counsellor's task under these circumstances would be a very ambiguous one.

This problem was discussed by the King's Fund Centre Counselling Committee in their report:

> Counselling in this situation may prove to be very difficult and is likely to be focused upon the distress and frustration flowing from a refusal to provide this available information. The limited provision of information to young adults born as a consequence of regulated infertility treatment is a source of concern to the Committee. It would appear to be inconsistent with a proper concern about the welfare of the child.
> (King's Fund Centre Counselling Committee Report, 1991, p. 19)

The Human Fertilisation and Embryology Authority

This chapter has reviewed how counselling in reproductive medicine has emerged historically and how different countries are likely to see its relevance. The examples used here have occurred in the UK, Australia and the USA. All the strands that were identified as emerging in the first part of this chapter have been encapsulated in one way or another in the Human Fertilisation & Embryology Act, 1990, in the UK, and in the consequent Code of Practice from the Authority which this Act estab-lished. The differences of opinions and controversies, however, have not been resolved in the UK, nor are they likely to be resolved for some time to come. The Authority, however, offers a framework within which these controversies can be debated and a policy of evolutionary change can be developed. This is made possible because the Authority has been set up to look two ways: to medical and scientific advances and devel-opments in the future, but also to the views and attitudes of con-temporary society and to the protection of potentially vulnerable participant individuals, of consequent children and any other children likely to be involved. Much will depend on how the HFEA resolves or keeps in balance these two perspectives.

Controversies in counselling practice in infertility programmes

The areas of discussion and controversy specific to counselling have already been mentioned in this chapter. Perhaps the first and most basic issue is whether doctors and nurses can do all the counselling tasks that have been identified, or do some of them require a training and orien-tation recognizedly different from the scientific/clinical and treatment skills that are part of good medical and nursing education and training.

Second, if infertility counsellors with a social science/behavioural and psychological orientation and training are used, are they to be seen as quite independent of the treatment programme or part of the multi-disciplinary team? In either case, how can their role, their knowledge and understanding of human situations and dynamics be used and incorporated into assessment and screening decisions? What contribution can they make to a heightened awareness in this whole area that, although the emphasis on all treatment and contacts is with adults, consideration must or should be given to the welfare of children who may be created as a result of these medical interventions?

Third, if counselling is accepted as beneficial, there emerge two possible and alternative scenarios. In one, counselling services would be available as a reactive provision to those who were perceived as experiencing emotional and psychological difficulties. In the alternative scenario it would be provided on a pro-active basis, potentially to all those experiencing the problems and anguish of infertility and facing the choices that this was presenting to them. In the former, it would be sited in or attached to centres providing reproductive medicine and infertility treatments. In the latter, a community health-care provision and approach would be called for.

Fourth, a corollary of the acceptance of counselling by those with a social science orientation is the question of how they should be trained. Guidelines for training in the USA have already been referred to. In the UK, work has started on this by the King's Fund Counselling Committee who produced a format for short courses as an interim measure (King's Fund Report, 1991, Appendix IV). The ideas presented there have taken root generally and form the basis for developing a long-term training pathway in counselling awareness and counselling skills appropriate to the specialism of infertility. A report is imminent from an HFEA working group on training for infertility counsellors.

Finally, there needs to be a wide-ranging debate about how far counselling, with its non-directive approach, can offer the 'safety check' that the Warnock Committee saw as important in this area. This was expressed as a fear or unease about 'what the medical scientists were up to'. There was also unease that medical science was moving too fast and that individuals might get caught up in new developments without being fully aware of the possible implications for themselves, and their immediate and wider kinship groups, of the processes that they were becoming involved with.

Conclusions – public view

Since the heated debates following the Warnock recommendations, public opinion appears to move 'moved on'. It seems that the 'community' in the UK accept IVF and GIFT as ethical and no longer problematical. Certainly, this is one of the findings of contemporary research into the perspective of parents who have had children in this way (McWhinnie, 1993), though it has to be pointed out that the research did not include a study of those who do not go on such programmes. How far does religious disapproval affect such choices? There still remains the certainty that some religious groups are totally opposed to these procedures.

Gifts of gametes have also slipped into social acceptance in a way that would not have seemed possible twenty years ago, although whether the full implications of these have been understood by the public at large is another matter.

The media has given these new developments a high profile and on the whole has been sympathetic to them. At what point, however, society will say 'thus far but no further' is for the future to answer. The need for counselling in this area, independent of the medical practitioner involved, has been established, certainly in UK and Australia. With new scientific developments around the corner, can it achieve for adults, children and the community all that is hoped of it? The earlier chapters describe some of the strategies already developed under its aegis, and no doubt others will follow in the future.

Appendix 1
Medical Acronyms and Important Word Glossary

Sammy Lee

Abortion   A term describing pregnancy loss. Sometimes described as miscarriage, when it has occurred spontaneously. Miscarriage occurs regularly when assisted conception is used (in up to 25% of all pregnancies). Sometimes pregnancies are deliberately aborted for medical (i.e. chromosomal) or social reasons. These are called termination of pregnancies (TOPs see below).

AC   Assisted conception, a term used to describe treatment methods collectively. Also known as assisted reproduction.

AIH   Artificial insemination by husband; an old technique that did not utilize sperm preparation nor intrauterine transfer. Now superceded by IUI (see below).

AH   Use of PZD technique to assist hatching of embryos. Sometimes, the outer covering (the zona) of the egg becomes hardened during time in the test tube. One way of overcoming this is to help the embryo hatch by using a sharp glass needle to lance the Zona.

Amenorrhoea/anovulation   Condition in women where there are no menstrual cycles at all (see Appendix 2).

Androgens   Male hormones e.g. testosterone. Testosterone in men helps to regulate FSH levels. It also has a direct action on sperm maturation. Poor motility may be treated with testosterone supplementation (but only if testosterone levels are proven to be low). Too much testosterone can cause low levels of FSH, which will inhibit spermatogenesis.

Asthenozoospermia   A condition in the male where less than 40% of the sperm show motility. It is also used sometimes to describe poor movement in motile sperm. Most cases are due to unexplained mechanisms. In some cases, where a blood test reveals low FSH or low testosterone, supplementation with the appropriate hormone may prove beneficial.

Azoospermia   Condition where a man has no sperm in the ejaculate. N.B. Even when there is no epididymal component (i.e. when the vas is blocked) the volume of semen will still be substantial, unless some of the accessory glands that contribute to the semen are also damaged. Azoospermia is only reversible if it is due to tubal blockage or absence of the vas deferens.

BBT   Basal body temperature/for prediction of ovulation. Body temperature is supposed to rise after ovulation.

Biopsy   Surgical procedure used to obtain tissue for analysis. In particular, in males, historically a testicular biopsy has been used to assess the status of the testis. These days, testicular biopsy may usually be avoided by the use of

253

blood assays for FSH. When the FSH levels are above 5 units per litre, testicular failure is imminent: above 10, failure has probably already occurred.

Chromosomes   Genes are to be found on chromosomes. In men and women there are 46 chromosomes in any one cell. One-half, 23 come from the egg and the other half from the sperm. One of the 23 chromosomes carried by egg and sperm will be the sex chromosome. In the case of eggs, the sex chromosome is an X one, each sperm will carry either an X or a Y chromosome. Of course, XX embryo is female, XY is a male. When damage occurs to even a small part of any one chromosome, the resulting abnormalities are usually so serious that pregnancy loss will occur. In cases where live birth occurs, common abnormalities are Trisomy 21 (Down's) or Trisomy 13 (cleft palate). When screening with PD for genetic diseases, gene probes are used to search for abnormalities occurring on these chromosomes.

Contraception   A global priority, not just a means of sex without reproduction in the West. Traditional methods involve monitoring the woman's menstrual cycle or using barrier devices. More recently, various types of progestagen pills have been used. Modern state-of-the-art methods use implants which contain progestagens. Contraception is supposed to be an aid in family planning i.e. those who do want to have children should use contraceptives. Those that want children should avoid contraceptives.

Cyclogest   Progesterone suppository to support the luteal phase. If the endometrium (lining of the womb) is not optimal, the embryo may not be able to implant. Progesterone supplementation may help the implantation procedure.

Delivery rate per cycle   There are arguments that this is the only way data should be presented. Other ways, e.g. pregnancy rate per transfer overstate the success rate, since some patients will not have transfer and some will also miscarry. So a 25% pregnancy rate per transfer may reduce to an 18% delivery rate per cycle.

Donor   A person who offers his or her gametes (eggs or sperm) for the use of an anonymous recipient. With sperm, the procedure is called donor insemination, donor IUI, donor IVF, or donor GIFT. With eggs, the procedure is called ovum donation.

DI   Donor insemination. Men with good sperm function donate samples for the use of infertile male factor couples. Donor samples must be frozen and quarantined before use. This ensures that no diseases will be passed from donor to recipient. Usually, the thawed sample is delivered to the female patient by artificial insemination. More recently, some units now carry out intrauterine insemination (DIUI) with prepared sperms.

DIPI   Direct intraperitoneal insemination. A method similar to IUI. Everything is done as with IUI, except that the prepared sperm sample is placed into the abdomen instead of the womb. The sperm then make their way into the tube in the same way as the egg does! Not done very often these days.

DOT   Direct oocyte transfer – like U-SET (see Appendix 2).

DOST   Direct oocyte sperm transfer (i.e. DOT).

Doxycycline   Antibiotic used in fertility, especially in PZD. Because the egg has been 'played with', it is thought that the resulting embryo will be more susceptible to infection; thus this antibiotic is used as a prophylactic agent guarding against infection.

Drug regimen For induction of ovulation or superovulation, the dose of gonadotrophins (FSH or FSH + LH) must be given in a planned and controlled manner, usually in conjunction with ultrasound monitoring and sometimes blood assays.

EC (Egg collection) The procedure by which eggs are removed from the body, being extracted from the follicles of the ovary. It may be done by laparoscopy, which requires general anaesthesia and surgery. More often, these days, it is done outside operating theatres. Here, the woman is mildly sedated and the eggs are usually recovered under ultrasound guidance, using an oocyte aspiration needle. It is a simple routine procedure.

Embryo A fertilized egg becomes an embryo; also called zygote (one-cell fertilized egg) or pre-embryo (embryo prior to implantation).

Embryo biopsy Taking one cell from an embryo for PD. It is now possible to manipulate an embryo, and to lance it, as in PZD. After this, a single cell from the embryo may be removed and taken for genetic testing.

Embryologist A highly trained, skilled individual (not a medical doctor) who is qualified to handle human gametes and the resulting embryos.

Endometriosis A condition where endometrial tissue is found outside of the uterus. (see also the Introduction).

Endometrium Lining of the womb. This changes throughout the cycle. During the woman's bleed, the lining becomes very thin. As follicles develop, it becomes thicker and thicker. After ovulation it becomes secretory, a stage at which implantation may occur.

Epididymal blockage Sperm are made in the testis and then stored in the epididymis prior to ejaculation. The epididymis is connected to the vas deferens. If the epididymis is blocked, azoospermia will result. Surgical correction is sometimes successful (see MESA).

ET Embryo transfer. A non-surgical procedure. A speculum is used to allow the specialist to see the cervix and to gain access to it. Then the embryos are picked up into a special catheter, which is then placed into the womb via the cervix. The embryos are then placed into the womb. This procedure usually happens two days after EC, see above, when the embryos will be between four and eight cells in development.

Fertilization The complex process whereby the egg is penetrated by the sperm. As the sperm approaches an egg, it must carve its way through the cloud of cells that nurture and protect the egg. Then, as it touches the zona pellucida (the outside membrane) of the egg, the sperm undergoes a remarkable process called the acrosome reaction (which may only happen once the sperm has undergone its epic journey to the egg). This reaction allows the sperm to sheer through the zona where it may then fuse with the egg membrane, thereby producing the final events of fertilization. The egg is now fertilized and may be deemed to be an embryo.

FET Frozen (thawed) embryo transfer. As with ET; except here the embryos have been frozen, stored a time and then been thawed prior to replacement. It is a useful method of making use of spare embryos from cycles where more embryos are available than may be used (a maximum of three embryos per transfer!

FISH   Fluorescent linked in situ hybridization carried out in conjunction with PD. This is a modern molecular biology method of doing genetic testing.

Follicular phase   Part of the cycle when follicles begin to grow, prior to ovulation. Ovulation ends this phase which is followed by the luteal phase.

Follicular tracking   Here ultrasound scans are used in a routine manner to monitor the progress of the ovary and endometrium during a woman's cycle, both natural or stimulated (see drug regimen, ovulation induction and superovulation).

FSH   Follicle stimulating hormone: this stimulates the ovary and testis. A strong commonly used fertility drug.

Fetus   When bodily organs form at about 5–7 weeks of pregnancy, the embryo develops into a fetus.

Gametes   A collective term for eggs and sperm.

GIFT   Gamete intrafallopian transfer see T-SET (see Appendix 2).

GnRH   Gonadotrophin-releasing hormone: used in AC. A drug which is used to switch off a patient's pituitary. This allows the specialist finer control when using FSH or HMG.

hCG   Human chorionic gonadotrophin or pregnancy hormone (cf LH). Although it is the hormone produced during pregnancy, hCG is exactly like LH, so it is used during fertility treatment to produce ovulation.

HMG   Human menopausal gonadotrophin: used as with FSH and contains LH.

HRT   Hormone-replacement therapy. Usually refers to the supplementation of oestrogen for post-menopausal women.

HSG   Hysterosalpingogram or tubal patency test. A test for tubal patency, which requires X-ray to image the womb and tubes, which are filled by a radio-opaque dye.

Hypogonadism   State in women or men where the sex hormones (FSH, LH, testosterone) may be deficient as shown by blood test.

Hypothalamus   The part of the brain which controls the pituitary, which releases FSH and LH (amongst many other hormones) in men and women.

ICSI   Intracytoplasmic sperm injection. A recent method which has caught both the public and the medical imagination. Single sperms may now be picked up and injected into eggs. This method needs fine glass needles as with PZD. (Seems to be giving encouraging results.)

IUI   Intrauterine insemination where semen must be prepared, cf SO (see Appendix 2).

Implantation   This occurs when the lining of the womb (the endometrium) is receptive and the embryo has been able to develop sufficiently to 'hatch' from its zona. The embryo must then invade the endometrium in order to implant and become a viable pregnancy. Embryos and wombs decide implantation not doctors and embryologists. Embryos are transferred not implanted.

Infertility counselling   Specialized area of counselling, and indeed treatment. Uptake of this resource continues to lag behind expectations.

IVF   *In vitro* fertilization or 'Test tube method' (see Appendix 2).

Laparoscopy   Surgical tubal patency test 'LAP & DYE'. Common method for determining tubal patency in women. It also allows specialists to assess the condition of the pelvis and overall anatomy of the tubes, womb and ovaries.

LH Luteinizing hormone: this produces ovulation in women and is a secondary hormone in men.

Luteal phase The part of a woman's cycle after ovulation has occurred. This phase ends at the onset of the period.

MIST-MICROINSEMINATION see ICSI.

MESA Microsurgical epididymal sperm aspiration (see Appendix 2).

Most fertile period of woman's cycle Ovulatory period, which should coincide with good mucus. This time is hard to define. May be defined by guessing, BBT, mucus, LH surge, or by follicular tracking.

Mucus Secretion found in the cervix. Good mucus is highly receptive to good active sperm. The best sperm are most able to penetrate mucus to arrive in the uterus, which is a useful way of assessing sperm function.

Normospermia Normal semen analysis, i.e. count, motility, abnormality rate are all alright.

OI Ovulation induction. This is a single follicular stimulation using HMG. Use of powerful fertility drugs to overcome amenorrhoea or oligomenorrhoea (anovulation or occasional ovulation).

OD Ovum donation. A controversial treatment option. Overcomes the lack of ovarian function in the recipient. Usually, the recipient is a woman who has undergone premature menopause. Sometimes the recipient may have eggs herself, but for some reason is willing to participate in this type of treatment. In other circumstances, some recipients are older women who have undergone natural menopause, yet still wish to overcome nature.

Oestrogen Follicular phase (preovulation) hormone in women. This hormone is produced by a healthy ovary. When blood levels are very high, it causes the pituitary to release high levels of LH, which triggers ovulation.

Oligozoospermia Term describing poor sperm count, i.e. less than 20 million sperm per ml.

Ovulation Is triggered by a mid-cycle LH surge. This produces release of the egg as well as having an effect on egg maturity.

Parthenogenesis Spontaneous activation of an egg. These may look just like embryos but lack the 23 chromosomes which the sperm contains. No parthenones are known to have been born in humans.

PCOS Polycystic ovarian syndrome which features abnormally high LH and androgens.

PCR Polymerase chain reaction. FISH relies on PCR.

PD Pre-implantation diagnosis, usually through FISH. This allows us to start screening embryos for genetic defects. This technology is now available, but is still in its infancy.

PID Pelvic inflammatory disease – a common cause of tubal disease.

Pituitary Organ just at the base of the brain which releases FSH and LH.

POST Peritoneal oocyte sperm transfer where the ova are not placed into the tube. This method is one step on from DIPI. Here the eggs are also recovered and then put back with the sperm into the abdomen. Not performed much these days.

Prednisone Steroid used for autoimmunity and also used in PZD. This steroid has an effect on the body's immune system, which is reduced to such an extent that the mechanisms causing the auto-immunity may be abolished or at least diminished. It will not work for everyone. When PZD is done, the steroid has been used in the hope that it will help the embryo implant. There is insufficient data yet regarding its efficacy in either use.

Preovulatory oocyte Term used to describe a fully mature egg.

Primary or secondary infertility Primary means never had a pregnancy. Secondary means has had a previous pregnancy, but not necessarily delivered.

Primary testicular failure Male infertility arising as a result of testicular failure routinely revealed by high FSH levels.

Progesterone Luteal phase (post-ovulation) hormone in women. The hormone is used as a test to determine whether a woman is ovulating or not. It is important for making the womb receptive to embryo implantation.

Prolactin Hormone that produces milk output and interferes with fertility. If there is a tumour (usually benign) in the pituitary, blood levels of this hormone become very high, which may then interfere with ovulation. Natural contraception when a mother is nursing a baby is thought to work through this mechanism.

Prost Pronucleate stage (embryo) transfer. Fertilization is proven with this method. Then the embryo is replaced directly into the body, either by embryo transfer or by ZIFT (into the tube, as per GIFT. The tubal environment is believed to be superior to embryo transfer at this stage.

PZD Partial zona dissection which assists the sperm's passage to the ovum. A sharp tiny glass needle is used to lance the outer covering (zona) of the egg. This allows motile sperms far easier access to the egg.

Reproduction technology (see AC). This arises from the reproduction revolution and means reproduction without sex. It is the opposite of contraception.

SA Semen analysis but not reliable for male factor diagnosis. A method for determining how many sperm there are in a sample and what percentage of them are moving. Less than 20 million per ml and/or less than 40% motile is thought to be infertile. The abnormality rate (morphology or how the sperms look) should also be less than 60%.

Sperm preparation Any treatment method relies on some form of sperm preparation. Most methods rely on the motile migratory properties of sperm. Most methods utilize centrifugation.

SO Superovulation/important for AC/multifollicular ovulation (Appendix 2)

SOTI Superovulation and timed intercourse/basic fertility treatment (see Appendix 2)

Sperm function/dysfunction Semen analysis reveals little about sperm function. A functional sperm will fertilize an egg, a dysfunctional one will not. IVF is useful as a diagnostic test therefore. Mucus penetration tests may be almost as good and also much cheaper.

Spontaneous pregnancy Pregnancies arising in patients without AC.

Surrogacy Used when uterus is absent. Paid surrogacy is illegal in UK. A woman agrees to carry a baby on behalf of a woman who has no womb or is at risk of death or illness if she were to become pregnant herself.

SUZI Sub-zonal insemination which is similar to PZD. The method uses a needle like ICSI. Again a single sperm may be picked up and injected. Instead of being injected directly into the egg, with SUZI, the sperm is placed inside the zona, next to the egg. This method is almost certainly going to be superceded by ICSI.

Testosterone   Male hormone with corresponding actions in males to that of oestrogen in females.

TEST   Tubal egg sperm transfer, i.e. by ultrasound or hysteroscope. This may be the future way of doing ET. Modification of PROST, ZIFT, GIFT and IVF.

Testis   Site of spermatogenesis. A man has two testes. One functioning testis is enough.

TET   Tubal embryo transfer/may be superior to normal ET.

T-SET   Ian Craft's name for GIFT.

TUDOR   Transvaginal ultrasound-directed oocyte recovery.

Turner's Syndrome   Situation where an X chromosome is missing in the woman's chromosomal make up. These people are primary patients for ovum donation.

U-SET   Like DOT/DOST.

Ultrasound   Used in all avenues of infertility, for diagnosis, monitoring and treatment. Also used for monitoring progress of pregnancy.

Unexplained infertility   All male and female tests completed with no abnormality detectable in either partner. No obvious cause for childlessness or involuntary infertility.

Varicocoele   Enlarged spermatic vein, which raises local temperature of scrotum. This is supposed to impair spermatogenesis.

Vas deferens   Joins the epididymis, where sperms are stored, to the urethra, where the sperms are emitted.

Vasogram   X-ray test used to check tubal patency of the vas deferens.

VISPER   Like DIPI.

ZIFT   Zygote intrafallopian transfer, much like PROST. Here the route of transfer is via laparoscopy.

Appendix 2
Treatment Options for the Infertile

Sammy Lee

For anovulation or oligomenorrhoea (problems with ovulation)

The treatment is simple and usually effective. Patients with low LH and FSH will benefit from injections of LH and FSH preparations (gonadotrophins). This therapy is effective for 70–90% of patients. For patients with normal FSH, LH and oestrogen, but low progesterone, follicular tracking (monitoring the stimulation of the ovary by means of periodic scanning by ultrasound) and hCG administration at the appropriate time should be successful in the vast majority of cases. When using gonadotrophins, hCG is also given when the follicle(s) are deemed to be mature. In all cases, once hCG is given, couples are advised to have sexual intercourse within the next 24–48 hours.

Patients with polycystic ovaries (PCO), a problem which may result in anovulation or oligomenorrhoea will benefit from FSH-only injections. Severe cases of PCO will benefit from down-regulation (the GnRH will stop the body from making its own LH and FSH, if it is used daily and in a high dose for a prolonged time period) first. A GnRH is therefore administered, usually by nasal spray. After 21–30 days, injections of LH and FSH may be given thereafter. As with normal gonadotrophin therapy, hCG is administered to time ovulation, which is followed by natural intercourse. Success with PCO patients is about 55–70% of all treated cases.

In all resistant (not responding to the drugs) cases of anovulation, down-regulation, using the nasal spray mentioned above may be offered. Failure with this treatment means progression to superovulation, IUI, GIFT or IVF.

In the old days, clomiphene, tamoxifen or rehibin, were given to such patients for up to six cycles. In the days when blood tests and ultrasound were not used routinely, this empirical therapy (i.e. treatment that has not been proven to be of value, but which is thought might be useful) was useful for up to half of those receiving the treatment. In others the treatment was either ineffective or made matters worse. Today, with the routine use of ultrasound, an argument may be made for the early use of gonadotrophins (LH and FSH), because of the high efficacy of the combination of follicular tracking, gonadotrophins and timing of ovulation by hCG administration. Some practitioners continue to use clomiphene and so on for cost and sometimes resource reasons.

Superovulation: the use of gonadotrophins to produce multifollicular development (up to four mature follicles per cycle)

The majority of patients with anovulation will succeed with ovulation induction with gonadotrophins. Those that fail may benefit from superovulation. Ovulation induction is the pursuit of one or two functional follicles. In superovulation, we are looking to develop between three to four follicles depending on the treatment option. In empirical superovulation (ES), we look to improve the couple's natural chances of success by simply producing more follicles, which should provide more eggs. We have learnt from IVF that more embryos = more likelihood of success. This maxim goes for eggs too. With empirical super-ovulation we must take care to avoid multiple pregnancies. Even a triplet could mean failure. The use of ES is particularly suited to couples who have failed with ovulation induction and for those with unexplained infertility. Three mature follicles is ideal with ES. When the follicles are mature, as with OI, hCG is given, after which the couple are advised to have sexual intercourse within the next 24–48 hours. Patients with endometriosis might also benefit from ES. About 30–40% of couples will succeed within six cycles of ES. Those that fail ES will progress on to IUI, GIFT, IVF (not necessarily in this order).

Intrauterine insemination (IUI) with ES

This is suitable for male factor infertility, though the therapy is not yet proven (neither is GIFT nor IVF.) Couples with the joint presence of male and female infertility factors should also be suitable for IUI and ES so long as tubal patency is demonstrable. Couples who have failed with ES may benefit from 3–6 cycles of IUI with ES. This treatment is also suitable for idiopathics (unexplained) who are not having sexual intercourse or who are not achieving penetration during sex.

Patients will be given ES, but instead of just having sexual intercourse, when hCG is given, the couple will attend the clinic 36 hours after hCG, in order to have the IUI. The male partner produces a semen sample, which undergoes preparation. The best sperms are then placed in the female partner's uterus by means of a transcervical catheter, thereby bypassing the cervix. The IUI is a simple procedure that is usually painless, quick and does not require general or local anaesthesia or surgery.

Patients failing ES and IUI

After six cycles of IUI with ES, only about 40% of couples will fail. Many will find themselves offered GIFT or IVF. More commonly these days they are offered IVF. In my opinion, IVF is for people with blocked tubes only. If there is tubal patency, ES alone should be sufficient, so long as male factors are absent. Thus GIFT should only be considered after ES failure at the earliest, since most couples may also benefit from IUI with ES. (up to six cycles). In some circumstances, where poor sperm or egg quality is suspected, a diagnostic IVF cycle may be useful before trying GIFT.

Gamete intrafallopian transfer (GIFT)

With GIFT, the female partner undergoes superovulation but after hCG, instead of sex or insemination, egg recovery takes place 36 hours afterwards; three eggs are then placed with prepared sperms directly into the fallopian tube, immediately egg recovery is completed. After three cycles 40–60% of couples will have delivered a baby.

Direct oocyte transfer (DOT)

This is a procedure just like GIFT. If differs only in the place that the eggs and prepared sperms are placed immediately after egg recovery. The site of transfer is the uterus. This technique is therefore suited to all couples who have tried and failed IUI with ES, as well as those with blocked tubes. An argument may be made that up to three cycles of DOT should be tried before IVF referral. The technique is used in very few clinics in the UK at present (as far as I am aware just by the author of this Appendix and his colleagues) and must still be considered to be experimental! After three cycles, 30–40% of couples will have succeeded in delivering a baby.

IVF

This is the first port of call for patients with tubal disease, if they are unsuitable for tubal surgery or choose not to consider it. It may also be suitable for some of the other categories of female infertility, after prolonged treatment with less stressful and invasive options such as IUI with ES or GIFT. IVF is contraindicated for severe male factors unless done in conjunction with sperm and egg manipulation (see below).

As with GIFT, IVF requires superovulation, egg recovery and semen preparation. However, the eggs and sperm are kept in a dish in the laboratory for 48 hours, instead of being transferred immediately after egg recovery. Therefore, with IVF, we may tell whether there has been fertilization or not (the sperm being able to penetrate the egg – failure of penetration means that nothing will be transferred and the IVF has failed). If fertilization has occurred, up to three embryos will be placed in the uterus transcervically, using a special catheter (similar to IUI). After three cycles 30–60% of couples will have delivered a baby.

Other treatment options

In severe cases of male infertility, none of the above-mentioned methods will be suitable. However, since 1991, new possibilities have been developed. All such new methods must be undertaken in conjunction with IVF.

MESA

Microepididymal sperm aspiration allows sperm to be obtained from azospermic men, with vasal (tube connecting epididymis to urethra) absence or blockage. This procedure requires surgery. A fine needle may be inserted into the epididymis allowing some motile sperm to be extracted. This sperm is then prepared and used for IVF.

ICSI

Intracytoplasmic sperm injection is carried out when the sperm count or motility is very poor. Sperm may be picked up using a very fine needle and injected into the egg direct. The injected egg is then subjected to IVF.

Biopsy-ICSI

This is the same as above, except that the sperm used are derived from testicular biopsy. Here a fine needle is inserted into the testes directly in order to extract sperm for injection.

Electroejaculation

This is used for men with impotence or who are spinally injured, usually the semen obtained in this way will be prepared and used for IVF.

However, if there is some evidence of residual sperm function (i.e. sperm swim up is just adequate or a few sperm are able to penetrate the cervical mucus), then IUI, IVF or GIFT may be offered, depending on the severity of dysfunction. The key to treatment lies in the quality of the preparation (the hunt and isolation of 'sperm troopers'). In my opinion, if there is no obvious female factor, IVF and GIFT are questionable treatment options for male factor infertility.

Empirical options

Other empirical treatments may be of value, but these have not been proven in controlled studies. Tamoxifen, mesterolone, FSH, hCG and vitamin supplements are popular supplementary therapies. Here the rationale is that they probably will not have any effect, but their use will not hurt. Courses of treatment are usually given for three months prior to assisted conception. Finally, more recently methods have relied on medium supplements. Pentoxyfylline and taurine have been used to 'supercharge' sperm (possibly converting some of the poorer sperms into 'sperm troopers') during semen preparation, whilst some specialists also add vitamin E to the preparation media.

Appendix 3
Useful Organizations and Addresses

Eric Blyth

British Association of Art Therapists (BAAT)
11A Richmond Road
Brighton BN2 3RL

A national organization for art therapists, arranging training and conferences. Publishes *Inscape*.

British Association for Dramatherapists (BADTh)
5 Sunnydale Villas
Durlston Road
Swanage
Dorset BH19 2HY

A national organization for dramatherapists, arranging training and conferences. Publishes *Dramatherapy*.

British Infertility Counselling Association
Ms F. Plowman
BUPA Alexandra Hospital
Impton Lane
Walderslade
Kent ME5 9GU

The major professional association in the UK for infertility counsellors.

Birthmasks
P.O. Box 32
Stratford-upon-Avon
CV37 6GU

Offers a diploma course in fertility counselling skills, supervision and short courses.

Birthright
27, Sussex Place
Regent's Park
London NW1 4SP
(Tel: 071-723 9296)

An organization funding medical research in areas affecting women and babies.

British Agencies for Adoption and Fostering (BAAF)
Skyline House
200 Union Street
London SE1 0LY
(Tel: 071-593 2000)

A national professional organization concerned with encouraging good practice in adoption, fostering and related work with children and families.

British Association for
Counselling
1, Regent Place
Rugby
Warwickshire, CV21 2PJ
(Tel: 0788 550899)

Provides a national voice on
issues related to counselling.
BAC promotes understanding
and awareness of counselling
and works towards raising the
standards in counselling
provision.

British Fertility Society
2nd. Floor, Room 2/62
Birmingham Maternity
Hospital
Edgbaston
Birmingham B15 2TG
(Tel: 021-627 2696)

An inter-professional
association promoting
increased knowledge and
practice in the field of fertility.

British Pregnancy Advisory
Service
Austy Manor
Wooten Wawen
Solihull
West Midlands B95 6BX
(Tel: 05642 3225)

National advisory service with
regional centres, providing
advice and a range of services
relating to conception and
pregnancy.

British Psychological Society
(BPS)
St Andrews House
48 Princess Road East
Leicester LE1 7DR

UK professional association
which regulates practice,
maintains membership and
organizes conferences and
publications.

CHILD
Suite 219, Caledonian House
98, The Centre
Feltham
Middlesex
(Tel: 081-893 7110)

A self-help organization for
those experiencing fertility
difficulties.

Childlessness Overcome
Through Surrogacy (COTS)
c/o Gena Dodd, Secretary
Loandhu Cottage
Gruids, Lairg
Sutherland IV27 4EF
(Tel: 0549 2401)

A self-help group for those
interested in surrogacy.

DI Network
P.O. Box 265
Sheffield S3 7YX

A network of people who
have used – or are thinking of
using – donor insemination.

Family Care
21, Castle Street
Edinburgh EH2 3DN
(Tel: 031-225 6441)

A voluntary agency providing services for vulnerable women and children, infertility and adoption counselling.

Family Planning Association
27, Mortimore Street
London W1N 7RJ
(Tel: 071-636 7886)

Provides nationwide family planning information service, education and training.

Foresight: Association for the Promotion of Pre-conceptual Care
The Old Vicarage
Church Lane
Witley, Godalming
Surrey GU8 5PN
(Tel: 042879 4500)

Aims to get couples into optimum health before conception to enhance the chances of delivering a healthy child.

Gay and Lesbian Foster Carers Assocation
c/o London Friend
86, Caledonian Road
London N1 9DN
(Tel: 081-854 8888 ext. 2088)

A support group for lesbians and gay men involved in fostering and adoption.

Human Fertilisation and Embryology Authority
Paxton House
30, Artillery Lane
London E1 7LS
(Tel: 071-377 5077)

The UK statutory body responsible for licencing and regulating certain forms of infertility treatment and embryo research.

Hysterectomy Support Group,
The Venture
Green Lane
Upton
Huntington PE17 5YE
(Tel: 081-690 5987)

A self-help organisation providing information, advice and support to women before and after hysterectomy.

Infertility Support Group,
c/o Women's Health and Reproductive Rights Information Centre
52–54, Featherstone Street
London EC1Y 8RT
(Tel: 071-251 6580)

Provides a telephone help-line and resource/library service on a range of health issues affecting women.

Issue (The National Fertility Association) Ltd
509, Aldridge Road
Great Barr
Birmingham B44 8NA
(Tel: 021-344 4414)

The largest UK self-help group for people with fertility difficulties.

Jewish Association for Fostering, Adoption and Infertility (JAFA)
P.O. Box 20
Prestwich
Manchester M25 5BY
(Tel: 061-773 3148)

A Jewish organization dealing specifically with Jewish problems associated with fostering, adoption and infertility.

Miscarriage Association
c/o Clayton Hospital
Northgate
Wakefield
W. Yorkshire WF1 3JS
(Tel: 0924 200799)

Provides support and information to women and their families during and after miscarriage.

Multiple Births Foundation
Institute of Obstetrics and Gynaecology
Queen Charlotte's Hospital
Goldhawk Road
London W6 0XG
(Tel: 081-740 3519)

Provides professional support for families with twins and higher order births, educational programmes for professional workers and undertakes research.

The National Endometriosis Society
35, Belgrave Square
London SW1X 8QB
(Tel: 071-235 4137)

Aims to raise the consciousness of the general public and health professionals to the condition of endometriosis; by education, the effective dissemination of information and by the stimulation of research, whilst providing support to women with endometriosis, and their friends and family.

National Foster Care Association
Francis House
Francis Street
London SW1P 1DE
(Tel: 071-828 6266)

Provides advice and information on foster care to carers, social workers and local authorities.

National Organization for
Counselling Adoptees and
Parents (NORCAP)
3, New High Street
Headington
Oxford OX3 7AJ
(Tel: 0865 750554)

Maintains a register and offers
advice, information and
counselling for adoptees and
parents wishing to make
contact with each other.

Parent to Parent Information
on Adoption Services (PPIAS)
Lower Boddington
Daventry
Northants NN11 6YB
(Tel: 0327 60295)

A self-help organization
providing support and
information for those
considering adoption or who
have already adopted
children.

Post Adoption Centre
8 Torrian Mews
Torriano Avenue
Kentish Town
London NW5 2RZ
(Tel: 071-284 0555)

Provides a counselling service
for adoptees, adoptive
parents and birth parents and
information and training for
professionals.

Pregnancy Advisory Service
11–13 Charlotte Street
London W1P 1HD
(Tel: 071-637 8962)

Provides general advice on
pregnancy as well as a
licenced donor insemination
service.

PROGRESS
27–35, Mortimer Street
London W1N 7RJ
(Tel: 071-436 4528)

The voluntary campaign for
research into human
reproduction which supports
and protects controlled
research into human
reproduction, the prevention
of infertility, miscarriage and
congenital handicap.
Activities include
parliamentary monitoring,
educational mailing and the
production of a quarterly
newsletter.

Stillbirth and Neonatal Death
Society
28, Portland Place
London, W1N 4DE
(Tel: 071-436 5881)

Provides support for bereaved
parents and information for
professional workers and the
general public.

STORK
Dan Y Graig Cottage
Balaclava Road
Glais
Swansea SA7 9HJ

A national association of parents who have adopted children from other countries, providing a focus for the interchange of information about inter-country adoption. STORK produces factsheets and first-hand information about adoption procedures for different countries.

Support around Termination
for Abnormality (SATFA)
National Office
29–30 Soho Square
London W1V 6JB
(Tel: helpline, 071-439 6124;
071-287 3753)

A national charity providing information and support to parents whose unborn baby has an abnormality.

Twins and Multiple Births
Association
P.O. Box 30
Little Sutton
Wirral L66 1TH
(Tel: 051-348 0020)

An umbrella organization for over 200 hundred local twins' clubs. Provides information and support for parents of twins and higher order births.

Women's Health
52, Featherstone Street
London EC1Y 8RT
(Tel: 071-251 6580)

Operates an enquiry service and reference library providing information on a wide range of health topics, including reproductive technology and infertility and aims to assist women make informed decisions about their health.

Appendix 4
Training Counsellors for Infertility Counselling

Sue Emmy Jennings

Although the HFEA (Human Fertilisation and Embryology Authority) requires that all infertility clinics should have independent counselling available for patients and clients, there is still a tremendous variety of opinion as to what constitutes 'independent counselling', who should do it and when. The HFEA are in no doubt about the need for implications counselling and the specific issues that should be covered under that heading – in particular the welfare of any children born as a result of donated gametes. They also recommend that support counselling and therapeutic counselling should be available where necessary, and that infertility counsellors should have access to social workers or psychologists as appropriate.

The HFEA are currently convening a working group which includes people from a range of professions to discuss the training needs for infertility counsellors. Their report will be published as this book goes to print (copies will be available from the HFEA – see Appendix 6).

Training courses

There is only one training course currently specializing in the training of fertility counselling. This has been running since 1989 at the London Hospital Medical College which offers a Diploma in Fertility Counselling Skills recognized by the Academic Board of the Medical College. Enquiries to:

BIRTHMASKS
P.O. Box 21
Stratford-upon-Avon
CV37 6GU

The Medical Counselling Unit, City University, Northampton Square, London EC1V 0HB offers an introductory certificate in Infertility Counselling Skills.

The British Infertility Counselling Association (BICA) has a newsletter in which short courses are announced. They also run workshops and conferences (see Appendix 5).

Appendix 5
The British Infertility Counselling Association (BICA)

Sue Emmy Jennings

The BICA organizes regular conferences, study-days and training events of interest and relevance to its membership (and a wider audience where possible), both on its own and in liaison with organizations.

Contact with other counsellors is facilitated through a directory of members, which also forms the basis of a nationwide referral system for those requiring liaison or referral to a counsellor. BICA publishes a regular newsletter as a forum for news and the exchange of ideas, as well as articles relating to infertility counselling.

Guidelines for the counselling of people with fertility problems, including those who are considering the donation of gametes, can be obtained from BICA at the address below:

BICA
White House
High Street
Campsall
Nr Doncaster
S. Yorks

Extract from the Guidelines for Practice:

Counselling for Assisted Conception
These procedures bring a heightened sense of personal inadequacy to many individuals. Women, in particular, often feel both physically and emotionally vulnerable and men may feel helpless and redundant during the medical procedures. Advances in reproductive technology have raised the expectations, not only of the recipients of the treatments but also of the multi-disciplinary team and society, for a successful outcome. Costs of private treatment and lengthy waiting lists on the NHS increase the stress associated with these procedures. Uncertainties about the long term effects of the drugs employed and general concern regarding the physical, social and emotional well-being of the mother and potential, or existing, children are relevant issues for discussion.

Counselling combines general infertility tasks with the special needs accompanying these procedures, in particular the demands associated with the investigations and medical interventions. Counselling will facilitate the making of decisions that arise about continuing or terminating treatments, and will address the ambivalence which is frequently experienced as a result of the procedures.

Despite available information regarding treatment outcome, success rates are frequently overestimated by clients, and the expectations for success of the treatments are often not met by reality. Additional expectations for an improved quality of life that accompany a much wanted child are sometimes not matched by the reality of the circumstances. The offering of counselling is particularly important when treatment has been withdrawn, or failed, and when a client experiences ambivalence if pregnancy is achieved, particularly when it is multiple.

Appendix 6
The Human Fertilisation and Embryology Authority

Carol Perkins

The Human Fertilisation and Embryology Authority (HFEA) was set up by the Human Fertilisation & Embryology Act, 1990 (HFE Act). The Act came about largely as a result of the findings of the 1984 Warnock Committee Report. This report was commissioned by the Government following the birth of the first baby from IVF in 1978. The Act makes provisions to regulate and monitor treatment centres and to ensure that research using embryos is carried out in a responsible way. This is done by means of a licensing system. Three areas of activity are covered by the Act:

- any fertilization treatment which involves the use of donated eggs or sperm (eg donor insemination) or embryos created outside the body (IVF)
- storage of eggs, sperm and embryos
- research on embryos.

The HFEA also has several other responsibilities, including:

- publishing a Code of Practice giving guidance to centres on how they should carry out licensed activities
- keeping a confidential register of information about donors, patients and treatments
- giving information and advice to people seeking fertility treatment, to donors, to people wishing to store their sperm, eggs or embryos and to the general public
- keeping the whole field of fertility treatment and research under review, whether the activities are licensed or not, and make recommendations to the Secretary of State for Health if asked to do so.

The value of infertility counselling was recognized when the HF&E Act was passed in 1990. The Act makes both information-giving and the offer of counselling compulsory parts of the treatment services provided by infertility clinics licensed by the HFEA. The HFEA's Code of Practice gives guidance to clinics on the provision of infertility counselling services.

The HFEA aims to promote high standards of care in all areas of infertility treatment, including counselling. It therefore facilitated the independent body known as the Working Group on Training for Infertility Counselling, which was set up to consider how training for those involved in infertility counselling might be developed, with the aim of generally improving standards. The

273

HFEA welcomed the Working Group's report which offered a basis from which a system of training and accreditation in infertility counselling might be developed.

Appendix 7
Summary of the History of Infertility Counselling

1984   Warnock Report published – identifying the role of counselling in infertility treatment.

1986   Government Consultation Document endorses Warnock proposals on counselling provision.

1987   Government White Paper proposes to formally regulate counselling in licensed treatment centres.

1988   Interim Licensing Authority recognizes confusion about counselling provision.

Inaugural Meeting of the British Infertility Counselling Association.

1989   Human Fertilisation & Embryology Bill laid before Parliament.

London Hospital Medical College launches Diploma Course in Fertility Counselling.

1990   Human Fertilisation & Embryology Act specifies legal duties of licensed centres to offer counselling.

King's Fund Centre Counselling Committee established at the request of the Department of Health to provide advice for the Human Fertilisation & Embryology Authority.

1991   Human Fertilisation & Embryology Act comes into force.

Report of King's Fund Centre Counselling Committee published.

1992   Human Fertilisation & Embryology Authority publishes its first Code of Practice, clarifying the counselling requirements under the Act.

Human Fertilisation & Embryology Authority publishes its first Annual Report, highlighting some deficiencies in counselling provision in licensed centres.

1993   Human Fertilisation & Embryology Authority publishes its second, revised, Code of Practice.

Human Fertilisation & Embryology Authority and BICA jointly organise a conference on Infertility Counselling Training resulting in the establishment of an Infertility Counselling Working Group.

1993/4   HFEA convenes Infertility Counselling Working Group chaired by Rabbi Julia Neuberger.

References and Further Reading

Introduction

Brearley, G. & Birchley, P. (1992) *Introducing Counselling Skills and Techniques*. Wolfe, London.

Brown, D. & Peddar, J. (1968) *Introduction to Psychotherapy*. Penguin, London.

Cambell, J. (1993) *Creative Art in Groupwork*, Winslow, Bicester.

Casement, P. (1985) On Learning From the Patient. Tavistock, London.

d'Ardenne, P. & Mahtani, A. *Transcultural Counselling in Action*. Sage, London.

Jennings, S. (1994) *Introduction to Dramatherapy*. Jessica Kingsley, London.

Masson, J. (1990) *Against Therapy*. Fontana, London.

Chapter 1

Erian, J. & Lee, S. (1990) J. Reprod Fertil, Abstracts **5** 66.

Chapter 2

Holden, P. & Littlewood, J. (Eds) (1991) *Anthropology and Nursing*. Routledge, London.

Egan, G. (1990) *The Skilled Helper*. Brooks & Cole.

Chaplin, J. (1988) *Feminist Counselling in Action*. Sage, London.

Human Fertilisation & Embryology Authority (1993) *Code of Practice*. HFEA, London.

Chapter 3

Aird, E. (1985) *From a Different Perspective: Change in Women's Education*. WEA, London.

Anyon, J. (1983) Intersections of Gender and Class: Accommodation and Resistance by Working Class and Affluent Females to Contradictory Sex Role Ideologies. In: Walker, S. & Barton, L. (Eds) (1983) *Gender, Class and Education*. Falmer Press, London.

Belotti, E.G. (1975) *Little Girls*. Writers and Readers Publishing Corporation.

Bishop, S. (1992) *A Study of Post-Abortion Syndrome in the Light of Recent Research to Consider How Social Work Might Better respond to this*

Area of Need. Unpublished MA, Social Work Thesis, University of York, York.

Brice, E. *Ready, Willing and Able. The Guardian*; 10 August 1993, London.

British Infertility Counselling Association *Infertility Counselling Guidelines for Practice*. BICA, London.

Bryan, B., Dadzie, S. & Scafe, S. (1985) *The Heart of the Race – Black Women's Lives in Britain*. Virago, London.

Chernin, K. (1984) *Womansize – The Tyranny of Slenderness*. The Women's Press, London.

Clothier Report (1992) *Report of the Committee on the Ethics of Gene Therapy*. **Cm 1788** HMSO, London.

Crawshaw, M.A. (1988) *It's Somewhere Else to Come. Learning for Mental Health*. WEA, London.

Dana, M. (1984) Abortion and The Emotions Involved. From: Channel 4 Television, London.

Dana, M. (1987) Abortion – A Woman's Right to Feel. In: Ernst, S. & Maguire, M. (Eds) (1987) *Living With the Sphinx*. The Women's Press, London.

Daniels, K.R. (1992) Management of the Psychosocial Aspects of Infertility. *Australia & New Zealand Journal of Obstetrics & Gynaecology* **32** (1) 57.

David, M. (1986) Morality and Maternity: Towards a Better Union than the Moral Right's Family Policy. *Critical Social Policy* **16**.

Davies, V. (1991) *Abortion and Afterwards*. Ashgrove Press, Bath.

Eichenbaum, L. & Orbach, S. (1983) *Outside In Inside Out. Women's Psychology: A Feminist Psychoanalytic Approach*. Penguin, Harmondsworth.

Eichenbaum, L. & Orbach, S. (1987) Separation and Intimacy: Crucial Practice Issues in Working with Women in Therapy. In: Ernst, S. & Maguire, M. (Eds) *Living With the Sphinx*. The Women's Press, London.

EOC (1992) *Some Facts About Women*. Equal Opportunities Commission Manchester.

Ernst, S. (1987) Can a Daughter be a Woman? Women's Identity and Psychological Separation. In: Ernst, S. & Maguire, M. (Eds) *Living With the Sphinx*. The Women's Press, London.

Goffman, E. (1963) *Stigma: Notes on the Management of Spoiled Identity*. Prentice-Hall, New Jersey.

Gorman, J. (1992) *Out of the Shadows*. MIND Publications, London.

Greil, A.L. (1991) *Not Yet Pregnant. Infertile Couples in Contemporary America*. Rutgers University Press, New Brunswick and London.

Hanmer, J. & Statham, D. (1988) *Women and Social Work: Towards a Woman-Centred Practice*. Macmillan Education, Basingstoke.

Hey, V., Itzin, C., Saunders, L. & Speakman, M.A. (Eds) (1989) *Hidden Loss. Miscarriage and Ectopic Pregnancy*. The Women's Press, London.

Houghton, D. & P. (1987) *Coping with Childlessness*. Unwin, London and Sydney.

Howe, D., Sawbridge, P., & Hinings, D. (1992) *Half a Million Women. Mothers Who Lose Their Children by Adoption*. Penguin, Harmondsworth.

Human Fertilisation and Embryology Bill Debate (1990), Hansard Report, London.

Jennings, S. (1991) Legitimate Grieving? Working with Infertility. In: Papadatos, C. & Papadatou, D. (Eds) *Children and Death.* Hemisphere, New York.

Kareem, J. & Littlewood, R. (1992) *Intercultural Therapy.* Blackwell Scientific Publications, Oxford.

Kohner, A. & Henley, (1992) *When a Baby Dies. The Experience of Late Miscarriage, Stillbirth and Neonatal Death.* Pandora Press, London.

Lawrence, M. (1992) Women's Psychology and Feminist Social Work Practice. In: Langan, M. & Day, L. *Women, Oppression and Social Work – Issues in Anti-Discriminatory Practice.* Routledge, London.

Leon, I.G. (1990) *When a Baby Dies. Psychotherapy for Pregnancy and Newborn Loss.* Yale University Press, New Haven and London.

Leroy, M. (1988) *Miscarriage.* Macdonald Optima, London.

Monach, J.H. (1993) *Childless: No Choice. The Experience of Involuntary Childlessness.* Routledge, London and New York.

Neustatter, A. & Newson, G. (1986) *Mixed Feelings. The Experience of Abortion.* Pluto, London.

Oakley, A., McPherson, A. & Roberts, H. (1990) *Miscarriage.* Penguin, Harmondsworth.

Oppenheim, C. (1993) *Poverty, The Facts.* Child Poverty Action Group, London.

Orbach, S. (1993) *Hunger Strike.* Penguin, Harmondsworth.

ParentAbility, Alexandra House, Oldham Terrace, London W3 6NH.

Parkes, C. (1986) *Bereavement: Studies of Grief in Adult Life.* Penguin, Harmondsworth.

Pfeffer, N. & Woollett, A. (1983) *The Experience of Infertility.* Virago, London.

Phillipson, J. (1992) *Practising Equality. Women, Men and Social Work.* Central Council for Training and Education in Social Work (CCETSW), London.

Pipes, M. (1986) *Understanding Abortion.* The Women's Press, London.

Raymond, J. (1987) Fetalists and Feminists: They are Not the Same. In: Spallone, P. & Steinberg, D.L. *Made to Order – The Myth of Reproductive and Genetic Progress.* Pergamon Press, Oxford.

Rich, A. (1984) *Of Woman Born. Motherhood as Experience and Institution.* Virago, London.

Sharpe, S. (1985) *Just Like a Girl. How Girls Learn to be Women.* Penguin, Harmondsworth.

Singer, I. (1993) *Infertility and Ethnicity.* Unpublished Paper given at British Infertility Counselling Association Study Day, York.

Spallone, P. (1989) *Beyond Conception.* Macmillan, London.

Warnock Report (1984) *Report of the Committee of Inquiry into Human Fertilisation and Embryology,* **Cmnd 9314** HMSO, London.

Williams, F. (1987) Racism and the Discipline of Social Policy *Critical Social Policy,* **20**.

Worden, J.W. (1991) *Grief Counselling and Grief Therapy.* Routledge, London.

Chapter 4

Jequier, A. & Crich, J. (1986) *Semen Analysis. A Practical Guide.* Blackwell Scientific Publications, Oxford.

Jequier, A. (1986) *Infertility in the male.* Churchill Livingstone, Edinburgh.

Lee, S. (1991) Biologists' involvement in the reproduction revolution. *Biologist* **38** 85–8.

Lee, S. (1991) *Andrology.* BUPA Hospital Press, Leicester.

Lee, S. (1991) *What it means to be a sperm trooper.* BUPA Hospital Press, Leicester.

Mason, M-C. (1993) *Male infertility – men talking.* Routledge, London.

Chapter 5

Britton, R. (1981) Re-enactment as an unwitting response to family dynamics. In: Box, S., Copley, B., Magagna, J. & Moustaki, E. (Eds) *Psychotherapy with families.* Routledge, London.

HFEA (1991) *Code of Practice.* Human Fertilisation and Embryology Authority, London.

Inglis, M. & Denton, J. (1992) Infertility nurses and counselling. In: Templeton, A. & Drife, J. (Eds) *Infertility.* Springer-Verlag, London.

Mattinson, J. (1992) *The reflection process in casework supervision* (2nd edn). Tavistock Marital Studies Institute, London.

Ruszczynski, S. (1993) *Psychotherapy with couples: theory and practice at the Tavistock Institute of Marital Studies.* Karnac Books, London.

Will, D. & Baird, D. (1984) An integrated approach to dysfunction in inter-professional systems. *Journal of Family Therapy,* **6** 275–90.

Wilson, S. & Wilson, K. (1985) Close encounters in general practice: experiences of a psychotherapy liaison team. *British Journal of Psychiatry* **146** 277–81.

Wirtberg, I. (1992) *His and her childlessness.* Karolinska Institute, Stockholm.

Woodhouse, D. & Pengelly, P. (1991) *Anxiety and the dynamics of collaboration.* Aberdeen University Press, Aberdeen.

Chapter 6

Berk, A. & Shapiro, J. (1984) Some implications of infertility on marital therapy. *Family Therapy* **11** 37–47.

Bresnick, E. (1981) A holistic approach to the treatment of the crisis of infertility. *Journal of Marital and Family Therapy* **4** 181–8.

Bresnick, E. and Taymor, M. (1979) The role of counselling in infertility. *Fertility and Sterility* **32** 154–6.

Burns, L. (1987) Infertility as boundary ambiguity: one theoretical perspective. *Family Process* **26** 359–72.

Burns, L. (1990) An exploratory study of perceptions of parenting after infertility. *Family Systems Medicine* **8** 177–89.

Colon, F. (1978) Family ties and child placement. *Family Process* **17** 289–312.

Edelmann, R. and Connolly, K. (1987) The counselling needs of infertile couples. *Journal of Reproductive and Infant Psychology* **5** 63–70.

Humphrey, M. and Humphrey, H. (1987) Marital relationships in couples seeking donor insemination. *Journal of Biological Science* **19** 209–19.

Jennings, S. (1991) Legitimate grieving? Working with infertility. In: Papadatos, C. & Papadatou, D. (Eds) *Children and Death*. Hemisphere, New York.

Jones, E. (1993) *Family Systems Therapy*. Wiley, Chichester.

Karpel, M. (1980) Family secrets: 1. conceptual and ethical issues in the relational context, 2. ethical and practical considerations in therapeutic management. *Family Process* **19** 295–306.

Matthews, R. and Matthews, A. (1986) Infertility and involuntary childlessness: the transition to nonparenthood. *Journal of Marriage and the Family* **48** 641–9.

McDaniel, S., Hepworth, J. & Doherty, W. (1992) *Medical Family Therapy*. Basic Books, New York.

McGoldrick, M. and Gerson, R. (1985) *Genograms in Family Assessment*. W.W. Norton, New York.

Mendelberg, H. (1986) Infertility and sexual dysfunctions: a family affair. *Family Therapy* **13** 257–64.

Penn, P. (1985) Feed forward: future questions, future maps. *Family Process* **24** 299–310.

Raphael, B. (1983) *Anatomy of Bereavement*. Basic Books, New York.

Rolland, J. (1990) Anticipatory loss: a family systems developmental framework. *Family Process*. **29** 229–44.

Schaffer, J. & Diamond, R. (1993) Infertility: private pain and secret stigma. In: Imber-Black, E. (Ed.) *Secrets in Families and Family Therapy*. W.W. Norton, New York.

Selvini-Palazzoli, M., Boscolo, L., Cecchin, G. & Prata, G. (1980) Hypothesizing, circularity, neutrality: three guidelines for the conductor of the session. *Family Process* **19** 3–12.

Shaw, P., Johnston, M. & Shaw, R. (1988) Counselling needs, emotional and relationship problems in couples awaiting IVF. *Journal of Psychosomatic Obstetrics and Gynaecology* **9** 171–80.

Tomm, K. (1987) Interventive interviewing. Part 1: Strategizing as a fourth guideline for the therapist. *Family Process* **26** 3–13.

Watzlawick, P., Beavin, J. & Jackson, D. (1967) *Pragmatics of Human Communication*. W.W. Norton, New York.

Watzlawick, P., Weakland, J. & Fisch, R. (1974) *Change: Principles of Problems Formation and Problem Resolution*. W.W.N Norton, New York.

Weinshel, M. (1990) Treating an infertile couple. *Family Process* **8** 303–12.

Chapter 7

Campbell, J. (1993) *Creative Art in Groupwork*. Winslow, Bicester.

Dalley, T. (1984) *Art as Therapy*. Tavistock, London.

Dryden, W. (1991) *Dryden on Counselling: Vol. 1, Seminal Papers*. Whurr, London.

Ehrenzweig, A. (1967) *The Hidden Order of Art*. University of California Press, California.

HFEA (Revised June 1993) *Code of Practice* Human Fertilisation & Embryology Authority, London.

Inscape (1990) Journal of the British Association of Art Therapy.

Jennings, S. (1992) The Importance of Fertility Counselling. Talk presented to the Association for Group and Individual Psychotherapy.

Jacobs, M. (1986) *The Presenting Past*. Open University Press, Milton Keynes.

Rhyne, J. (1961) *The Gestalt Art Experience*. Magnolia St Publishers, Chicago.

Rogers, C. (1970) Creativity, (Vernon, P. Ed) Penguin, London.

Rogers, C. (1961) *On Becoming a Person*. Houghton Mittlin, Boston.

Milner, M. (1950) *On Not Being Able to Paint*, Heinemann, London.

Nowell-Hall, P. (1987) *Images of Art Therapy*, (Ed. T. Dalley) Tavistock, London.

Schaverien, J. (1990) The Triangular Relationship: Desire alchemy and the picture. In: *Inscape Journal of the British Association of Art Therapists* 14–19.

Waller, D. (1991) *Becoming a Profession*, Routledge, London.

Weir, F. (1987) *Images of art therapy* (Ed. by T. Dalley) Tavistock, London.

Winnicott, D. (1971) Playing and Reality. Tavistock, London.

Wood, C. (1990) The Triangular Relationship: The beginnings and endings of art therapy relationships. In: *Inscape Journal of the British Association of Art Therapists* 7–13.

Chapter 8

Bannister, D. & Fransella, F. (1986) *Inquiring Man*. Penguin, Harmondsworth.

Bloch, M. & Parry, J. (Eds) (1982) *Death and the Regeneration of Life*. Cambridge University Press, Cambridge.

Brinton-Perera, S. (1981) *Descent to the Goddess*. Inner City Books, Toronto.

De Coppet, D. (Ed) (1992) *Understanding Rituals*. Routledge, London.

Grainger, R. (1988) *The Message of the Rite*. Lutterworth Press,

Grainger, R. (1990) *Drama and Healing: the Roots of Dramatherapy*. Jessica Kingsley, London.

Jennings, S. (1990) *Dramatherapy with Families, Groups and Individuals*. Jessica Kingsley, London.

Jennings, S. (1991) Legitimate Grieving? Working with Infertility and Loss In: Papadatou, D. & Papadatos, C. (Eds) *Children and Death*. Hemisphere, London.

Jennings, S. (1993) An Operating Theatre of Healing? Dramatherapy in the Surgical Setting *Dramatherapy* **14**(2)

Jennings, S. (1993) The Counsel in Drama and the Drama in Counsel *Journal of the British Association for Counselling* **4**(3)

Jennings, S. (1993) Implications Counselling: Case History Example 'Shakespeare's Theatre of Healing' *Dramatherapy* **15**(2)

Jennings, S. (1993) Birth Masks in: *The Independent Magazine*, 8 May.

Jennings, S. (1994) *Theatre Ritual and Transformation: The Senoi Temiar* Routledge, London.

Jennings, S. (1995) Introduction to Dramatherapy, Jessica Kingsley, London.
Jennings, S. & Minde, A. (1993) Dramatherapy and Art Therapy: Masks of the Soul, Jessica Kingsley, London.
McLaren, A. (1984) *Reproductive Rituals* Methuen, London.
Shakespeare, W. *King Lear*. New Penguin Editions, Harmondsworth.
Silman, R. (Ed) (1993) *Virgin Birth* WFT Press, London.
Van Gennep, A. (1960) *The Rites of Passage*, Routledge, London.
Winnicott, D. (1971) Playing and Reality. Tavistock, London.

Chapter 9

Kareem, J. & Littlewood, R., (Eds) *Intercultural Therapy – Themes, Interpretations and Practice*. Blackwell Scientific Publications, Oxford.
Pipes, M. (1986) *Understanding Abortion*. Womens Press, London.
Zolese, G. & Blacker, C.V.R. (1992) The Psychological Complications of Therapeutic Abortion. *British Journal of Psychiatry* **160** 742–9

Chapter 10

Appleton, T. (1990) IVF (Host) Surrogacy. *BICA Newsletter* **4**(Winter). 7–15.
BICA (1989) Minutes of Executive Committee Meeting, 27th April.
BICA (1990) Survey on Some Issues Related to Donor Insemination, *BICA Newsletter* **3** (Spring).
BICA (1991) Infertility Counselling Guidelines, *BICA Newsletter* **5** (Winter).
Blyth, E. (in press) *Infertility and Assisted Reproduction: Practice Issues for Counsellors*. British Association of Social Workers and Essex County Council, Birmingham.
Blyth, E. (1993) Section 30: The Acceptable Face of Surrogacy? *Journal of Social Welfare and Family Law*, 1993 **4** 248–60.
Bydlowski, M. & Dayon-Lintzer, M. (1988) A Psychomedical Approach to Infertility. *Journal of Psychosomatic Obstetrics and Gynaecology* **9** 139–51.
COTS (1993) Infertility Counsellors, *COTS Newsletter* **22** (August) 10.
Crawshaw, M. (1990) Having Difficulty Conceiving? *BICA Newsletter* **4** (Winter) 23–7.
Crawshaw, M. (1993) Results of Questionnaire sent to all BICA members working in a counselling capacity in a licensed clinic. *BICA Newsletter* **9** (Spring) 2–4.
Department of Health (1992) *Review of Adoption Law – Report to Ministers of an Inter-Departmental Working Group: A Consultation Document*. Department of Health, London.
Department of Health and Social Security (1984) *Report of the Committee of Inquiry into Human Fertilisation and Embryology. (The Warnock Report)*. **Cmnd 9414** HMSO, London.
Department of Health and Social Security (1986) *Legislation on human infertility services and embryo research*. **CM 46** HMSO, London.
Department of Health and Social Security (1987) *Human fertilisation and embryology: a framework for legislation*. **Cm 259** HMSO, London.

Department of Health and Social Security (1988) *Checklist for the Training of Infertility Counsellors.* HMSO, London.

Donaldson, M. (1991) *The sixth report of the Interim Licensing Authority for Human* In Vitro *Fertilisation and Embryology.* Medical Research Council with Royal College of Obstetricians and Gynaecologists, London.

Dustin, G. & Waugh, S. (1991) *Review of Counsellor Training Courses,* British Infertility Counselling Association, London.

Frew, J. (1989) Counselling in IVF Clinics: statement on behalf of the Interim Licensing Authority. *The British Infertility Counselling Association Newsletter* **2** (Autumn) 4–5.

Harman, H. (1990) *Trying for a baby: a report on the inadequacy of NHS infertility services.* House of Commons, London.

Human Fertilisation & Embryology Authority (1991) *Code of Practice: Explanation.* HFEA, London.

Human Fertilisation & Embryology Authority (1992a) *Code of Practice.* HFEA, London.

Human Fertilisation & Embryology Authority (1992b) *Annual Report.* HFEA, London.

Human Fertilisation & Embryology Authority (1993a) *Code of Practice.* HFEA, London.

Human Fertilisation & Embryology Authority (1993b) *Second Annual Report.* HFEA, London.

Inglis, M. (1989) Counselling in Infertility Clinics, *BICA Newsletter* **2** (Autumn) 9.

ILA, (1990) *The fifth report of the Interim Licensing Authority for Human* In Vitro *Fertilisation & Embryology.* Medical Research Council and Royal College of Obstetricians and Gynaecologists, London.

ILA, (1991) *The sixth report of the Interim Licensing Authority for Human* In Vitro *Fertilisation & Embryology.* Medical Research Council and Royal College of Obstetricians and Gynaecologists, London.

King's Fund Centre (1991) *Counselling for Regulated Infertility Treatments: the report of the Counselling Committee.* King's Fund Centre, London.

Latarche, L. (1992) Annual Report, *BICA Newsletter* **7** (Summer) 1–5.

Matthews, A.M. & Matthews, R. (1986) Beyond the Mechanics of Infertility: Perspectives on the Social Psychology of Infertility and Involuntary Childlessness. *Family Relations* **35** 479–87.

Mathieson, D. (1986) *Infertility services in the NHS: what's going on?* House of Commons, London.

NAIC (1988) The National Association for Infertility Counselling's Response to the DHSS Checklist for the Training of Infertility Counsellors, NAIC, London.

Owens, D.J. & Read, M.W. (1984) Patients' experience with and assessment of subfertility testing and treatment. *Journal of Reproductive and Infant Psychology* **2** 7–17.

Pfeffer, N. & Quick, A. (1987) *Infertility services: a desperate case.* The Greater London Association of Community Health Councils, London.

Pfeffer, N. & Woollett, A. (1983) *The experience of infertility.* Virago Press, London.

Spallone, P. & Steinberg, D.L. (1987) *Made to Order: The Myth of Reproductive and Genetic Progress*. Pergamon Press, Oxford.

VLA (1986) *The first report of the Voluntary Licensing Authority for Human* In Vitro *Fertilisation & Embryology*. Medical Research Council and Royal College of Obstetricians and Gynaecologists, London.

VLA (1987) *The second report of the Voluntary Licensing Authority for Human* In Vitro *Fertilisation & Embryology*. Medical Research Council and Royal College of Obstetricians and Gynaecologists, London.

VLA (1988) *The third report of the Voluntary Licensing Authority for Human* In Vitro Fertilisation & Embryology. Medical Research Council and Royal College of Obstetricians and Gynaecologists, London.

Chapter 11

Adler, N., Keyes, S. & Robertson, P. (1991) Psychological issues in new reproductive technologies: pregnancy-inducing technology and withdrawal of life prolonging treatment in neonatal medicine. In: Adler, N., Keyes, S., & Robertson, P. (Eds) *Women and New Reproductive Technologies: Medical, Psychological, Legal and Ethical Dilemmas*. Lawrence Erlbaum, Hillsdale, New Jersey.

Brazier, M. (1990) The challenge for Parliament. In: Dyson, A. & Harris, J. (Eds) *Experiments on Embryos* Routledge, London.

Brazier, M. (1992) *Medicine, Patient and the Law*. Penguin, Harmondsworth.

De Marco, D. (1987) *In My Mother's Womb: The Catholic Church's Defense of Natural Life*. Trinity Communications, (Manassas, Va) 156–7.

Doyal, L. (1990) Medical ethics and moral indeterminacy. *Journal of Law and Society* **17** (1) 1–16.

Doyal, L. (1993) Access to IVF: what should be available to whom? In: Silman, R. (Ed.) *Virgin Birth* 93–9. WFT Press, London.

Doyal, L. (1993) Needs, rights and the moral duties of clinicians In: Gillon, R. (Ed.) *Principles of Health Care Ethics* 217–30. Wiley, London.

Doyal, L. & Wilsher, D. (1994) Towards guidelines for withholding and withdrawal of life prolonging treatment in neonatal medicine. *Archives of Disease in Childhood* **70** 66–70.

Doyal, Lesley (1994) *Self-insemination and the politics of regulation*. Policy and Politics, London.

Dyson, A. (1990) At Heaven's command?: the churches, theology, and experiments on embryos. In: Dyson, A. & Harris, J. (Eds) *Experiments on Embryos* 65–81. Routledge, London.

Greil, A., Leitko, T. & Porter, K. (1988) Infertility: his and hers. *Gender and Society* **1** (2) 172–99.

Harris, J. (1990) Embryos and hedgehogs: on the moral status of the embryo. In: Dyson, A. & Harris, J. *Experiments on Embryos* 65–81, Routledge, London.

HFEA (1990) Human Fertilisation and Embryology Act. HMSO, London.

Human Fertilisation & Embryology Authority (1993) *Code of Practice*. HFEA, London.

Kennedy, I. (1988) *Treat Me Right*. Clarendon Press, Oxford.

Lee, S. (1986) Re-reading Warnock. In: Byrne, R. (Ed.) *Rights and Wrongs in Medicine*, King's Fund, London.

Lesser, H. & Pickup, Z. (1990) Law, ethics and confidentiality. *Journal of Law and Society* **17** (1) 17–28.

Lorber, J. (1989) Choice, gift, or patriarchal bargain? Women's consent to *in vitro* fertilization in male infertility. *Hypatia* **4**(3) 169–80.

Marshall, J. (1990) The case against experimentation. In: Dyson, A. & Harris, J. (Eds) *Experiments on Embryos* 65–81. Routledge, 1990.

Morgan, D. & Lee, R. (1991) Human Fertilisation & Embryology Act. 2–3/2, Blackstone, Oxford.

Oldfield, S. (1983) *The Counselling Relationship: A Study of The Client's Experience*. Routledge, London.

Overall, C. (1991) Access to *in vitro* fertilisation: costs, care and consent. *Dialogue* **XXX** 383–97.

Reidy, M. (1982) Ethical issues in reproductive medicine: from the perspective of moral theology. In: Reidy, M. (Ed.) *Ethical Issues in Reproductive Medicine* 118–45. Gill & Macmillan, Dublin.

Report of the King's Fund Centre (1991) *Counselling for Regulated Infertility Treatments*, King's Fund, London.

Singer, P. & Dawson, K. (1990) IVF technology and the argument from potential. In: Singer, P., Kuhse, H., Buckle, S., Dawson, K. & Kasimba, P. (Eds) *Embryo Experimentation* 76–90. Cambridge University Press, Melbourne.

Scritchfield, S. (1989) The infertility enterprise: IVF and the technological construction of reproductive impairments. *Research in the Sociology of Health Care* **8** 72–3.

Shaw, P. (1991) Infertility counselling. In: Davis, H. & Fallowfield, L. (Eds) *Counselling and Communication in Health Care Reproductive Choices* 161–75. Wiley, London.

Trounson, A. (1990) Why do research on human embryos. In: Singer, P., Kuhse, H., Buckle, S., Dawson, K., & Kasimba, P. (Eds) *Embryo Experimentation* 14–25.

Warnock, M. (1985) *A Question of Life*. Blackwell, Oxford.

Warren, M.A., (1990) Is IVF research a threat to women's autonomy? In: Singer, P., Kuhse, H., Buckle, S., Dawson, K. & Kasimba, P. (Eds) *Embryo Experimentation* 14–25. Cambridge University Press, Melbourne.

Chapter 12

Human Fertilisation & Embryology Authority, Code of Practice, **6.4**.

HFEA Code of Practice, **6.2**.

HFEA Code of Practice, **6.7**.

HFEA Code of Practice, **6.4**.

HFEA Code of Practice, **6.3**.

Chapter 14

Chang, M.C. (1959) Fertilisation of rabbit ova in vitro. *Nature*, **184**: 466–467.

Craft, I.L., Djahanbakhch, O., McCleod, F., Bernard, A., Green, S., Twigg, H., Smith, W., Edmunds, D.K. & Lindsay, K.S. (1982) Human pregnancies following intrauterine transfer of pre-ovulatory oocytes and sperm. *Lancet*, **ii**: 1031–1033.

d'Ardenne, P. & Mahtari, A. (1989) *Transcultural counselling in action*. Sage Publications Ltd, London.

Kareem, J. and Littlewood, R. (Eds) (1992) *Intercultural therapy: themes, interpretations and practice*. Blackwell Scientific Publications, Oxford.

Steptoe, P.C. & Edwards, R.G. (1978) Birth after re-implantation of human embryo. *Lancet* **1178**: 366.

Chapter 17

Asche, A. (1985) *Creating Children. Report of the Family Law Council of Australia*. Australian Government Publishing Service, Canberra.

British Medical Association Working Group on *in vitro* Fertilisation (1983). Interim Report on human *in vitro* fertilisation and embryo replacement and transfer. *British Medical Journal* **286** 1594–1595, London.

Covington, S.N. (1988). Psychosocial Evaluation of the Infertile Couple: Implications for Social Work Practice, p. 26. In: Valentine, D. (Ed.) *Infertility and Adoption: A Guide for Social Work Practice*. The Haworth Press, New York.

Daniels, K.R. and Taylor, K. (1993) Secrecy and Openness in Donor Insemination. *Politics and the Life Sciences*. **V12**(2) 155–70.

Gunning, J. and English, V. (1993) *Human in vitro Fertilisation: A Case Study in the Regulation of Medical Innovation*. Dartmouth Publishing, Aldershot.

Hansard (1988) 4 February 1988, House of Commons, **column 1204**, London.

Human Fertilisation & Embryology Act (1990) Sections 13(5), 13(6), 31(5) and Schedule 3, para 3(1) (a). HMSO, London.

Code of Practice of the Human Fertilisation & Embryology Authority (1991) (revised June 1993) HFEA, London.

Infertility (Medical Procedures) Act 1984. Parliament of the State of Victoria, Australia, Melbourne.

Report of the King's Fund Centre Counselling Committee (1991), *Counselling for Regulated Infertility Treatments*. Terms of Reference, Section 5, p. 19 and Appendix IV. King's Fund Centre, London.

McWhinnie, A.M. (1992a) Creating Children: The Medical and Social Dilemmas of Assisted Reproduction, *Early Child Development and Care*, Vol 81, pp 39–54.

McWhinnie, A.M. (1993b) Findings of ESRC-funded project entitled, 'A Study of Parenting in Families Created by Artificial Insemination and IVF' (Ref R/000/23/1463.

Mahlstedt, P. (1980). The Psychological Component of Infertility. *Fertility and Sterility*, **43**(3) 335–46.

Menning, B.E. (1980) The Emotional Needs of Infertile Couples. *Fertility and Sterility*, **34**(4) 313–19.

National Bio-ethics Consultative Committee: *Reproductive Technology Counselling* (1991) Final Report for the Australian Health Ministers Conference, Commonwealth of Australia, Section 3, paras 3.1 and 3.3, Section 4, paras 4.4.1 to 4.4.4.

Personal communication from Dr Howard W Jones, The Howard and Georgeanna Jones Institute for Reproductive Medicine, Eastern Virginia Medical School, Norfolk, USA, dated 25 October 1993.

Personal communication from Dr Linda Hammer Burns, PhD, Licensed Psychologist, Center for Reproductive Health, University of Minnesota, Minneapolis, USA, dated 1 November 1993.

Ramsay, P. (1971). Shall we reproduce: the Medical Ethics of *in vitro* Fertilisation, *Journal of the American Medical Association* **220** (10) 1346–1350 in Gunning, J. and English, V. (1993) *Human in vitro fertilisation: a Case Study in the Regulation of Medical Innovation* 8–9. Dartmouth Publishing, Aldershot.

Randall, J.M. and Templeton, A.A. (1991) Infertility – The Experience of a Tertiary Referral Centre, *Health Bulletin 49/1, Scottish Home and Health Department*, January 1991.

Valentine, D. (Ed) (1988) *Infertility and adoption: A Guide for Social Work Practice*, The Haworth Press, New York.

'Virgin Birth' headlines in *The Times*, 12–15 March, 1991.

Waller Report – Committee to consider Social, Ethical and Legal Issues arising from *in vitro* fertilisation (1984), *Report on the disposition of embryos produced by* in vitro *fertilisation*. Parliament of the State of Victoria, Melbourne.

Warnock Report – Department of Health and Social Security (1984) *Report of the Committee of Inquiry into Human Fertilisation & Embryology*, HMSO, London.

Warnock. Mary (1985) *A Question of Life*. Report of the Committee of Inquiry into Human Fertilisation & Embryology, with two new chapters by Mary Warnock. Introduction, xiii. Blackwell, Oxford.

Index

289